Traumatic Brain Injury
and Neuropsychological Impairment

Rolland S. Parker

Traumatic Brain Injury and Neuropsychological Impairment

Sensorimotor, Cognitive, Emotional, and
Adaptive Problems of Children and Adults

With an Appendix by Arthur Greenspan

With 23 Illustrations

Springer-Verlag New York Berlin Heidelberg
London Paris Tokyo Hong Kong

Rolland S. Parker, Ph.D.
Diplomate of the American Board of Professional Psychology
(Clinical Neuropsychology; Clinical Psychology)
Consulting Neuropsychologist
50 West 96th St. (9C)
New York, New York 10025
and
Assistant Professor
Department of Psychiatry
New York Medical College
Valhalla, New York 10595

Library of Congress Cataloging-in-Publication Data
Parker, Rolland S.
Traumatic brain injury and neuropsychological impairment: Sensorimotor, cognitive,
emotional, and adaptive problems of children and adults / Rolland S. Parker.
p. cm.
Includes bibliographical references.
ISBN 0-387-97239-0 (alk. paper)
1. Brain damage. I. Title.
[DNLM: 1. Brain Injuries—physiopathology. 2. Neuropsychology.
WL 354 P242t]
RC387.5.P37 1990
617.4'81—dc20
DNLM/DLC
for Library of Congress   90-9492
Printed on acid-free paper.

© 1990 Springer-Verlag New York Inc.

Typeset by Publishers Service, Bozeman, Montana.
Printed and bound by Edwards Brothers, Ann Arbor, Michigan.
Printed in the United States of America.

9 8 7 6 5 4 3 2 1

ISBN 0-387-97239-0 Springer-Verlag New York Berlin Heidelberg
ISBN 3-540-97239-0 Springer-Verlag Berlin Heidelberg New York

For Irmgard, with appreciation for her support and forgiveness when this task took me away.

Preface

The brain is a delicate, complex, and easily disrupted organ. Unfortunately, the frequency of brain injury and the impairing effects of even seemingly minor injury is generally unknown to the public, the media, and, surprisingly, even many health professionals. It is hoped that this book will make a contribution to the welfare of brain-damaged people through a comprehensive and detailed statement concerning their impairment and how to recognize it. *Increased understanding of impairment, and the significant symptoms that reveal it, will enhance treatment planning, and aid in avoiding the error of assuming that symptoms are emotional, malingering, or exaggerations.*

In writing this book I have drawn on my experience in assessing individuals of all ages who have undergone traumatic brain injury, in order to alert the public, their families, concerned professionals, teaching physicians, psychologists, and attorneys to the clinical and technical issues that will aid in understanding and serving these people. Experience as a psychotherapist and career counselor offered a clinical perspective from which to document the conclusion that traumatic brain damage frequently impairs adaptive capacity of children and adults after even relatively "minor" injury.

To some extent, the problems of the brain-damaged victim have been ignored and misunderstood. One of the most insidious qualities of brain damage is the inability of victims to describe fully their impairment and suffering, since both comprehension and communications may be impaired. In addition, symptoms may occur years after the injury. *The victim's ability to communicate the full quality of their distress is usually not understood. No wonder! The brain, the very organ of experience, communication, and understanding has been damaged.* The causes and signs of this communication loss, that is, "expressive deficits," are detailed here, enabling the reader to help the victim to express the suffering and impairment.

Professional people who serve victims of traumatic brain injury need considerable information to understand this complex, frequent, and disabling condition. Sufficient technical information is provided to enable the practitioner (treatment, teaching, assessment, counseling, rehabilitation, attorney, etc.) to understand research, clinical literature, and clinical reports. Topics include the anatomical and physiological basis for brain functioning, neuropsychological concepts emphasizing the integration of the brain, a comprehensive taxonomy of neuropsychological deficits, symptoms, including emotional reactions, and victims' experiences of being brain damaged. There is an extensive list of contemporary references

Failure to appreciate the extended effect of "minor" trauma leads to ascribing legitimate deficits to failure of will, "compensation neurosis," malingering, or "unconscious processes." Clinical and research information will overcome common misinformation concerning etiology and prognosis. It is not true that concussion symptoms are largely emotional, or that concussion and whiplash are temporary. The consequences of this ignorance are plain: The victim, family, friends, teachers, and employers are perplexed by the impairment of a person who may have no scars or loss of limbs to prove that a serious accident or illness took place. Dependents (in the family, or employers) are confronted by a familiar and loved person who has become nonfunctional, irritable, withdrawn, and unable to work, concentrate, or assume family responsibilities. This person has suddenly become a burden instead of a functional member of the community. Moreover, through lack of information, *there is little pressure to reduce the danger to the community through careless automobile driving, construction accidents, poorly maintained buildings, etc.*!

Ability to recognize brain damage, and understanding how impairing relatively minor injuries are, will be useful to professionals in psychotherapy, counseling, rehabilitation, teaching, the law, and other aspects of public and personal service. The brain-injured person has special characteristics, which are ill served by concluding that their reactions are due to emotional and other symbolic causes. Awareness of neuropsychological concepts can aid psychotherapists and rehabilitation counselors by clarifying adaptive functions that are impaired as a result of traumatic brain injury.

Proper emphasis is given to the emotional stress consequent to an injury. Posttraumatic stress disorders (in various forms) are probably universal. Accidents are frightening and unexpected events, e.g., vehicular injuries, falling ceilings, assaults, falling objects, or long falls. Sometimes people wake up in a hospital with tubes coming out of them, or in a damaged car, not knowing what happened to them. Anxiety and depression become constant companions. The victim soon learns that he or she is unable to perform at the level expected. There may be pain and loss of body mobility. Income, social support, and self-esteem are reduced. Many experience their lives as shattered, and this assessment can be accurate.

Throughout, the unity of the brain and the requirements for understanding a wide range of neuropsychological functions are emphasized. It is my belief that brain trauma is a gross injury requiring considerable focus of attention, breadth, and empathy from the practitioner.

I would like to express deep appreciation to certain colleagues who offered support, advice, and detailed comments on this manuscript. First, to Arthur Greenspan, M.D., a neurologist with whom many cases were shared, who taught me much, and who is a leader in understanding the needs of brain-damaged victims and the complexity of assessing their condition. Second, to Barbara Bess, M.D., director of Resident Training at Metropolitan Hospital Center, and professor, New York Medical College, who offered the opportunity of training and exchanging professional experiences with psychiatric residents. Other professional colleagues to whom appreciation is due include: Harold Hall, Ph.D., who reviewed the entire manuscript, Richard Winters, M.D., Harold Hubbard, M.B.A., Rafael Cilento, M.D., Jerry Solk, M.A., J. Lawrence Thomas, Ph.D., Danella Schiffer, Ph.D., Paul Gunser, Ph.D., Morris Zedeck, Ph.D., Margaret Strahl, M.D., and Pat Murphy, M.A.

Finally, I am happy to acknowledge the great support and cooperation of the staff of Springer-Verlag.

Contents

1
The Hidden Epidemic

Injuries are the leading cause of death for most categories of age, race, or sex, and the leading cause of preretirement years of lost life (Frankowsky, Annegers, & Whitman, 1985). The result is suffering by individuals, medical and rehabilitation care, disability and relief payments, and loss of income and service from the victim. In particular, the cost to the community of impairment due to brain damage is enormous. This major public health problem exists because lack of information discourages unified social action.

It is not generally understood that brain damage is so impairing, and that it has such long-lasting effects. Kraus and Arzemanian (1989) observe how little epidemiologic information can be found in the scientific literature on mild and moderate brain injuries, although these account for most of the brain trauma in the industrialized world. This volume will document that this follows from the lack of recognition of brain injury by many physicians. In particular, head injury victims' emotional distress is commonly ignored, particularly if focal signs of neurological damage are minimal or missing.

The intention of this work is to make the concerned professional and the general public more aware of the generally impairing consequences of brain damage. One outcome can be a broader and more sophisticated examination of accident victims as they seek assistance at different phases after an accident. The more thorough the examination the more likely the detection of positive findings (Hart & Faust, 1988). With an accurate estimate of the social cost of brain damage and of the number of individuals suffering from brain damage, changes can be made in the present short-sighted social policy that causes the toll to go needlessly on and on. Research into more effective rehabilitation and therapeutic procedures will be encouraged.

What Is It Like to Have an Accident?

The following case histories offer subjective statements concerning the experience of being in an accident, and the quality of life afterward.

1

Case 1. A dancer was sitting in his car near the curb when it was hit from behind by another car, impelling it forward to strike another car. His head cracked the windshield. "I heard a loud noise, like something popped inside my head. I opened up my eyes and discovered that my windshield had been cracked. I discovered I was hit from behind. I was dazed for at least 2 days. I was not incoherent, it was like a film around me and I just couldn't get out. I felt encased in something. My speech was very slow." After a considerable period, he is still unable to work. Medication has been prescribed for pain and anxiety. He cannot execute any dance movements or gestures due to stiffness and pain. It makes his body feel as though it refuses to move. "Pain in the head makes me afraid to turn, jump, move quickly."

Case 2. One woman when asked about her identity stated: "I can't deal with people, and feel uncomfortable in my own body. My vehicle was struck from behind while I was stopped waiting for the light to change. My head was turned to the left. I didn't know what happened. Due to the impact my car was knocked through the intersection. It spun, I don't know how much. I managed to gain control and stop it and went to a nearby house for assistance. I don't think I passed out. When I went to get out of the car I realized I felt stunned. My entire head just hurt." The pain was concentrated in the left occipital and right frontal area. She does not believe that she struck her head but there were bruises on her hands. She went to the ER where they kept her for 4–5 hours. She had a few drinks prior to the accident, which may significantly compound the effects of head injury (Bakay, Glasauer, & Alker, 1980, p. 357). She was in a wheelchair in the hospital and left on somebody's arm. "I feel I'm encapsulated. Something is around me. I'm not part of the world. Most people don't realize I have a problem. I have this space, this personal little fog that separates me from everybody else."

Case 3. Another woman was driving within the city, and a car coming from the opposite direction turned and hit the front of her car on the driver's side. She had her seatbelt on, but flew forward and hit her head against the windshield. She remembers only the accident, going forward, and her head smashing against the glass. "I opened my eyes and saw the front of a car smashed. I saw him coming and started to turn." She was dazed until the ambulance got there. "I don't know how long it took. After my head hit, everything was foggy and sparkling. Now its just a scary memory." There is no retrograde amnesia, but memory gaps occur later on. "I will be thinking of something and totally lose track of what I am talking about. I could do something and forget I did it and do it again. I don't want to socialize. I stumble over my words. I can't think of what to say. I can't express myself. I'll be thinking of something and can't put it into words. I'm embarrassed at my scar. I feel ugly. Yes. I used to be a lot happier. Now I am a lot more tired. I used to be alert. I was more self-confident. I can't work, write, read, or sleep. It feels like my whole life is in a bubble. I don't understand it. I feel people have to lead me. I don't feel in control."

Case 4. A woman described the experience of tripping on a protrusion from the floor of her office, and hitting her head on a desk: "I thought I was dead. I felt my skull shaking. I thought my brain was out of my skull. I thought I would go insane. There was a loud noise, the whole room heard it." She was aware that somebody picked her up. "I was crying because my first thought was I would go crazy. I was throwing up, dizzy. I thought I was dead. I let them do what they had to do. I was not aware of everything." Since then she has not returned to work because of confusion, weakness of her right hand grasp, and ringing in the ears. She cannot turn her head to the right. There is spontaneous locking of her jaw. Numbness makes her feel as if there is a stone on the right part of her face. She takes Librium for nervousness and insomnia, a medication for headaches, and physical therapy.

Varied Meanings Ascribed to an Accident

Brain damage is characteristically a consequence of a frightening experience. It is typically followed by some variety of anxiety reaction (e.g., posttraumatic stress disorder), and causes people to give profound consideration to the meaning of their life and what has happened to them.

"As quickly as life can come it can go." "When I didn't die, I said my mother was watching over me." Being spared meant to one man that he should return to a certain charismatic figure whom he had left in a rage and who had cursed him for that reason. "Did I do something wrong. Was this my destiny?" One woman felt ecstatically happy after an accident that she anticipated, when she knew that she would live.

A man was in an industrial accident in which a platform he was riding on fell freely more than 400 feet. Almost 10 years later he still has nightmares and is frightened of cranes, elevators, etc. He drank for 10 months after the accident: "It was a way to kill myself. I gave up on life. I didn't know what to do with my life. I drank and drugged for 10 months."

Another man who was in the same accident stated: "The accident destroyed my life. I tried to put my life together after the drinking. On the anniversary, it intensifies the feelings. I'm very depressed so I can't be around my family. I have nothing to look forward to. Arthritis and nerves create apprehension."

Causes of Traumatic Brain Injury (TBI)

The contents of this book will emphasize accidents, and not medical conditions, although the conceptual foundation of brain structure and function, and the range of deficits that occur will prove useful in understanding the patient suffering from diseases of the central nervous system. Brain damage may be classified according to the context within which it occurs, and the physiological and mechanical trauma. For orientation, the following direct sources of damage will be listed, but will be discussed in detail in Chapter 4 on Trauma and Brain Damage.

Some Types of Accidents Resulting in Traumatic Brain Injury

1. *Anoxia* (restricted blood circulation). Traumatic events include fires and inadequate ventilation (e.g., carbon monoxide release preventing oxygenation of the blood), but also ensues after arterial spasm (stroke), embolism, fetal and birth injury, migraine and epilepsy. Shock, drowning, pulmonary insufficiency, suffociation or strangulation cause metabolic derangements in the brain sufficient to produce coma (Trauner & James, 1985).

2. *Neurotoxins* (see Chapter 17 on Environmental Neurotoxins). A variety of industrial, medical substances cause brain damage. Exposure can be in the workplace, home, roadside, etc. Although miners and industrial workers are particularly exposed to metallic neurotoxins, the general population of industrialized societies is exposed to significant amounts of several of these metals (Bondy & Prasad, 1988, preface). The fetus is susceptible to neurotoxins during pregnancy, e.g., cocaine (Washton & Gold, 1987). See also Chapter 4 on Trauma and Brain Damage. General references include Hartman (1988), Klaasen, Amdur, and Doull (1986), and Tilson and Sparber (1987). Deficits tend to be progressive for considerable periods after exposure (Singer and Scott, 1987) (see Chapter 4 on Trauma and Brain Damage). Alcohol (Goodwin, 1989) and psychoactive substances (Jaffe, 1989) cause considerable damage.

3. *Penetrating head injuries.* These can result from bullets, other flying objects, and sharp weapons.

4. *Closed head injuries.* These can result from impact in an auto accident, sports, falls, explosions, and falling objects.

5. *Acceleration/decelleration.* Rapid change of movement causes the brain to stretch and bounce back and forth within the skull, sometimes becoming scraped (lacerations) or impacting (contusions).

6. *Depressed skull fractures.* These can result in pressure on the brain from bone and possible bleeding (hematoma).

7. *Birth injury* (prenatal and perinatal), including seizures (Fenichel, 1988, pp. 1–41), anoxia, trauma, and infectious diseases (Fenichel, 1985; Zimmerman, 1985). The brain is considered to be the organ most vulnerable to anoxia during gestation and delivery (Towbin, 1987).

Epidemiology

Estimates of the number of traumatic brain injuries in the United States tend to be low and even vague. As noted, many people do not have a medical examination, or, if they do, this injury becomes unrecognized in emergency rooms or private offices. Therefore, these injuries do not become a part of health survey statistics. The rate of injury is impressive, but cannot be precisely defined, as will be observed.

According to Dacey and Dikmen (1987), 5–10% of head injuries are fatal; of people with nonfatal head injuries 50–70% received medical care, an estimated 20–40% do not receive medical care, and 30–50% are hospitalized. Although only 5–10% are estimated to have neuropsychological sequelae (Frankowski et al., 1985), this is probably a gross underestimate.

It is estimated that head injuries in the United States are in excess of 8 million per year, of which 200 per 100,000 of the population (approximately 400,000) are hospitalized according to Rimel, Giordani, Barth, Boll, and Jane (1981), citing the National Center for Health Statistics. Another estimate is that between 400,000 and 500,000 Americans suffer head injuries severe enough to cause death or admission to a hospital (National Institutes of Health, 1984). Brain injuries, directly calculated, are estimated to be 700,000 per year, including 70,000–90,000 who suffer coma and extreme loss of bodily functions (according to the National Head Injury Foundation; Hinds, 1989). According to other sources (Frankowsky et al., 1985; Hinds, 1989; Marshall and Marshall, 1985):

1. Injuries are the leading cause of death for most age–race–sex categories, and the leading cause of preretirement years of lost life. There is a tendency for younger, i.e., more athletic and/or aggressive, individuals to be at greater risk for traumatic brain injury (TBI).

2. Head injury is a cause of secondary epilepsy.

3. In the United States, the rate of head injuries is 0.2–0.3% per year. This involves 500,000 new cases, with 30–50% as moderate, severe, or fatal. Head injury mortality rate is about 25/100,000.

4. Analysis: One study of head injuries lists their causes in order as road accidents (47%), accidental falls (23%), work accidents (14%), assaults (11%), sports accidents (3%), and miscellaneous (1%). Of these 71% occurred to men (Cartlidge and Shaw, 1981, p. 180). Another offered this breakdown: traffic and transport (20–50%), gunshot wounds (20–40%), falls (20–30%), sports and recreation (10%), other blunt forces (7%).

5. Half of all mild and moderate brain damage cases occur in motor vehicle accidents, particularly to passengers. In San Diego County (1981), mild and moderate brain injury incidence was 131/100,000 and 15/100,000, respectively (Kraus and Arzemanian, 1989).

It is estimated that 100 injuries occur for every 10,000 skier visits, including 6 head injuries. Of 23 skiing deaths in Vermont, 19 involved head injuries, including 4 with other complications as well. There is considerable participant resistance to using helmets in hazardous activities such as skiing and motorcycling. Some states do not require the use of helmets.

6. Each year 290,000 people suffering minor head injury are hospitalized in the United States.

7. Approximately 150,000 individuals who suffer a minor head injury will be disabled for at least 1 month.

8. Moderate head injuries, defined as a Glasgow Coma Scores (GCS) of 9–12 are estimated at 60,000–75,000.

9. Of pediatric hospitalizations due to trauma 75% occur to the head. Mortality rate estimates vary from 9 to 35% (James, 1985). Ten of every 10,000 children die each year from head injury, exceeding leukemia (Luerssen, 1985).

10. Neurological injury to the spine, peripheral nerves, or autonomic system may accompany head trauma. More than 200,000 people in the United States are paralyzed as a consequence of spinal cord injury; these people, mostly young, are victims of automobile and motor cycle accidents (Livingston, 1985, p. 1238). This topic is discussed in two sections of the volume by Becker and Povlishock (1985).

Why the Ignorance of Brain Damage?

1. *The victim does not relate a symptom to the accident.* When symptoms occur years later, or even when they occur immediately, their importance and relationship to the accident may not be realized (see Chapter 16 on Expressive Deficits).

2. *False information perpetuates incorrect conclusions:*

• If it is believed that brain damage during infancy is later overcome, then early effects are not documented, and subsequent learning and behavioral problems are not attributed to the accident.

• Superficial recovery, involving a belief that the residual symptoms will disappear, discourages follow-up, with its educational advantages, and discourages informing the patient of the potential seriousness and permanence of the injury.

3. *Lack of information by diagnosticians.* It has been asserted plainly that "behavioral derangements that stem from diffuse axonal injury are beyond the recognition of most neurologists let alone the average practitioner (Cytowic, Stump, and Larned, 1988). Normal neurological findings lead to the false conclusion that postinjury problems (cognitive and emotional) are psychogenic (Uzell, Langfitt, and Dolinkas, 1987). The following facts concerning TBI are sometimes ignored.

• *"Simple concussion" may represent permanent brain damage.* Some physicians believe that a mild concussion (e.g., headaches and dizziness), although irritating, is only temporary (see Minor head injury in Chapter 18). Not all physicians know that symptoms of a mild concussion can exist without loss of consciousness (Genarelli, 1987). I have seen numerous neurological reports after severe impact, or rapid deceleration without impact (whiplash, see below), in which the patient was assessed as neurologically normal in the presence of classical signs of brain damage, such as problems of memory and concentration.

• *Brain damage can occur without loss of consciousness* (LOC). An injury not affecting the brainstem or its cortical connections may not be accompanied by immediate or subsequent unconsciousness (Gennerelli, 1987). A bullet wound may ultimately be fatal, but the victim may not be immediately unconscious. Slow bleeding from an undetected hemorrhage can also lead to coma weeks later. See Chapter 4 on Trauma and Brain Damage.

• *Underestimating the morbidity of head injury.* As Alves and Jane (1985) stated: "We cannot consider mild brain injury as a simple and self-limiting disorder." Consequently, an evaluation of recovery based solely on the resolution of acute deficits and focal neurologic signs underestimates the deficits of higher mental functions or adaptability produced by diffuse brain damage.

• *Ignorance of the natural history of brain damage.* Psychologists who believe that early brain damage causes relatively little impairment (the "Kennard Principle") tend to underpredict the amount of impairment and may make the error of attributing to "functional causes" deficits such as attention and concentration.

• *Utilizing stereotypes.* Some neurologists assert that a claim of sensory deficit must be wrong because it is not an agreement with "known" pathways. However, the pattern of damage corresponding to a particular sensorimotor symptom can vary considerably with the location of an injury, considering the complexity of the nervous system, as well as unknown injuries, lack of knowledge, etc.

Livingston (1984, p. 1153) states that it is a mistake to "disregard or discredit [the patient's] experiences that seem improbable in the light of current physiological knowledge." In addition, the impaired person's statement is conditioned by what he or she considers reasonable, and by what he or she believes that the professional needs to understand. Thus, there are far more patients accused of malingering than there are malingerers.

One of the most familiar concepts, i.e., the frontal lobe syndrome of poor motivation, apathy, and disinhibition, has recently been described as "based more on preconceived notions of frontal lobe behavior than on firm localizing evidence" (Stuss & Benson, 1986, p. 48).

4. *Not recognizing injurious events.* The occurrence of prior injuries is often ignored by examiners and psychotherapists, whether or not the immediate referral related to a particular injury. Childhood injuries, high fevers, damage that did not lead to coma, etc., are not known. The vulnerability to a high level of impairment after a prior injury is not taken into account in assessing the current adaptation.

• When a woman was 2 she had a high fever requiring her to be immersed in cold water. She went to a special school for 2 years. At that time she would write letters and words backward, and had spelling problems. She appears to have met all educational milestones without delay (graduation from high school, college, and professional school). However, this required more study time than other students, and she believed that she did not achieve as much as those who put in less effort.

• A man had fevers when he was 6 months old (102–105°F) causing convulsions. At 3 he was hit by a car. At 5 he fell and broke a collar bone. He was a well-behaved child at home, but in school, to his parents' surprise, was described as poorly disciplined. He states that he always had problems in concentration and in reading instructions.

5. *Overestimating the diagnostic value of focal neurological procedures.* I have heard many stories of patients who were diagnosed as being unimpaired after a "neurological examination" lasting from less than 5 to about 15 minutes. Diffuse brain damage may not be accompanied by focal neurological deficits. Yet focal neurological examinations are not designed to detect diffuse axonal injury or diffuse brain damage, but rather to diagnose neurological illness. In one study, only 2% of patients with minor head injury had positive neurological findings 3 months later. These were cranial nerve deficits (a primary focus of the traditional neurological examination), including pupillary dysfunction, although 78% complained of headaches, 59% of memory deficits, and about 15% of difficulties with

activities of daily living or transportation (Rimel et al., 1981). Impairment can be overlooked if "soft signs" are ignored (see below).

6. *Overestimating EEG and imaging techniques.* Apart from screening for posttraumatic epilepsy, the EEG has not proved useful for predicting neurological or behavioral recovery patterns. The EEG abnormalities are usually no longer in evidence by a time a recording is made, or disappear in weeks or months. The EEG is of prognostic value only concerning epilepsy (Adams and Victor, 1989, p. 25). However, quantified EEG, also known as neurometric testing, is sensitive to deficits of cognitive performance (Randolph and Miller, 1988). Magnetic resonance imaging (MRI) and CT scans may be negative in the presence of reliable signs of brain damage, e.g., cognitive or emotional impairment, anxiety, depression, distractibility, and impulsivity, which can be assessed by neuropsychological procedures (Dean, 1986). Imaging and other techniques may not detect small or diffuse injuries caused by diffuse axonal damage, petechial hemorrhages, torsion, shearing forces too small to create hemorrhage, tears in long fibers, etc., which can cause considerable distress.

7. *Insensitivity to "soft signs."* In the absence of localized or focal neurological deficits, ignoring vaguer deficits can prevent detection of diffuse or generalized brain damage (Tupper, 1987). Ignoring complex functions also blinds the examiner to diffuse brain damage and stress. The definition of "soft" signs is somewhat controversial. For example, Touen (1987) raises the question of the contribution of minor signs to diagnosis, but defines "soft signs" as mild symptoms that can be observed reliably and consistently during an appropriate neurological assessment carried out by a well-trained examiner. He specifically excludes complex operations used in everyday behavior, i.e., concentration, attention, motivation, and understanding. I believe that deficits in these "higher functions" are precisely those that invite further exploration, while presenting significant problems of recognition and documentation. A familiar example is the "frontal lobe syndrome" (see Chapter 13 on Cerebral Personality Disorders and Frontal Lobe Syndromes), in which judgment, inability by children to achieve maturity, inability to learn from experience, etc., are implicated.

8. *Reduced mental level may not be recognized.* Even a generalized reduction of ability corresponding to an IQ loss of 10–30 points does not impair simple conversations, and can be missed (see Chapter 21 on Assessment). Examiners do not carefully assess "higher" cognitive functions if they so primitive a techniques as "count backward by 7 from 100").

9. *The use of an inappropriate criterion of recovery* (see Chapter 18). Assessment recovery depends on the viewpoint of the provider. As a neurologist told me, a neurosurgeon reported that a patient was doing well, when in fact the patient was totally aphasic. The neurosurgeon who has repaired a broken skull and removed a hematoma from a crash victim has achieved a great deal when the person survives and can walk. Rimel, Giordani, Barth, and Jane (1982) observe that patients may be deemed to have made a good recovery at the time of discharge from the hospital, while still being disabled. However, the injured per-

son's spouse, children, friends, and employer may see the survivor as a completely impaired and different individual.

10. *Misjudgment by emergency personnel*. Two types of errors are common:

a. *Stating that there was no loss of consciousness*. By the time emergency personnel comes, the victim was awake, and therefore the medical record is noted inaccurately as "no loss of consciousness." Sometimes, the victim forgets that he or she was unconscious, also leading to a false statement.

b. *Not encouraging hospital admission*. I have examined many individuals who have never had a single examination after an injury, yet, after a head trauma, or whiplash, together with emotional shock and possible injury to other parts of the body, were permitted to leave the scene of the accident. The victim is in no position to make significant decisions about treatment or examination, but the police or medical personnel often let them decide whether or not to seek treatment, or go to the hospital for an examination. They ignore that the injured person is in a state of shock, or dazed, unable to use proper judgment. The person is sent home in an impaired condition and may remain unaware of his or her injuries.

The emergency personnel's lack of urgency is often compounded by the victim's confusion and desire to proceed where they were going when injured (job interview, for example!) or wish to see one's personal physician, etc.

• A physician, an accident victim, stated: "It is unfair to ask the person 'Are you injured? Are you OK?' They may not know it, or be able to know they are injured, or they may not be willing to admit they're injured."

• A woman, obsessed with proceeding to a job interview, did so 20 minutes after her car was violently struck from the rear. After being ignored by police, she continued on foot to her destination unaware of having suffered a brain injury!

• Another woman hit her head against the dashboard. She felt achy for a few days but had not seen a physician, and did not go to the hospital. Bad headaches and blurry vision developed a considerable time after the accident. She will have a problem in establishing a valid insurance claim for her treatment, since over 1 year has elapsed since the accident.

11. *The emergency room may not recognize brain damage*. When a head injured person reaches the ER examination may be poor. Medical personnel look for soft tissue and orthopedic injuries, but may ignore brain damage. An X ray will be ordered, which is insensitive to diffuse injury, small hematomas, etc. Zimmerman (1985) states that ER radiological evaluation is usually limited to a cursory examination of the skull and cervical spine. It may be concluded that no serious injury has occurred because there is no fractured skull (which is actually uncommon). The victim is discharged, and may be told that there is nothing wrong, and not instructed to return.

One boy's mother saw him 2 hours after the incident. He was complaining about his leg and his head. "Nobody really checked his head." A woman, hospitalized after a car accident, was pressured by her physican and her husband to leave almost immediately. The hospital wanted the bed, and her husband wanted her to take care of the kids. After a week of pressure to have her leave, a physician-relative convinced them to give her a CT scan (which was negative). Then a hospital MD wanted to state in the discharge report that "She might need home care." Actually, she could not walk up steps or take care of herself. He had to be prevailed on to request more comprehensive convalescent care!

I have personally observed a woman, brought to an ER after an accident, gradually lose consciousness. Her son was making futile and repeated telephone calls drawing attention to his mother's injury. Finally he showed up in person and demanded that she be seen. She had been ignored, although possibly dying of a cerebral hemorrhage, since she was quiet while others were crying and bleeding.

12. *Expressive deficits.* Brain damage is often ignored because of the victim's inability or reluctance to describe impairment, due to deficits of communication, reduced ability to manifest distress due to cerebral injury, and loss of self-understanding (see Chapter 16 for a detailed description of Expressive Deficits).

13. *Believing that emotional symptoms are all in the mind.* The extent of distress following an accident is poorly appreciated. A study of "posttraumatic stress disorder in the general population" (Helzer, Robins, & McEvoy, 1987) does not even list injury as a source. See Chapters 13 on Cerebral Personality Disorders and 15 on Anxiety, Stress and Psychodynamic Reactions.

Consequence of Neglect

1. *Epidemiological reports minimize the extent of traumatic brain damage.* The community estimate of the actual level of impaired and dead is much less than reality. Consequently, little action is taken to prevent reckless and drunken drivers, negligent landlords and employers, careless parents, etc.

2. *Victims are not properly compensated.* The determination of "no neurological damage" leads to seriously impaired people being characterized as malingerers or "compensation neurotics" (a term used by defense lawyers and insurance companies to deny impairment), and causes them to receive insufficient or no compensation, or be refused social security disability.

3. *Physicians, policemen, and other medical personnel do not receive proper orientation to head injury.* Nonneurologically trained physicians do not take "concussion" seriously, or follow through properly on accident cases generally. As an indirect consequence, the training of policemen, paramedics, emergency room physicians and nurses, and ER medical personnel is often not sensitive to this type of injury. This is not universal, since I have found some to be well trained to observe "soft" signs of brain damage, and handle accident victims well.

2
Neuroanatomy and Organization from a Behavioral Viewpoint

This chapter (and Chapter 4 on Trauma) has multiple purposes for the concerned professional in traumatic brain injury:

1. Increased ability to understand professional reports and research;
2. Appropriate treatment planning and assessment;
3. Increased understanding of the effects of traumatic stress;
4. Illustration of the integrated functioning of the nervous system;
5. Combatting the idea that slight brain trauma has little effect;
6. Understanding consequent illness and impaired development;
7. Using neurological findings to estimate prognosis.

The chief sources for neuroanatomy and physiology include Barr and Kiernan (1983, 1988), Brodal (1981), Livingston, (1985), Carpenter and Sutin (1983), DeGroot and Chusid (1988), Kandel and Schwartz (1985), Pansky, Allen and Budd (1988), and Trimble (1988a,b). Wilson-Pauwels, Akesson, and Stewart (1988) offer a comprehensive, well-illustrated summary of the cranial nerves.

The topics are anatomical (neural masses and fiber tracts) and neurochemical substances and their relationship to particular structures, pathways, and functions, and the functions served by the above. To avoid redundancy, points are not completely discussed at first mention. This chapter presents an overview of the subject; the reader will find references to further information about particular topics, which will give a further understanding to the issues in this chapter, elsewhere in the text, and in related professional sources. For readers who still require further neuropsychological information, a general neuroscience textbook would be useful.

The Neuron

The neuron is the basic unit of the nervous system. *The cell body* contains genetic and metabolic structures, manufactures neurotransmitters, and utilizes glucose as the brain's chief energy source (see Kandel & Schwartz, 1985, Chapters 2–18). Some useful definitions include the following:

Dendrites (branch-like extensions) convey impulses from other neurons to the cell body.

Axons lead nerve impulses and neurotransmitters away from the cell body to the synapse (gap between neurons) or the end organ. Certain cells secrete neurohormones that are transported in the local blood circulation to other cerebral areas.

Myelin is a fatty substance that surrounds the long extensions of cell bodies (axons) that convey impulses, and that insulates the depolarization passing along the axon. Myelinization is a process of maturation that occurs normally at different stages of development and thus is a measure of maturity. At birth many neurons lack myelin sheaths. Larger axons are surrounded by myelin, whose loss contributes to the symptoms of various degenerative diseases including multiple sclerosis.

Neurotransmitters are chemical substances, often created in the cell body, transported to a target neuron and released into the synapse. Important examples are *acetylcholine*, released in the autononomic nervous system, and also in the neuraxis (more details are given below), and *catecholamines*, a significant group of neurotransmitters including dopamine, norepinephrine, and epinephrine. Alterations in their availability have been found in depression, schizophrenia, and other significant aspects of behavior.

Presynaptic terminals (branches of the axon) transmit information to another neuron or organ.

Postsynaptic cells receive impulses within a ganglion or nucleus and then extend to a target organ or other neuron.

Endorphins are a variety of substances manufactured in various areas of the brain, and elsewhere in the body, that bind to opioid receptors, i.e., have opiate-like effects (sleep inducing). They are involved in pain reduction and stress control.

Peptides are groups of amino acids that form substances such as hormones (ACTH), endorphins, oxytoxin and vasopressin. These are behaviorally and physiologically significant, and are found in many brain areas.

Neuromodulators are peptides that modulate the activities of other neurons and nonneuronal cells.

Nucleus (nuclei) is a mass of gray matter or cells, usually controlling one or more definable functions.

Classification of Neurons

Afferent: Neurons or fiber tracts that are sensitive to stimuli from the environment (e.g., various sensations), or that bring stimulation to a central nucleus or ganglion.

Efferent: Neurons, pathways, and/or nerve impulses leading into muscles, glands, or other nerve centers, thus initiating activity, leaving a nucleus.

Internuncial: Found in the spinal cord they interconnect afferents and efferents, i.e., integrating various functions.

Neurons Are Considered to Be Secretory Cells
(Schwartz, 1985)

Chemical messengers mediate cell-to-cell communication at the synapse, in circulating body fluids, and in the interstitial fluid (surrounding the neurons), without entering the bloodstream. Although given substances may have multiple functions in different parts of the body, in terms of (overlapping) ability to stimulate neuronal activity, one may utilize these definitions (Ganong, 1986):

Neurotransmitters: present in nerve endings
Neurohormones: hormones secreted by neurons that diffuse in the fluid surrounding the cells, i.e., paracrine communication
Hormones: secreted by endocrine cells, that enter the circulation.

Although particular neurosubstances may be identified with particular nuclei and pathways, these nuclei may also connect with other terminals, and particular neurosubstances can be secreted in many other anatomical regions by nonneurological tissue. So significant neurotransmitters such as dopamine and norepinephrine actually occur in all three categories.

Neurostimulation Involves the Entire Cell

The requirement for transport of neurotransmitters, cytoskeletal, and other metabolic substances and their by-products by round-trip along the axon adds additional vulnerability to neural functioning in injury in which the axons are damaged, cut, or stretched.

Anterograde transport. Neurotransmitters are manufactured in the cell body and transmitted in synaptic vesicles (small sacs) down the the axon (anterograde transport) to the synaptic membrane to be stored and then released during stimulation of an end organ or postsynaptic neuron.
Stimulation. Neurotransmitters are released at specific places on the axon (boutons) and taken up (bind) on specific proteins on the outer surface of the cell membranes. Certain tracts of great behavioral significance transport particular neurotransmitters (see below).
Retrograde transport. The membrane of the vesicle returns along the axon to be recycled. Retrotrade transport has many functions: it provides to the nerve cell information about conditions at the end of the axon to the nerve; and moves worn-out neutransmitter materials from terminals to the cell body for degradation, restoration, and reuse; and moves nerve growth factor, tetanus toxins, and herpes simplex viruses, and probably rabies and polio viruses (Schwartz, 1985, pp. 42–44).

Synapse

The synapse is a gap between two neurons, i.e., between the nerve membranes, which functions as a link. It may be bridged by either electrical impulses (depolarization) or chemical substances (neurotransmitters). The postsynaptic influence may be inhibitory or excitatory. Simultaneous stimulation by more than one presynaptic neuron simultaneously has a cumulative effect on a post-synaptic neuron. Summation in space or time enhances the integration of the nervous system.

Blood–Brain Barrier

The brain has the ability to selectively permit certain substances to permeate the cerebrospinal fluid and brain substance. This affects which natural substances and drugs can enter neural tissue. Permeability is determined by the characteristics of the capillaries, the nature of the dissolved substances in the blood, and the presence or absence of disease and/or pathology of the brain and body.

Circulating peptides modulate neuronal function in different portions of the brain (not through the blood brain barrier, but through the more permeable circumventricular organs within the ventricles (Carpenter, 1985, pp. 18–19). These include thyroid-releasing hormone, luteinizing hormone-releasing hormone, somatostatin (growth hormone-release inhibiting hormone, or GH-RIH), opioid peptides, cholecystokinin, angiotensin II, Substance P, Adenohypophysial hormones, and Neurohypophysial hormones.

Embryological Development

Neural Tube

Understanding this structure enables visualization of the organization of the brain and the spinal cord.

The most anterior bulge of the neural tube is the prosencephalon or forebrain. The forebrain divides into the telencephalon (cerebral hemispheres) and diencephalon (thalamus and hypothalamus). Next posteriorly is the midbrain (mescencephalon), whose structure is relatively unmodified in the adult. The rhombencephalon divides into the metencephalon anteriorly, and the myelencephalon posteriorly (just before the spinal cord). The metencephalon forms the cerebellum dorsally, and the pons ventrically. The myelencephalon forms the medulla.

The Ventricles (Figures 2.1 and 2.15)

Ventricles are the bulges from the hollow central canal situated as follows:

The lateral ventricles (1,2) are within the frontal (anterior horn), temporal, and occipital lobes (inferior horn). They communicate with the centrally located third ventricle via the *interventricular foramen*.

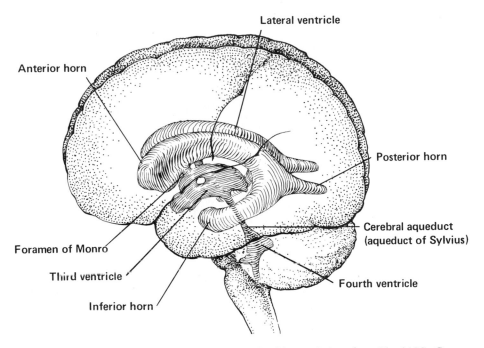

FIGURE 2.1. The ventricular system. Reproduced, with permission, from Chusid JG: *Correlative Neuroanatomy and Functional Neurology*, nineteenth edition, copyright © 1985, Lange Medical Publications, Fig. 3.54.

The third ventricle is central within the cerebral hemispheres. Its medial wall is the *septum pellucidum*, which contains some of the *septal nuclei*, which are important within the limbic system (see Netter, 1986, pp. 27, 208). It is surrounded by the diencephalon, i.e., the thalamus dorsally and the hypothalamus ventrally. It communicates with the lateral ventricles. It leads to the fourth ventricle via the cerebral aqueduct.

The cerebral aqueduct connects the third and fourth ventricles, and is surrounded by the "central gray matter" (see mesencephalon). It extends the length of the midbrain (mesencephalon), and opens up as the fourth ventricle.

The fourth ventricle is underneath the cerebellum (metencephalon) and anterior portion of the medulla (myelencephalon). This canal is continuous with the central canal of the spinal cord. (For excellent diagrams see Carpenter and Sutin, 1983. pp. 72–73) (Table 2.1).

Cerebrospinal Fluid

Cerebrospinal fluid (CSF), secreted within the ventricles, serves these purposes: cushioning the brain against shock, distributing oxygen and other nutrients, and maintaining the balance of sodium and potassium for nerve transmission.

TABLE 2.1. Embryological and anatomical features.

Primary vescicles	Mature derivatives
Prosencephalon (forebrain)	Telencephalon (cerebral cortex, basal ganglia, olfactory bulb)
	Diencephalon (thalamus, hypothalamus)
	Ventricles: (two lateral, and the third central).
Mesencephalon (midbrain)	Mesencephalon
	Tectum roof (superior, inferior collicul),
	Tegmentum floor (red nucleus)
	Ventricles: aqueduct of Sylvius
Rhombencephalon (hindbrain)	Cerebellum
	Pons
	Medulla
	Ventricle: fourth
Caudal part of neural tube	Spinal cord
	Ventricle: central canal

The CSF plays a role in integrating brain and peripheral endocrine functions insofar as hormones or hormone-releasing factors from the hypothalamus are secreted into the extracellular space or into the CSF (Carpenter, 1985, 18–19).

The spinal canal is the continuation of the ventricular system into the spinal cord.

Reference Planes and Orientation

Reference planes and orientation are horizontal (parallel to the floor), coronal (right angles to the horizontal (side to side), sagittal (dividing the body into left and right halves), parasagittal (parallel to the midsagittal plane), transverse (cross sections, e.g., of the brain stem) (DeGroot & Chusid, 1988, p. 113), ventral (oriented in the nervous system toward the front of the body), and dorsal (oriented toward the back).

The direction of long tracts is described as *rostrally* (toward the cortex from below) or *caudally* (away from the cortex in the direction of the spinal cord), with relays; tracts or reference points confining themselves to the same side of the CNS are *ipsilateral*, and those involving the opposite side to some reference point are *contralateral*. Layers or masses of cells are considered "gray matter" and fibers tracts are "white matter." Groups of cells having an integrative or transmission function are called ganglia or nuclei. The area of interaction between one neuron and the next, or between a neuron and an effector cell of an end-organ, is called the synapse. Since many cells are usually involved in transmission, a synapse is more of an abstraction than a specific anatomical location.

Fiber tracts are named from the point of origin to point of termination, e.g., corticospinal indicates the cell body is in the cerebral cortex, and the tract terminates in the spine. A *funiculus* is a fiber bundle whose neurons have the same origin, course, and termination. *Cranial nerves* exit the nervous system from the brain, i.e., within the skull. They are both motor and sensory. Spinal nerves serve sensory and control functions, and originate from the spinal cord. The autonomic nervous system (ANS) controls physiological supportive functions, and is anatomically independent of the sensory and muscular tracts, outside the CNS. The cerebellum's tracts enter and exit from the neuraxis at the level of the lower brainstem, and primarily influence strength and integration of movement. A *ganglion (ganglia)* is a group of nerve cell bodies.

The Central Nervous System (CNS): Neuraxis

The neuraxis involves tracts completely within the brain and spinal cord. Some important skull landmarks include the *foramen magnum*, the gap at the base of the skull through which the medulla connects with the spinal cord and the *fossa (cranial)*, a hollow or depressed area. *Anterior:* Supports the frontal lobes and orbital cavities; a significant transverse feature is the crista galli, supporting the dura mater, both structures creating vulnerability during acceleration/deceleration trauma. *Middle:* Supports the temporal lobes of the brain, and contains the sella turcica, which contains the pituitary gland. *Posterior:* Contains the cerebellum, pons, and medulla, and has at its center the CNS exit, i.e., foramen magnum.

Meninges

The neuraxis is surrounded by three layers or meninges, i.e., membranous coverings of the brain and spinal cord.

1. Outer: *The dura mater*. This is applied directly to the skull, and is comprised of two layers with a hard texture. It envelopes the cerebral hemispheres and cerebellum. It is applied to the skull, and its inner surface is the outermost of the brain coverings. It sends folds into the cavities of the brain, which cover and separate the cerebral hemispheres, the cerebellum, occipital lobe, and the stalk of the pineal gland (Lewis, 1936, pp. 866–868). The *falx cerebri* is a double fold separating the two cerebral hemispheres, with its edge over the corpus callosum. The *falx cerebelli* is in a similar midline position between the cerebellar hemispheres. The *tentorium cerebelli* is a doubled fold separating the occipital lobe and the cerebellum. The *diaphragama sellae* is a double layer forming the roof of the sella turcica (a cavity in the floor of the cranial cavity, into which the pituitary gland is inserted). *Subdural hemorrhages* occur between the inner layer of the dura and the brain, i.e., more directly on the brain surface than epidural hemorrhages between the two layers of the dura and the skull, i.e., separated by the inner layer of the dura from contact with the brain.

2. Middle: *arachnoid*. This is a delicate transparent network of fibers containing blood vessels that may hemorrhage during trauma.

3. Inner: *pia mater.* The pia is applied directly to the brain; it follows its contour closely.

Periostium

The periostium is a fibrous membrane covering the entire surface of the bone except its articular cartilage. It is significant as a protection that may be breached by penetrating wounds, making the brain vulnerable to infection. That portion surrounding the skull is the *pericranium.*

The Spinal Cord

Subdivisions

The spinal cord (Fig. 2.2) is divided into cervical (C1–C8), thoracic (T1–T12), lumbar (L1–L5), sacral (S1–S5), and coccygeal (1) divisions. Within the spinal cord, ascending (afferent) and descending (motor) tracts are generally isolated. The cord is protected by the spinal column. Each segment, corresponding to a single vertebra, innervates embryological segments of skin (dermatomes) and muscular areas (myotomes) that are consecutive and perpendicular to the body axis. This orderly arrangement becomes disturbed in human beings due to the vertical rather than horizontal position of the body in ambulation. In other vertebrates, limbs are perpendicular to the ground, with the body axis horizontal. The arrangement of nerve roots and innervated areas seems more logical. In humans the limbs are extensions of or are parallel to the body axis.

Dermatome

The dermatome is an area of skin innervated by a single spinal root (Fig. 2.3). The dermatomes of the trunk are parallel and circular, but the dermatomes of the arms and legs are long strips extending the length of the limb. The sensory nerves for each dermatome have their cell bodies adjacent to the spinal column in the *dorsal root ganglion* (see spinal nerves). The dermatomes generally correspond to the vertebrae, although each section of the skin is served by several dorsal nerve roots, and the degree of overlapping differs with the test stimulus. Pain is most specific for localization, compared to touch (Kandel & Schwartz, 1985, p. 302).

In the spinal cord, the arrangement of cell bodies (gray matter) and axons (white matter) is reversed compared to the cerebral cortex and cerebellum, i.e., cell bodies surround the central canal, and axons are located externally.

Spinal Nerves

Spinal nerves are the union of the dorsal and ventral roots of the spinal cord outside the vertebral column, extending to the periphery, but excluding the autonomic trunk (Fig. 2.4). Spinal nerves enter the cord through dorsal (sensory)

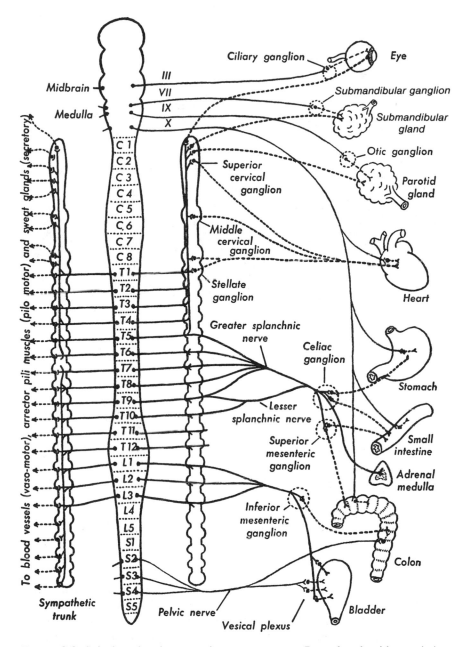

FIGURE 2.2. Spinal cord and autonomic nervous system. Reproduced, with permission, from Carpenter MB and Sutin J: *Human Neuroanatomy*, Eighth Edition, copyright © 1983, Williams and Wilkins Co., Baltimore, Fig. 8.1.

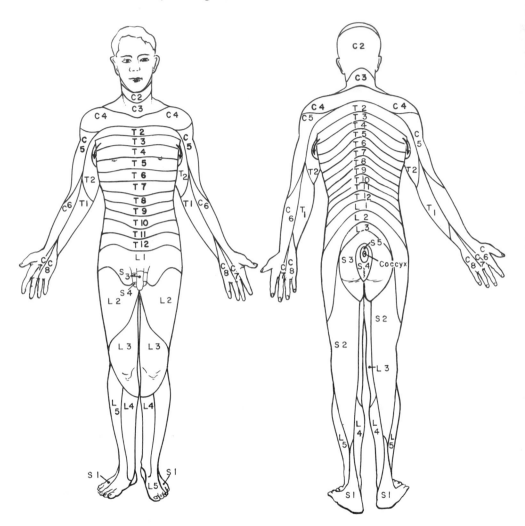

FIGURE 2.3. Spinal nerves and dermatomes From Barr ML and Kiernan JA (1988), Fig. 5.13, with permission.

roots and leave it through ventral (motor) roots. Spinal roots actually serve overlapping dermatomes. These roots are composed of smaller units (radicles) that exit the spinal cord through gaps between the vertebrae (intervertebral foramena), making them vulnerable to being cut and pinched by impact trauma to the vertebrae (see radiculitis in Chapter 7 on Sensorimotor Functions).

Root, Dorsal

The dorsal root is composed of sensory nerve fibers entering the spinal column.

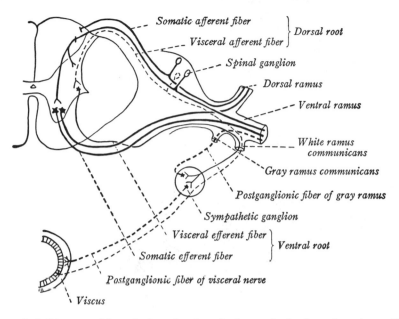

Somatic afferent fiber

Visceral afferent fiber } Dorsal root

Spinal ganglion

Dorsal ramus

Ventral ramus

White ramus communicans

Gray ramus communicans

Postganglionic fiber of gray ramus

Sympathetic ganglion

Visceral efferent fiber

Somatic efferent fiber } Ventral root

Postganglionic fiber of visceral nerve

Viscus

FIGURE 2.4. Diagram of the spinal cord and a spinal nerve in the thoracic region to illustrate the chief functional types of peripheral nerve fibers. From Ranson SW and Clark SL (1959), Fig. 109, with permission.

Root, Ventral

The ventral root is composed of action (motor, efferent) fibers leaving the spinal column, including innervation for organs, glands, blood vessels, and muscles. Occasional sensory fibers also enter through the ventral root.

Functions of the Spinal Cord

Sensory Input

Sensory fibers originate as peripheral nerves. As they approach the spinal cord, they join with motor fibers into spinal nerves. Then they separate, into primarily sensory and motor tracts (still outside the spinal cord). Sensory fibers cell bodies of each nerve occur at one location, i.e., the dorsal root ganglion, alongside the vertebrae. Almost all sensory fibers enter the spinal cord via the dorsal root and synapse in the dorsal horn (Chusid, 1985, pp. 224–226). Some enter via the ventral root (Brodal, 1981, p. 60). Visceral sensory fibers (Autonomic Nervous System) also enter via the dorsal roots. Sensory fibers ascend upwards in the spinothalamic or medial lemniscus system (Fig. 2.5).

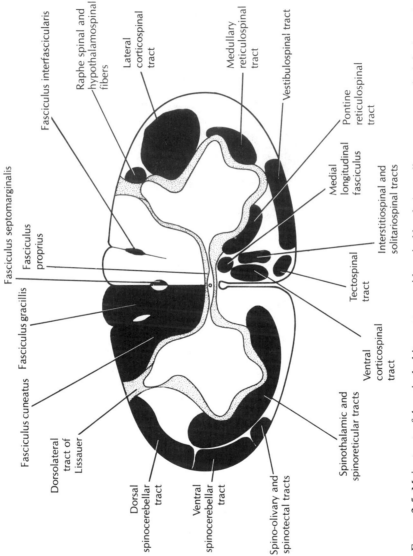

FIGURE 2.5. Major tracts of the spinal white matter at midcervical level. Ascending tracts are on the left; descending tracts are on the right. From Barr ML and Kiernan JA (1988), Fig. 5.9, with permission.

Light Touch, Pain, and Temperature

Light Touch

Impulses are carried centrally by the *anterior spinothalamic tract*, and are also transmitted centrally by the posterior white columns. Anterior spinothalamic pathways decussate to the opposite side of the CNS at the level of sensory input, or over several segments, making localization difficult; they then ascend in the lateral lemniscus (see spinothalamic lemniscus, below) toward the sensory nuclei in the thalamus.

Pain

Pain ascends in the *spinotectal tract* in association with the anterior spinothalamic tract, i.e., lateral lemniscus, terminating in the contralateral superior colliculus (visual integrative nucleus of the midbrain) and periaqueductal gray (reticular activating system of the midbrain), where it stimulates analgesia through opiate receptors (Weber & Pert, 1989).

Heat, Cold, Pain

These cross to the opposite side, or within one segment of entering the dorsal root, and enter the *lateral spinothalamic tract*. Damage to this tract causes contralateral anesthesia (pain and heat) one segment below the lesion. A lesion in the midbrain or medulla can cause loss of pain and thermal sense over the face, neck, trunk, and limbs on the opposite side of the body (Fig. 2.6).

Proprioception (Kinesthesis, i.e., Stimuli from Muscles and Tendons)

These fibers enter the posterior white column, i.e., the fasciculus gracilis and fasciculus cuneatus. Rostrally, they synapse in the medulla in the nucleus fasciculus and cuneate nucleus fasciculus, then decussate to form the contralateral medial lemniscus. Some fibers have reflex connections within the spinal cord. Other fibers ascend to the reticular formation (brain stem) and reenter the spine. Some fibers connect ipsilaterally (same side of the CNS) with stretch reflex motor fibers at a lower level (enhancing sensory integration). Fibers enter the ventral spinocerebellar tract ipsilaterally and contralaterally (see medial lemniscus, below).

Somesthesis, Touch, Pressure, and Vibration

These fibers ascend via the posterior columns of the spinal cord to the medulla, decussate, and ascend via the medial lemniscus (see below) to the thalamus, and then to the parietal lobe (see below) (Fig. 2.7).

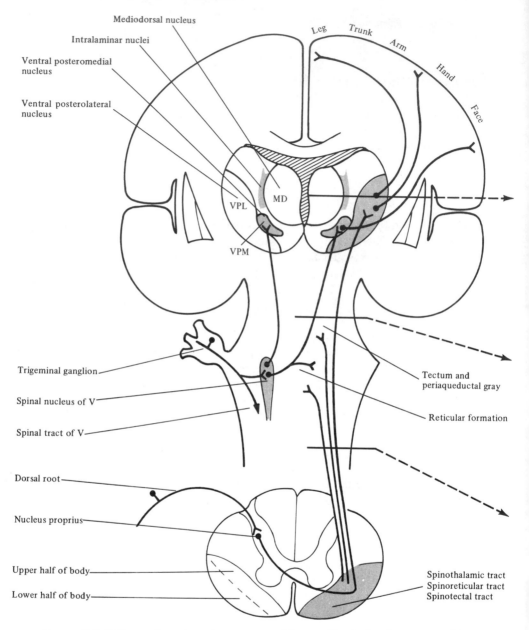

FIGURE 2.6. Pathways for pain and temperature. Diagram illustrating the course and termination of the main pathways for pain and temperature, i.e., the spinothalamic and trigeminothalamic tracts. Many of the ascending fibers in the anterolateral system of the spinal cord as well as from the trigeminal system terminate in the reticular formation, periaqueductal gray, and tectum. From Heimer L: *The Human Brain and Spinal Cord: Functional Neuroanatomy and Dissection Guide*, 1983, Springer-Verlag, New York, Fig. 102, with permission.

Descending Efferent Pathways

Fibers from higher motor centers (see Upper Motor Neuron and Lower Motor Neuron, below), after integrating with sensory centers and with interneurons at the spinal level, synapse with neurons directly controlling muscles and viscera, then exit via the ventral root.

Descending Sensory Control Pathways

Cortical and lower level centers modulate sensations such as pain, vision, and hearing. They affect somatic and visceral reflexes through direct synapses, and indirectly via interneurons (internuncials), which synapse on afferent and efferent cells.

Spinal Reflexes (see Figure 2.4)

Some sensory neurons (dorsal root) terminate directly on motor neurons (ventral root). However, in most reflex arcs there is an interneuron between sensory and motor neurons. These send axons to motor cells of the same, higher, or lower levels, or decussate to the other side. Thus, the motor response need not be at the level as the sensory input.

Pain Suppression

Pain and defensive reflexes are suppressed by corticospinal fibers that terminate near the cells of origin of the spinothalamic tract (reciprocal effect). The analgesic effect occurs through a circuit from the periaqueductal gray matter (around the aqueduct of Sylvius connecting the third and fourth ventricles, in the midbrain), to the raphe nucleus of the reticular formation of the medulla (enkephalin sensitive or opioid receptors), to the raphe spinal tract (centrally located ganglia of the midbrain, that utilize the neurotransmitter serotonin).

Autonomic Nervous System (ANS)

The ANS (see Fig. 2.2) controls the internal milieu of the body, adjusting it to global demands for action, and needs of specific organs. It operates continuously in support of muscular and organ requirements in times of danger, ongoing and appetitive functional requirements, emotions, and anticipated activity. The ANS controls and alters output, providing support for physiological activities and demands, including cardiac output, vascular tone, blood pressure, metabolic requirements, and sexual functions. Sexual functioning can be impaired after trauma to fiber tracts within the spinal cord or autonomic pathways.

Control over the ANS is expressed via the frontal lobe cortex, the limbic lobe, amygdaloid nuclei, and the hypothalamus (Adams & Victor, 1989, p. 428). The

ANS is represented by tracts leaving the brainstem and spinal cord, and having pathways separate from the spinal nerves into the viscera, glands, blood vessels, sexual organs, and organs of elimination (Brodal, 1981, p. 688). An exception is the cranial division of the parasympathetic nervous system, in which some sensory and motor fibers may be mixed in the same nerve root. Nerve pathways of the ANS are outside the CNS, and the mass of cell bodies is a ganglion (ganglia). The efferent pathways are composed of two neurons. The preganglionic neuron has its cell body within the CNS; the postganglionic neuron has its cell body outside the CNS. Sympathetic ganglia are in the body cavity; parasympathetic ganglia are in the organ or closely applied to it.

Acetylcholine is the principal neurotransmitter for all autonomic ganglia. Since its effects are like nicotine, the frequent description is nicotonic. In the craniosacral division (parasympathetic NS), its postganglionic fiber effects are like muscarine, which is derived from some species of mushroom (muscarinic).

Visceral afferent fibers are not considered part of the autonomic nervous system.

The ANS is divided into the sympathetic nervous system (SNS) and parasympathetic nervous system (PSNS). In general, these two divisions of the ANS control in opposite directions.

Parasympathetic (PSNS)

Control is either by the vagus nerve (X) or the sacral division. The two divisions are not so much antagonistic, as cooperative, in controlling internal organs, glands, and blood vessels, and coordinating them with the activity of the voluntary muscle systems. The ANS is influenced by many structures in the brain, including the cerebral cortex and the hypothalamus. At higher levels, integrative centers for visceral functions cannot be differentiated from somatic functions. The postganglionic fiber utilizes the neurotransmitter acetylcholine.

Sympathetic Nervous System (SNS)

The predominant postganglionic neurotransmitter (at the stimulated organ) is norepinephrine, which has a prolonged and generalized effect. It tends to act as

▶

FIGURE 2.7. The spinocervicothalamic pathway for touch and pressure. Diagram illustrating the second major pathway mediating impulses for tactile discrimination. Following a relay in the nucleus proprius, the impulses ascend in the dorsolateral fasciculus to the lateral cervical nucleus, which is located in the upper cervical region. Axons from the lateral cervical nucleus cross over to the other side and ascend in close relationship to the spinothalamic tract. From Heimer L: *The Human Brain and Spinal Cord: Functional Neuroanatomy and Dissection Guide*, 1983, Springer-Verlag, New York, Fig. 106, with permission.

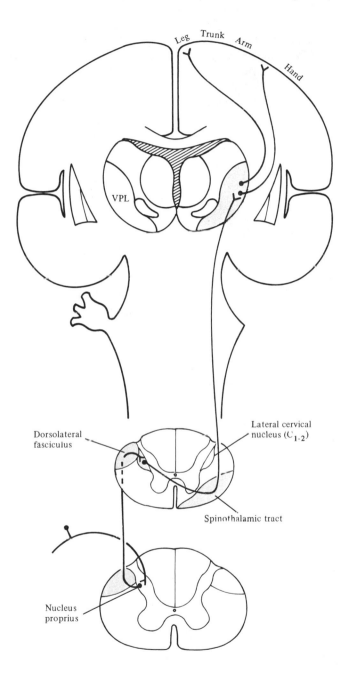

VPL

Dorsolateral
fasciculus

Lateral cervical
nucleus (C$_{1-2}$)

Spinothalamic tract

Nucleus
proprius

an integrated unit since preganglionic neurons synapse with up to 30 or more postganglionic neurons, which end on many effector cells (Pansky et al., 1988, p. 230). Its action is magnified by stimulating the core (medulla) of the adrenal gland to secrete epinephrine and norepinephrine, which contribute to energy utilization. Stimulation of the SNS as a whole results in emotional expression, acceleration of the heart, increased blood pressure, elevated blood pressure, erection of hairs, sweating, dilation of the pupil, release of epinephrine and norepinephrine from the medulla of the adrenal gland, liberating glucose, increasing metabolism, inhibiting insulin secretion, reducing blood clotting time, increasing red and white cell count, inhibiting activities of stomach, intestines, and constricting intestinal sphinctors. These characterize the "fight-or-flight" response.

Levels of Spinal Cord and ANS Functioning

The cranial branch of the parasympathetic nervous system leaves the brain and skull from the midbrain and medulla (see Barr & Kiernan, 1983, p. 78; Carpenter & Sutin, 1983, pp. 186–187, p. 215; Livingston, 1985, p. 1238; Kandel & Schwartz, 1985, pp. 472–473). Some spinal segments have no autonomic outflow.

Parasympathetic Branch (Craniosacral)

The PSNS is divided into two branches: the craniosacral, which leaves the midbrain and medulla and the sacral, which leaves the spinal cord from S2 to S4.

Cranial division (bulbar outflow): The predominant neurotransmitter is acetylcholine.

Midbrain: oculomotor nerve (III)
Medulla: facial nerve (VII)
            glossopharyngeal nerve (IX)
            vagus nerve (X)

Sacral division: The preganglionic fibers are in S2–S4.
This innervates organs of the pelvis, i.e., lower colon, elimination, and sex.

Sympathetic Nervous System (Thoracolumbar)

The SNS has pre-ganglionic cells in the ventral horn of the spinal cord. Fibers leave via the ventral root (T1–L3), and then join to become a chain of nerve cells (ganglia) on each side of the spinal column. These run up and down the visceral cavity, extending into the neck as the stellate ganglion, middle cervical ganglion, and superior cervical ganglion. Postganglionic neurons innervate the bodily organs, glands, and muscles of the eye pupil.

Sacral Division of Parasympathetic: S2–4

The pelvic nerve and pelvic plexus serve pelvic viscera, carrying inhibitory impulses to the internal anal, vescical, and uterine sphincters, and dilator impulses to blood vessels of the bladder, rectum, and genitalia. They control tumescence of the labia, clitoris, and penis (Livingston, 1985, p. 1217).

Spinal Levels of Innervation (see Figures 2.2 and 2.3)

The section of the spinal cord at C2 results in quadriplegia, with survival requiring permanent artificial respiration.

Movements of the head by neck muscles: C1–C4.
Movements of the diaphragm: C3–C5.
Sensation of clavicle: C4.
Abductor of fifth finger: C8.
Sensation of fifth finger: C8.
Brachial plexus, innervating the upper limbs, C5–8, T1.
Diaphragm: C3–5.
C5: deltoid and biceps muscles.
Upper extremity: C5–T2.
Thoracic segments: position sense of upper limbs are in dorsal funiculi above the
    level of T1.
Movements of the trunk: T1–T12.
Spinal transaction at T10 results in motor and sensory disconnection at the level
    of the umbilicus, including loss of voluntary use of both legs, bowel, and blad-
    der. The patient is paraplegic.
Movements of the lower extremity: L1–S2.
Sensation of anterior surface of the thigh: L3.
Lumbar: L3–L5 innervate large muscle groups in the lower extremities.
Sensation of great toe: L5.
Quadriceps muscle and knee jerk: L2–4.
Long extensor of great toe: L5.
Plantar flexor reflex, gastrocnemius muscle, ankle jerk: S1.
Sensation from lateral aspect of foot: S1.
Sacral segments: S2–S4 innervate the parasympathetic nervous system (pelvic
    nerve).
Cremasteric reflex (elevation of scrotum on striking inner aspect of thigh):
    T12–L2.
Sensation from genitals: S2–4.
Genital center for ejaculation: L1,L2 (smooth muscle); S3–4 for skeletal muscle.
Retention of urine: T12–L2.
Descending colon and rectum: sympathetic, T12–L3; parasympathetic S2–4.
Genital center of erection: sympathetic, T10–L2; parasympathetic, S2–4.

Evacuation of bladder: S2–5 (sites vary with the source).
Sensation from perineum: S3–5.
Anal reflex: S4–5 and coccygeal.

Sensory Routes to the Cortex

Sensory input (see Figs. 2.5–2.7) involves interaction between ascending and descending pathways. Sensory pathways have several synapses between the receptor and the cortex. Different pathways converge at particular nuclei, permitting integration of sensory information and activation of motor reflexes for life-preserving and other physiological activities. Ascending sensations are modified by descending information from the first sensory area of the cerebral cortex (postcentral gyrus), and other sensory cortical areas and intermediate nuclei (vestibular, visual, auditory, see Livingston, 1985).

Direct Route

Specific sensory information proceeds with relatively few synapses from the spinal cord via the medulla to the posterior sensory nuclei of the thalamus (see Livingston, 1985, p. 1142 for comparison of direct and indirect routes to the cortex).

There are three important sensory pathways within the brain, which terminate in the ventral posterior nucleus of the thalamus: the spinothalamic lemniscus, which decussates within the spinal cord (pain, temperature, touch); the medial lemniscus, which decussates within the medulla (discriminative touch, proprioception, vibration); and the trigeminal lemniscus, whose origin is the fifth cranial nerve. The trigeminal nerve is the principal sensory nerve for the head (pain, temperature, and light touch), and is partially crossed and uncrossed.

Medial Lemniscus System

This mediates proprioception (sensation from joints and ligaments), which contributes to position sense and thus to muscular control and movement and kinesthesis (sensations from muscles and ligaments), kinesthesis (awareness of the position and of parts of the body), 2-point touch, tactile detection of shapes and objects, textures, and the position of stimuli moving across the surface of the skin. It is the shortest, most accurate, and modality-specific path to the cortex (sometimes two synapses).

Primary fibers enter the cord through lumbar and sacral roots, divide into long ascending and short descending branches (Carpenter and Sutin, 1983, p. 267), and terminate in spinal gray matter, where they establish connections for spinal reflexes. Most ascending fibers terminate at various levels of the cord.

Fibers of the lower limb and lower portion of the body ascend as the fasciculus gracilis, which is bilateral on both sides of the dorsal midline, and terminate ipsilaterally in the medulla in the nucleus gracilis. Since these continue from the lower portion of the spinal cord upward, this fasciculus is present throughout the spinal cord. It contains the ascending branches of the sacral, lumbar, and lower six thoracic dorsal roots. Upper limb and body fibers give rise to the fasciculus cuneatus higher in the spinal cord, just lateral to the fasciculus gracilus, which terminates in the medulla as the nucleus cuneatus. The fasciculus cuneatus, lateral to the fasciculus gracilis, contains long ascending branches of the upper six thoracic and all cervical dorsal roots.

Some fibers of the cuneate fasciculus synapse in the accessory cuneate nuclei and enter the cerebellum via the inferior cerebellur peduncle (see spinocebellar, below).

These nuclei give rise to fibers that decussate ventromedially around the central gray matter, and contralaterally form an ascending bundle, the medial lemniscus. This ascends through the medulla, pons, and mibrain to terminate somatopically in the ventral posterolateral nucleus of the thalamus, providing kinesthetic and tactile sense to the parietal cortex for the contralateral portion of the body.

Spinothalamic System: Pain, Temperature, Light Touch

This provides less accurate and less modality-specific information than the above-discussed lemniscal system. Pain fibers ascend in the spinothalamic and spinoreticular tract, then enters the dorsolateral tract of Lissauer, ascends or descends for one to four segments, then crosses the midline in the ventral gray and white commissures, and ascends in the spinothalamic tract (ventral and lateral funiculus) to the thalamus. Damage to tracts of the spinal cord close to the ganglion of entry will hamper ipsilateral sensation, but contralateral sensation at lower levels.

Light touch, in contrast to other senses, is not much interrupted by hemisection of the spine, since it is bilateral (Barr & Kiernan, 1983, p. 80).

These sensations are processed apparently at the thalamus, where they may enter consciousness. They can be experienced even after complete destruction of the sensory areas of the cortex (Carpenter & Sutin, 1983, p. 664). The spinothalamic system at the medulla and pons gives off fibers to the reticular formation (spinoreticular path) and to periaqueductal gray matter of the midbrain. In the medulla, the spinothalamic tract moves laterally, and forms the spinal lemniscus, which is lateral to the medial lemniscus.

Spinocerebellar

This tract provides information required for coordination and balance. Spinocerebellar stimulation does not enter consciousness. The posterior (dorsal) spinocerebellar tract (not part of the lemniscus) carries stimuli for proprioception and kinesthesis ipsilaterally and enters the cerebellum through the inferior cerebellar peduncle. The anterior spinocerebellar tract forms from fibers that cross the midline (contralateral) and ascend, mostly entering the cerebellum through the superior peduncle. (A few fibers recross to the side of origin.)

Indirect Route

Indirect pathways to the cortex may be considered under two headings, i.e., the spinoreticular tract, which participates in the ascending reticular activating system (ARAS), and visceral afferents.

Spinoreticular Tract

This pathway is mostly uncrossed, and terminates in various medullary nuclei, from which stimuli are transmitted rostrally (intrathalamic nuclei and hypothalamus), back to the spinal cord, and to the cerebellum. This path transmits somesthetic and visceral information, which widely influences much of the cerebral cortex through thalamic relays. The spinoreticular system participates in the ascending reticular aystem, which is significant in maintaining consciousness. The ARAS is discussed in more detail below.

Ascending Visceral Projection System

Afferent fibers from the visceral organs, suspensory tissues, lung, and organ surfaces are sensitive to shearing forces, tension, pressure, dilation, peristalsis against an obstruction (gallstones), inflammation, etc. (Livingston, 1985, 1137–1140, 1142). They are phylogenetically the oldest, slowest, most multisynaptic, and least modality-specific path. More than half of the fibers decussate. They pass through autonomic nerve trunks and plexes, and reach the central nervous system through the vagus nerve (X) and autonomic nerve roots entering through the spinal dorsal root and brainstem analogues.

The gray matter sensorimotor network serving visceral functions is almost continuous through the spinal, brainstem, and diencephalic levels. There is a multisynaptic succession of relays contributing to gray matter along the central core of the neuraxis, including the floor of the fourth ventricle and midbrain periaqueductal gray. This joins the medial forebrain bundle, projecting to the diencephalon and basal forebrain. Other relays contribute to spinothalamic projections, and via thalamic relays to the cerebral cortex. These signals ascend a few segments at a time, are repeatedly relayed, and therefore are diffused over time and space. Ordinarily they do not reach consciousness, except when there is a massive afferent activation. Visceral locations are poorly localized (e.g., may be "referred"), have feeling tone, and command attention.

Efferent Actions of the Spinal Cord

Descending Motor Pathways

Upper Motor Neuron

Upper motor neurons originate in the cerebral cortex and extend into the spine (corticospinal or pyramidal, corticobulbar), and those which participate in other descending brainstem pathways (Fig. 2.8). These descending pathways of the

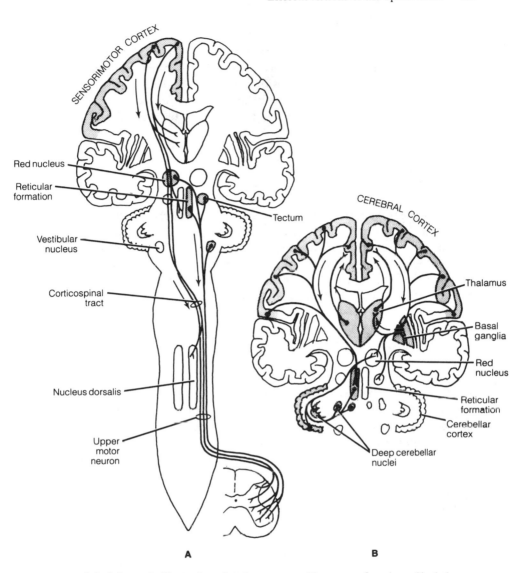

FIGURE 2.8. Schematic illustration of pathways controlling motor functions. Shaded areas denote gray matter actively involved in the circuits. *A*: Arrows denote descending pathways. *B*: Arrows denote cerebellar and basal ganglia circuit. Reproduced, with permission, from deGroot J, Chusid JG: *Correlative Neuroanatomy*, twentieth edition, copyright © 1988, Appleton & Lange, East Norwalk, CT, Fig. 12.2.

brain and spinal cord are involved in volitional control of the musculature (see "Integrated Sensory and Motor Functioning"). Properly coordinated movements depend on the cerebral cortex, basal ganglia, thalamus, subthalamic nuclei, red nucleus, substantia nigra, reticular formation, vestibular nuclei, and cerebellum (Barr & Kiernan, 1983, p. 331).

Lower Motor Neuron

Lower motor neurons originate in the ventral (anterior) horn of the spinal cord, i.e., the last unit in the motor response. These innervate muscles, glands, and viscera for action. One branch serves the muscles. Complete lesions result in a loss of all motion. The other branch enters the autonomic ganglia of the parasympathetic nervous system and also the sacral branch of the sympathetic nervous system (see above).

The Brainstem

The brainstem is defined as that part of the brain between the spinal cord and the cerebral hemispheres, exclusive of the cerebellum, including the medulla, pons, midbrain, and diencephalon (Carpenter and Sutin, 1983) (Fig. 2.9). Some authorities (Walton, 1985, p. 19) do not include the diencephalon. The brainstem includes ascending, descending, and decussating tracts, nuclei of the cranial nerves, vital centers for survival, and other nuclei affecting movement (*substantia nigra* and *red nucleus* of the midbrain, and *inferior olivary nuclei* of the medulla). It is vulnerable to severe or fatal damage from rotation, compression, etc.

Reticular Formation (RF)

This RF system is a bilateral structure extending from the midbrain to the medulla (see Carpenter & Sutin; 1983; Pansky et al., 1988). It is part of a primitive reticulum of cell groups and fibers extending along the neuraxis from the spinal cord through the brain stem. It was formerly thought to have diffuse connections with the cerebral cortex. It is now conceived to have widespread rather than diffuse projections, i.e., neurons that make specific cortical connections and utilize particular neurotransmitters. Particular fibers may transmit both rostrally and caudally, or only to one destination. For example, a locus ceruleus neuron can have collateral branches to the neocortex, hippocampus, cerebellum, and spinal cord (Watson, Khachaturian, Lewis, and Akil, 1986). RF pathways project to the orbitofrontal surface, frontal convexity, sensorimotor cortex (Carpenter & Sutin, 1983, p. 442), hypothalamus, mamillary body of the hypothalamus, spinal column, and cerebellum (chief references: Carpenter & Sutin, 1983, p. 332; Kandel & Schwartz, 1985, pp. 556–561; Pansky et al., 1988, pp. 258–263).

The key integrating area appears to be essentially in the medulla, pons, and midbrain, i.e., the periaqueductal gray matter, which has an integrating and arousing function. Further, it contains opiate receptors that suppress the immune system (Weber & Pert, 1989, see further Chapter 15 on Stress). It has a facilitating and inhibiting effect on spinal and cranial motor activity. The medullary reticular formation projects to the cerebellar cortex and nuclei. It receives topographically arranged input from the spinal cord via spinoreticular pathways, motor input from rubrobulbar pathways, and vaginal input related to sexual behavior (Carpenter & Sutin, 1983, p. 326).

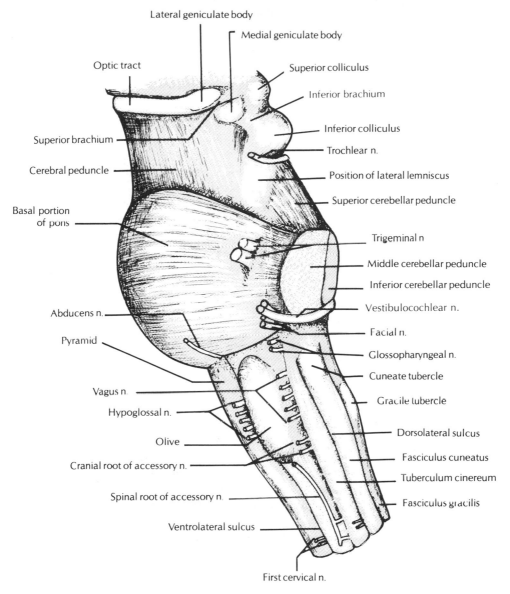

Lateral geniculate body

Medial geniculate body

Optic tract

Superior colliculus

Inferior brachium

Superior brachium

Inferior colliculus

Trochlear n.

Cerebral peduncle

Position of lateral lemniscus

Superior cerebellar peduncle

Basal portion
of pons

Trigeminal n

Middle cerebellar peduncle

Inferior cerebellar peduncle

Vestibulocochlear n.

Abducens n.

Facial n.

Pyramid

Glossopharyngeal n.

Cuneate tubercle

Vagus n.

Gracile tubercle

Hypoglossal n.

Dorsolateral sulcus

Olive

Fasciculus cuneatus

Cranial root of accessory n.

Tuberculum cinereum

Spinal root of accessory n.

Fasciculus gracilis

Ventrolateral sulcus

First cervical n.

FIGURE 2.9. Lateral aspect of the brain stem. From Barr and Kiernan (1988), Fig. 6.2, with permission.

General Functions

• Monitoring environmental and bodily information;
• Processing of information that is further transmitted to the thalamus and to the spinal cord;

• Maintaining consciousness (ascending fibers);
• Influences the level of motor functioning (descending).

Reticular Formation Output

The RF sends out ascending projections in the direction of the cortex (ascending reticular activating system, or ARAS), and descending projections to the spinal cord (descending reticular activating system, or DRAS).

Input to Reticular Formation

Afferents originate from the cortex (sensorimotor motor areas primarily), spinal column, and from all the cranial nerves [chiefly visual, auditory and vestibular (balance)], except for olfaction, whose input is indirect (Livingston, 1985, p. 1267); globus pallidus, and, hypothalamus. Sensory stimulation from a wide variety of sources converges on the medulla. Thus, the RF can monitor "virtually all that is going on in the body and in the environment and to contribute to priority decision making with respect to ongoing behavior" (Livingston, 1985, p. 1207).

Ascending Reticular Activating System

The ARAS stimulates more general areas of the cortex, in contrast to specific sensory or motor projections. It includes fibers from the spinal cord (a poly-synaptic extralemniscal route) to the intralaminar group of thalamic nuclei, where it influences levels of consciousness. Its route to the cortex is separate from the various sensory tracts.

Sensory stimulation reaching the RF is relayed as the ascending reticular activating system (ARAS) to the cortex, causing *desyncronization* of neurons (characteristic of alertness), as opposed to the high voltage, synchronized pattern found in sleep and seizures. This process maintains consciousness.

ARAS stimulation can create activation (arousal) even when the sensory tracts are destroyed. It is not involved with any sensory modality, rather it appears to "sharpen the attentive state of the cortex and create optimal conditions for the conscious perception of sensory impulses mediated by the classical pathways" (Carpenter & Sutin, 1983, p. 443).

Descending Reticular Activating System

• Modifies muscle tone (see Magnocellular Nucleus, below);
• Modifies breathing and cardiac function through input from the autonomic nervous system, hypothalamus, and prefrontal association cortex;
• Influences the sense of pain through pathways to the dorsal horn of the spinal cord (sensory input);
• Integrates sensorimotor activities.

Behaviorally Significant Brainstem Nuclei, Tracts, and Neurotransmitters

Many nuclei and pathways of the brainstem, and reticular formation in particular, are implicated in functions that are impaired after TBI. Nieuwenhuys (1985) is a detailed source, including characteristics of particular classes of neurotransmitters and their pathways. Cells manufacturing, or being stimulated by, particular neurotransmitters are frequently bunched together into behaviorally identifiable systems. Chemical aspects of neural transmission are found in Trimble (1988a, pp. 63–86). Some behaviorally significant neurotransmitters are discussed below.

The pathways of neurons that secrete and carry particular neurotransmitters differ from pathways established through gross anatomical studies (Watkins et al., 1986). They have great importance for both brain damage and many psychiatric disorders.

Catecholamines (Synthesized from the Amino Acid Tyrosine)

Catecholamines include epinephrine, norepinephrine, L-tyrosine, L-DOPA, dopamine, isoproterinol. Catecholamine neurotransmitters are synthesized in the brainstem locus ceruleus, and its receptors are found in the cortex, limbic system, basal ganglia, and hypothalamus.

Dopamine receptors are significant in movement-related neurons [the basal ganglia (subcortical) and substantia nigra (pons)], and are implicated in psychosis and Parkinsonism. Dopamine is transported from the brainstem to the striatum and limbic system. Its influence is primarily motor, and is greater in sensory association areas than in primary sensory regions, and in auditory areas than in visual association areas. Dopaminergic fibers are found in circuits of the midbrain, substantia nigra, and hypothalamus. They project to the basal ganglia, hypothalamus, limbic system, and neocortex.

The *nigrostriatum*, i.e., reciprocal connections between substantia nigra and striatum (see Basal Ganglia below; see Carpenter & Suton, 1983), modulates responsiveness to the environment through a gating function. Input from all areas of the cortex, and the ascending reticular activating system through the nonspecific thalamic nuclei, converges on it. Dopamine is a significant neurotransmitter. The nigrostriatal system protects the organism against the effects of stress by hyperarousal, i.e., increasing sensory responsiveness. The adverse effects of stress are compensated for through behavioral change, which also overcomes the effects of neurological deficits, e.g., in Parkinson's disease (Antelman & Caggiula, 1980). Other dopaminergic cells are part of the circuitry of the median eminence of the hypothalamopituitary axis.

Noradrenergic fibers emanating in the locus ceruleus have an excitatory function, and run to the entire forebrain, including diencephalon, telencephalon, hippocampus, cerebral cortex, and cerebellar cortex. Lesions create a decrease in cortical activation (Kales & Kales, 1984, p. 16).

Serotonin

This is manufactured in the floor of the brainstem (raphe nuclei). It is transported *rostrally* to the frontal cortex, basal ganglia, limbic system, thalamus, hypothalamus, entorhinal cortex of the temporal lobe, and, *caudally*, to the cerebellum, reticular formation of the lower brainstem pons, and medulla (Carpenter & Sutin, 1983, 415–416). It affects mood and ability to sleep.

Raphe nuclei are behaviorally significant cell masses in the midline, extending from the diencephalon to the medulla (see the diagram, Carpenter & Sutin, 1983, p. 330; Watson et al., 1986). Raphe nuclei of the anterior pons and above project to the diencephalon, thalamus, amygdala, hippocampus, limbic cortex, reticular formation, and neocortex. Ascending fibers are widespread, and are implicated in aggressive behavior, sleep, and neuroendocrine regulation. Lesions of serotonergic cells create irreversible insomnia (Carpenter & Sutin, 1983, p. 409; Kales & Kales, 1984, p. 15). Posterior nuclei project to the spine, where they modulate pain-related neurons, and inhibit sympathetic preganglionic neurons.

Acetylcholine (ACH)

ACH is the principal transmitter for all autonomic nervous system (ANS) ganglia (nicotonic), and many neurons of the parasympathetic craniosacral division (muscarinic) of the ANS. ACH is primarily used by motor neurons in the spinal cord and preganglionic autonomic neurons, postganglionic parasympthathetic neurons, and caudate nucleus and hippocampus.

Magnocellular Nuclei (Pons and Medulla)

1. Affect muscle tone: Predominantly crossed fibers from the sensorimotor area of the cerebral cortex terminate in the region where fibers from the reticular formation originate to the spinal cord. Fibers originating in the medulla inhibit, and those of the pons facilitate muscle tone.
2. Regulate sleep phase. During REM sleep there is reduced inhibition by serotonergic and noradrenergic fibers. These cells fire during the REM phase, only to be inhibited at the next phase of the cycle (Kales & Kales, 1984, p. 16).

GABA

γ-Aminobutyric acid (GABA) is usually inhibitory. Its receptors are closely associated with the benzodiazepine receptor (known for its tranquilizing effect), and are found in the cortex and midbrain.

Releasing Factors

These are chemical substances, found in the hypothalamus and elsewhere, that are released into the local capillary circulation to influence hormonal release from the anterior pituitary gland. (See Pituitary Gland, below.)

Enkephalins

These are peptides that have opiate-like activity. Their neurons and receptors have been identified in the limbic system and striatum.

Hindbrain

Medulla Oblongata (Myelencephalon)

Anatomical

The medulla oblongata is the most posterior portion of the brainstem, located below the posterior floor of the fourth ventricle, in turn underneath the posterior portion of the cerebellum (see Figs. 2.1, 2.9, and 2.10). It extends from the entry of the spinal cord into the skull (foramen magnum) to the pons. It has a structure similar to the spinal cord. Significant features include fourth ventricle, continuation of the central gray matter of the spinal cord into the reticular formation, decussation of the corticospinal tracts (pyramids), termination of ascending spinal sensory tracts (fasciculi gracilis and cuneatus), formation of the significant ascending sensory tract, the medial lemniscus, and nuclei of cranial nerves VIII—vestibulocochlear (in part), IX—glossopharyngeal, X—vagus, XI—spinal accessory, and XII—hypoglossal.

Physiological

It is influenced by higher level neurons from the hypothalamus, cerebral cortex, and other central areas that integrate vasomotor activity. Its activity is also influenced by respiratory input and the chemical composition of the blood. Its vasomotor center controls arterial and capillary dilation, constriction, cardiac output, the constriction of peripheral blood vessels, etc.

Inferior Olivary Complex

Situated in the medulla (Fig. 2.9), this group of nuclei is a characteristic landmark. It receives fibers from all cerebral lobes, the red nucleus of the midbrain, and the gray matter surrounding the aqueduct (important for consciousness) and projects to all sections of the cerebellum. It is also significant for coordination, projecting to the cerebellum (Carpenter & Sutin, 1983, p. 331). The inferior olive is believed to be part of the informational input circuit for motor learning, whose tract is located in the cerebellum (Thompson, 1988).

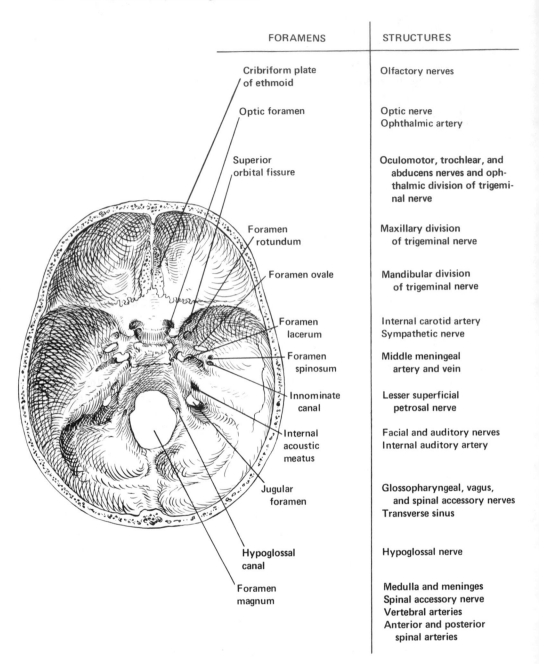

FORAMENS	STRUCTURES
Cribriform plate of ethmoid	Olfactory nerves
Optic foramen	Optic nerve Ophthalmic artery
Superior orbital fissure	Oculomotor, trochlear, and abducens nerves and ophthalmic division of trigeminal nerve
Foramen rotundum	Maxillary division of trigeminal nerve
Foramen ovale	Mandibular division of trigeminal nerve
Foramen lacerum	Internal carotid artery Sympathetic nerve
Foramen spinosum	Middle meningeal artery and vein
Innominate canal	Lesser superficial petrosal nerve
Internal acoustic meatus	Facial and auditory nerves Internal auditory artery
Jugular foramen	Glossopharyngeal, vagus, and spinal accessory nerves Transverse sinus
Hypoglossal canal	Hypoglossal nerve
Foramen magnum	Medulla and meninges Spinal accessory nerve Vertebral arteries Anterior and posterior spinal arteries

FIGURE 2.10. Emergence of cranial nerves from the brain. Reproduced, with permission, from Chusid JG: *Correlative Neuroanatomy and Functional Neurology*, nineteenth edition, copyright © 1985, Lange Medical Publications, Fig. 6.1.

Pons (Mesencephalon)

The pons extends from below the anterior portion of the fourth ventricle (Figs. 2.1, 2.9, and 2.13), and underneath the anterior cerebellum, to the cerebral aqueduct (passageway connecting the third and fourth ventricles). It is identified by a broad band of fibers that projects between the two cerebellar hemispheres (middle cerebellar peduncle). The ventral part contains descending fibers. The dorsal part (tegmentum) contains a portion of the reticular formation and ascending sensory fibers.

The pons is significant for states of consciousness and sleep. Fibers from the locus ceruleus (noradrenergic) and the raphe nuclei of the midline (serotonergic) project to the cortex and hippocampus. It contains the nuclei of cranial nerves V, VI, VII, and VIII (in part) – see below. Projections of the locus ceruleus uniquely project directly to the neocortex without synaptic relays in the thalamus.

Vestibular Nuclei

The vestibular nuclei are of great significance because of the frequency of balance problems following trauma. Balance and motor control are maintained through the medial longitudinal fasciculus to the motor nuclei for the eyes (III, IV and VI), spinal cord, cerebellum, and reticular formation (Livingston, 1985, p. 1032). Trauma may also affect balance through injury to the inner ear, which is innervated via the vestibular nuclei.

Trapezoid Body

The fiber tracts for hearing are separate from those concerning movement of the body in space, although both are part of cranial nerve VIII. The trapezoid body represents fiber tracts that convey most auditory stimuli contralaterally (although some auditory stimulation is ipsilateral) to the opposite side of the pons, then rostrally via the lateral lemniscus to the inferior colliculus (see below).

Midbrain or Mesencephalon (Figures 2.1, 2.9, 2.13)

This is penetrated by the narrow cerebral acqueduct (aqueduct of Sylvius).

The Tectum

The roof contains two pairs of bulges, the *corpora quadrigemina*, i.e., the colliculi.

Superior colliculus (anterior). This is concerned primarily with detection of the direction of movements in the visual field, facilitating visual orientation, searching, and tracking. It receives inputs from relay nuclei of the somesthetic and auditory systems, various cerebellar and brainstem nuclei, and the reticular formation.

Inferior colliculus (posterior). This is an auditory stimulation relay station that projects to the medial geniculate body of the thalamus, which projects in turn to the auditory cortex of the temporal lobe (Heschl's gyrus). The inferior colliculus receives feedback from the auditory cortex, lateral lemniscus, and opposite inferior colliculus.

The central gray substance (significant in arousal) surrounds the aqueduct.

The medial lemniscus, an ascending sensory tract, is found at about the level of the aqueduct.

The posterior commissure is between the mesencephalon and the anteriorly situated diencephalon. It contains fibers of significance for pupillary reflexes, eyelid retraction, and vertical eye movements.

The Tegmentum

The floor (below the aqueduct of Sylvius) is the ventral region of the midbrain.

Red nucleus is anterior and medial (bilateral) and extends to the diencephalon. It receives ascending cerebellar fibers.

Substantia nigra is a dopamine-producing nucleus that projects to the basal ganglia, thalamus, and superior colliculus. It is significant in motor control, and is implicated in Parkinson's disease. The substantia nigra is believed to inhibit the globus pallidus, which when unopposed has an excitatory motor effect (tremor). Then incorrect stimuli are transmitted via the thalamus to the motor cortex (Pincus & Tucker, 1985, pp. 219–220).

The tegmentum contains the *superior cerebellar peduncle*, which contains ascending tracts from the cerebellum and decussates at the midbrain. It extends diagonally across the tegmentum.

The *crus cerebri* are descending tracts from the cortex, and comprise the external section of the lower mesencephalon.

Forebrain

Cerebral Hemispheres

These are the most visible, large paired structures, at the anterior end of the central nervous system comprising the cerebral cortex or gray matter (cell bodies), white matter (fiber tracts connecting the cells), and basal ganglia. In common usage, this refers to bilateral structures (cortex, fiber tracts, and basal ganglia), and not the brainstem, which is considered to be a distinctive structure (Figs. 2.11, 2.12, and 2.13).

Cerebral Ventricle

These important landmarks inside the cerebral hemispheres are interconnecting cavities that are continuous inside the spinal cord (see Fig. 2.1). They are filled

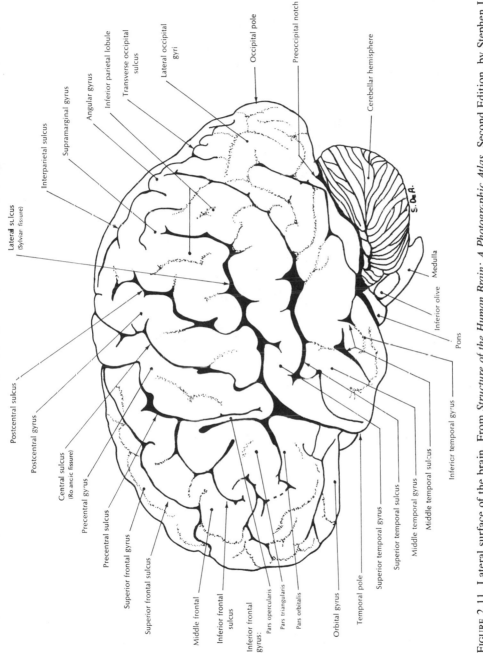

FIGURE 2.11. Lateral surface of the brain. From *Structure of the Human Brain: A Photographic Atlas*, Second Edition, by Stephen J. DeArmond, Madeline M. Fusco, and Maynad M. Dewey, copyright © 1974, 1976 by Oxford University Press, Inc., Fig. 2, reprinted by permission.

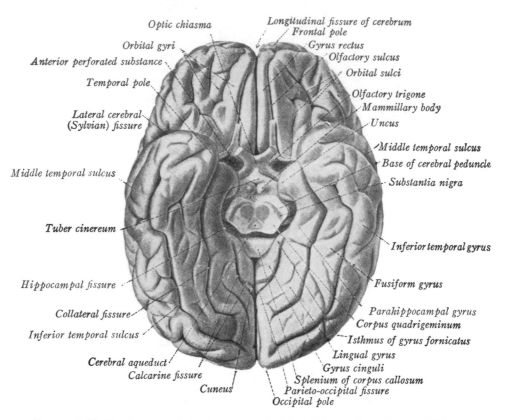

Optic chiasma
Orbital gyri
Anterior perforated substance
Temporal pole
Lateral cerebral (Sylvian) fissure
Middle temporal sulcus
Tuber cinereum
Hippocampal fissure
Collateral fissure
Inferior temporal sulcus
Cerebral aqueduct
Calcarine fissure
Cuneus

Longitudinal fissure of cerebrum
Frontal pole
Gyrus rectus
Olfactory sulcus
Orbital sulci
Olfactory trigone
Mammillary body
Uncus
Middle temporal sulcus
Base of cerebral peduncle
Substantia nigra
Inferior temporal gyrus
Fusiform gyrus
Parahippocampal gyrus
Corpus quadrigeminum
Isthmus of gyrus fornicatus
Lingual gyrus
Gyrus cinguli
Splenium of corpus callosum
Parieto-occipital fissure
Occipital pole

FIGURE 2.12. Basal aspect of the human cerebral hemisphere. From Ranson SW and Clark SL (1959), Fig. 51, with permission.

with cerebrospinal fluid, and are important in the circulation of oxygen, nutrients, and waste products. Various pathological conditions (e.g., hydrocephalus from interference with circulation, swelling, hematoma, tumors) cause them to expand, shrink, or be displaced from their symmetrical position in the center and/or bilaterally in the cerebrum.

Thalamus

This major nucleus has complex functions (Fig. 2.14). A table of input, output, and functions is found in Kandel and Schwartz (1985, p. 234).

▶

FIGURE 2.13. Medial surface of the brain. From *Structure of the Human Brain: A Photographic Atlas*, Second Edition, by Stephen J. DeArmond, Madeline M. Fusco, and Maynad M. Dewey, copyright © 1974, 1976 by Oxford University Press, Inc., Fig. 4, reprinted by permission.

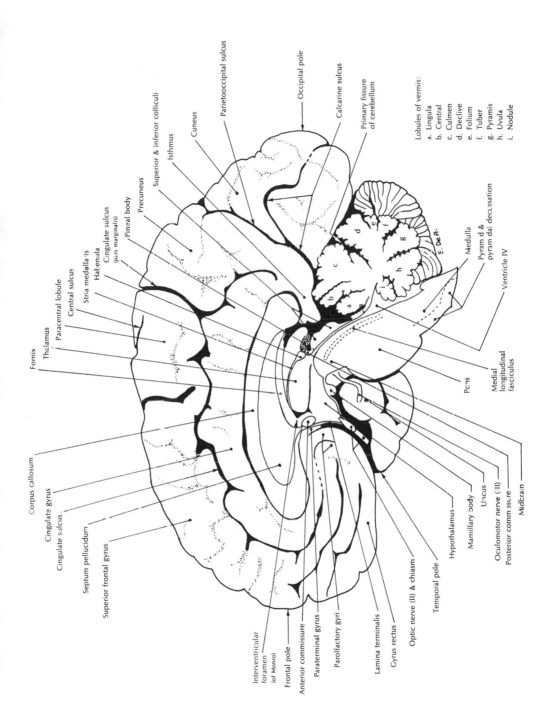

Lobules of vermis:
a. Lingula
b. Central
c. Culmen
d. Declive
e. Folium
f. Tuber
g. Pyramis
h. Uvula
i. Nodule

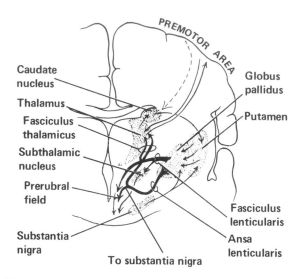

FIGURE 2.14. Diagrams of principal thalmocortical projections showing relation of corti-cal areas to thalamic nuclei. Reproduced, with permission, from Chusid, JG: *Correlative Neuroanatomy and Functional Neurology*, nineteenth ed., © 1985, Lange Medical Publi-cations, Fig. 3.25. (Adapted from an original painting by Frank H. Netter, M.D. from *The Ciba Collection of Medical Illustrations* copyright by CIBA-GEIGY Corporation, with permission.)

1. Relaying sensory and integrating sensory information from the spinal cord, and all cranial nerves except the olfactory nerve.
2. An association or relay system for other forebrain mechanisms, i.e., within nuclei of the limbic system, between basal ganglia and cerebral cortex, between cerebellar and cerebral cortices, between the superior colliculi and cortex, for limbic functions and emotional expression, etc.
3. Influencing various cognitive functions (Brodal, 1981, pp. 836–837), although the temporal cortex is best known for its vulnerability to verbal deficits.
4. Integrating reticular formation, cortex, and other thalamic nuclei with limbic functions and other thalamic nuclei.

Hypothalamus

The hypothalamus (Figs. 2.10, 2.12, and 2.13) lies in the lower portion of the walls of the third ventricle, and is continuous across its floor. It is an integrating system between the thalamus, the cerebral cortex, the brain stem, and the spinal cord. It is concerned with visceral, autonomic, and endocrine functions, and affective behavior. The hypothalamus is sensitive to the physiological status of the body as reflected in blood (temperature, dissolved particles, water concentra-tion, hormones, etc.). Through efferent pathways to autonomic nuclei in the brainstem and spinal cord, and to the pituitary gland, it maintains a constant internal environment (homeostasis).

The regulatory activity of the hypothalamus is accomplished through the hypothalamic–pituitary axis and via direct descending spinal tracts to the autonomic nervous system.

It influences behavioral adjustments to changes in the internal or external environment, e.g., aggression, defense, etc. (see Neuroactive Peptides, above). Functionally, it responds to emotional changes, hunger, thirst, etc., integrates the behavioral expression of emotional states (Kandel and Schwartz, 1985, p. 623) (e.g., sex and anger), and exercises homeostatic control over food and water intake, and temperature control (pp. 626–635).

Behaviorally significant hypothalamic landmarks include the following:

Optic Chiasm

Just below the anterior hypothalamus, the optic nerve (II) reaches the midline, where fibers from the nasal retina decussate, and temporal fibers remain ipsilateral.

Infundibulum

This is the stalk of the pituitary gland that extends from the floor of the third ventricle (hypothalamus). An extension is the posterior pituitary gland (composed of neural tissue). A bulge slightly posterior to it is the *tuber cinereum*.

Median Eminence

The median eminence (the floor of the third ventricle) is part of the hypothalamopituitary axis, involved in control of the pituitary gland. It is of considerable significance in the stress response as a way station for releasing hormones. Pathways from the central nervous system converge here on the peripheral endocrine system, as the interface between the brain and the anterior pituitary gland.

Preoptic Region

This is part the periventricular gray matter, in the wall of the third ventricle. It plays a role in regulating release of gonadotropic hormones from the anterior lobe of the pituitary gland. Fluctuating levels in the female regulate the length of the menstrual cycle. In the male, gonadotropins are released tonically without regular fluctuations.

Supraoptic Region

This structure is located immediately above the optic nerve. It contains the paraventricular nucleus, which secretes vasopressin and oxytocin; the functions of these hormones are described under Posterior Pituitary Gland, below. These peptide hormones are formed in the cell bodies, and carried by axoplasmic transport along the axon to the posterior lobe of the pituitary gland (see below).

Mammillary Bodies

These are a pair of bulges immediately posterior to the optic chiasm. They are part of the limbic circuit. The mammillary bodies are a nucleus significant in emotional and visceral patterning. They receive input from the hippocampus via the fornix and the brainstem reticular formation. Mammillary efferent output is to the thalamus (accompanied by hippocampal stimuli), which feeds in turn to the cingulate gyrus, to the entorhinal cortex, and back to the hippocampus.

Hypophyseal Portal System

This consists of capillaries in the floor of the third ventricle (above and within the median eminence) that pass down the pituitary stalk into the anterior pituitary, carrying releasing hormones for that body.

Efferent and Afferent Connections of the Hypothalamus

The hypothalamus receives input primarily from the phylogenetically oldest areas of the cortex (pyriform cortex and hippocampus), which are each reinforced by subcortical projection from the amygdala and septum. These subcortical nuclei are reciprocally connected with the overlying cortical area. In addition, the orbital cortex (frontal lobe) also passes into the hypothalamus. A newer portion of the cortex (the cingulate gyrus, which is also a portion of the limbic area), has input into the hypothalamus through the entorhinal cortex (temporal lobe) and hippocampus. In turn, the hypothalamus influences the cingulate cortex through the anterior nuclear group of the thalamus (Carpenter & Sutin, 1983, pp. 563–564).

Hypothalamic circuits are reciprocal with connected nuclei (Carpenter & Sutin, 1985, p. 564).

- The famous *Papez circuit*, significant for emotional behavior, goes from the hippocampus to the mammillary body to the anterior nucleus of the thalamus to the cingulate gyrus to the cingulate pathway to the the the entorhinal cortex (medial temporal lobe) and back to the hippocampus. Other pathways lead to the reticular formation.
- The medial forebrain bundle conveys incoming impulses from the olfactory region, periamygdaloid region, and septal region to various hypothalamic regions. Efferent fibers go to the septal nuclei (in the wall subdividing the third ventricle, and in the frontal lobe just rostral to the anterior commissure), then via the fornix to the hippocampus, to the central gray, and tegmentum of the midbrain.
- *Dorsal longitudinal fasciculus* is a tract that is distributed to the central gray of the midbrain and the tectum. After synapsing in the reticular formation, impulses are relayed to the medulla and spinal cord.
- *Hypothalamicospinal:* Direct pathways to the medulla and spinal cord.
- *Hypothalamicocortical:* Fibers project to the motor cortex, perhaps influencing the corticospinal system.

Epithalamus

This is found on the dorsal surface of the diencephalon, including the pineal body (see below) and habenular nuclei and tracts (posterior and lateral portion of the thalamus).

Pineal Gland

This gland is located in a median dorsal position, behind the diencephalon. Changes in amount of light are transmitted neuronally to the pineal via norepinephrine-secreting cells that stimulate enzymes to synthesize melatonin. This occurs in a marked daily rhythm. Other secretions include serotonin (released into the extracellular space, not to nerve endings), norepinephrine, TRH, LHRH, and somatostatin (Carpenter and Sutin, 1983, p. 497).

Hypothalamic–Pituitary–Adrenal Axis

This is presented in some detail in Chapters 8 and 15 on Neurophysiological functions and Stress. The essential point to be covered here is that the pituitary gland is connected by a stalk (infundibulum) from the floor of the hypothalamus to its nesting place in the skull at the base of the brain (*sella turcica*). Various hypothalamic and other nuclei create neurohormones that are transported via the *median eminence* (floor of the third ventricle) directly to the pituitary gland by neural tissue, or through blood circulation directly or via the posterior pituitary gland (portal system) to the anterior pituitary (glandular tissue). These exercise considerable somatic control through hormones secreted into the general circulation.

Cerebral Lobes and Cortex

The landmarks known as cerebral lobes are covered by a layer of neurons or cortex ("gray matter") (Figs. 2.15 and 2.16). Corticocortical and corticosubcortical interconnecting axons are known as "white matter." The cortex has evolved in different stages. The oldest, or *archipallium*, is the hippocampal formation and dentate gyrus. Next is the *paleopallium* or olfactory cortex. The remainder is the *neopallium* or neocortex. These layers are accreted on the mesencephalon, which was the level of development of birds and reptiles, to which the thalamic nuclei were added as way stations to aid in processing.

Gyri

The richness of the cortex and its connections cause the surface to be thrust upward into various elevations, which are separated by sulci. Some localization

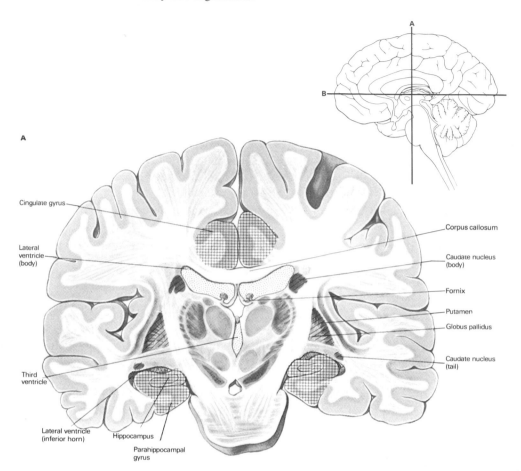

FIGURE 2.15. Coronal section of the brain. Reprinted by permission of the publisher from Development as a guide to the regional anatomy of the brain by Kandel ER and Schwartz, JH: *Principles of Neural Science*, Second Edition, (p. 256), Fig. 21.14A. Copyright 1985 by Elsevier Science Publishing Co., Inc.

of function is associated with particular gyri. In cases of cortical atrophy, the cells composing the gyrus are dead or have lost internal components or liquid.

Sulcus (Sulci)

These important landmarks are grooves in the surface of the cerebrum that separate the gyri (see Figs. 2.11, 2.12, and 2.13).

The central sulcus (fissure of Rolando), i.e., its anterior surface, is called "the motor area" (precentral gyrus, which has some sensory cortex). The posterior wall of the central sulcus is the somatosensory area (postcentral gyrus) which receives touch sensation.

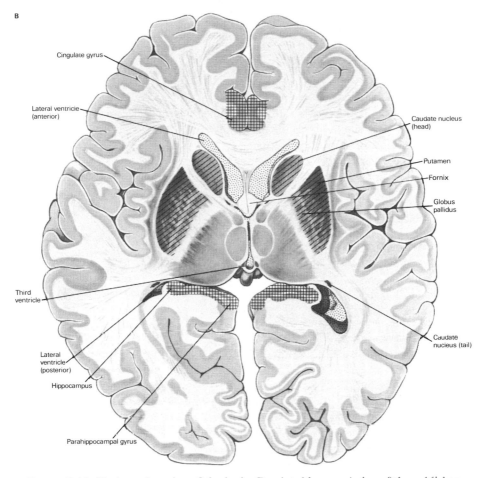

FIGURE 2.16. Horizontal section of the brain. Reprinted by permission of the publisher from Development as a guide to the regional anatomy of the brain by Kandel ER, and Schwartz JH: *Principles of Neural Science*, Second Edition, (p. 257), Fig. 21.14B. Copyright 1985 by Elsevier Science Publishing Co., Inc.

The lateral sulcus (Sylvian fissure) separates the frontal and parietal from the temporal lobe.

The parietal-occipital sulcus separates parietal and occipital lobes.

The Cerebral Cortex

The terminus of the neuraxis is a sheet of nerve cells covering the cerebral hemispheres. Brodal (1981, p. 847) observes that there is no clearcut distinction between "motor" and "somatosensory" cortical areas. The combined sensory and motor functions probably involve about 20% of the total cortex (Livingston,

1985, p. 1256). The remaining 80% of the cortex and the remaining volume of the brain represent additional "decision-making capacity."

Some Functions of the Cortex

Receives and analyzes sensory information
Secondary sensory areas integrate and give meaning to sensations
Makes plans for, and modifies, motor action
Modulates sensory input at the periphery
Input creates alterations of consciousness
Verbal and non-verbal comprehension and communication

Organization of the Cortex

The Basic Unit

A vertically arranged column of cells that processes tasks between input and output.

Input

Local (collateral), contralateral (commissures), or *projection (long vertical tracts)* fibers. Projections from reticular nuclei of the thalamus and locus ceruleus of the brainstem are concerned with general state conditions such as attention, sleep, and arousal (Livingston, 1985, p. 1148). Vertical columns fire back reciprocally to the same nuclei that provided cortical input (Livingston, 1985, pp. 1148–1149), influencing sensory relay nuclei, subcortical visceral and somatic motor control systems, cortical motor fields, and cortical sensory fields (contributing to higher order motor command and processing of sensory integration).

Incoming information is finely analyzed as to source, quality, and amount. It enters memory, is offered meaning and associations from the memory bank, and various types of sensory information are integrated.

The primary sensory areas are as follows:

• Parietal (somesthetic area of postcentral gyrus; gustatory of the post ventral part (operculum, see below) of the postcentral gyrus.
• Occipital (striate area—not the striatum, so named because a fine stripe in the cortex is visible even without a microscope).
• Temporal lobes (auditory area; olfactory areas on the interior surface, i.e., prepyriform and periamygdaloid).

A vestibular projection to the cortex is not yet known.

Secondary sensory areas exist in the parietal (somesthetic), temporal (acoustic), and occipital (visual) lobes. These project to adjacent cortex and to each other, and to association areas of the frontal lobe (Brodal, 1981, p. 801). The posterior portion of the brain is sometimes referred to as the parietal–temporal–occipital region (PTO), and is significant for integrating vision, somatic sensation, audition, etc.

Secondary areas do not analyze stimuli as precisely as the primary areas, and lesions create relatively minor deficits (Carpenter & Sutin, 1983, pp. 657–658). Luria (1980, pp. 47–48) states that stimuli for secondary areas receive subcortical integration through relays in the associative nuclei of the thalamus. Lesions create deficits of orientation to the outside world, and in the complex relationships between different stimuli impinging on the cortex.

Although particular functions may be primarily associated with a given lobe, they usually have multiple cortical representation. Of cortical connections 80% are considered intracortical (Livingston, 1985, p. 1269), e.g., the secondary sensory areas.

Anterior Posterior

It is often stated that the anterior portion of the cortex (rostral to the central sulcus) is involved with planning and motor execution and organization of movement, whereas the posterior portion is involved with reception of stimuli, forming associations to input, and verbal and nonverbal processing.

Somatotopic Localization

The structure of a nucleus (sensory or motor) is related to the structure of the body. Examples would include the motor cortex, i.e., the anterior wall of the central sulcus and adjacent precentral sulcus (Carpenter & Sutin, 1983, p. 686), sensory cerebral cortex, i.e., the postcentral gyrus (pp. 660–664), cerebellar cortex (p. 475), thalamic sensory nuclei, and visual cortex of the parietal lobe.

A representation of the human figure, with its proportion determined by the extent of cortical representation, is called a "homunculus." A representation of sensory stimuli and motor initiation has been drawn (Carpenter & Sutin, 1983, p. 660). The face points down, followed by the hand, with the body on the superior surface of the cortex, with genitals and lower limbs extending into the medial cortex. There may be multiple representations of the body in different portions of the motor cortex.

The auditory cortex is organized according to sensitivity to successive tones (as is the cochlea), which is referred to as "tonotopic."

Frontal Lobe

The frontal lobe serves many functions directly, and also integrates many aspects of behavior, e.g., control (see Chapters 11, Efficiency and Control and 13 Cerebral Emotional Disorder).

The Motor Cortex

An area, which if electrically stimulated, leads to relatively discrete movements in the extremities lies immediately in front of the central sulcus. These depend on the position of a limb, the state of the organism, etc. Damage is more associated with skilled action than particular movements. It is possible that the motor cortex is associated with "images" of action representing plans for future behavior (Davidson, 1980).

The corticospinal tract forms the pyramidal system. Motor impulses for each hand originate in the contralateral motor cortex. The corticospinal tract gives off branches to the thalamus, the striatum (see below), and particularly the corticospinal tract. There are fibers from cortex to the red nucleus, reticular formation, pontine nuclei, and inferior olivary complex (see projection pathways, below). Corticobulbar fibers project to motor nuclei of the cranial nerves. This area projects through the *pyramidal tract* (e.g., corticospinal fibers), and also receives sensory input *(secondary sensory area)*.

The Premotor Cortex

This is a motor area just anterior to the primary motor area. It runs along the lateral aspect of the brain, and is continued on the medial surface to the cingulate gyrus. Electrical stimulation of the area adjacent to the motor area produces similar responses, although stronger currents are required, i.e., it probably discharges through the corticospinal tract. Stimulation of the area rostral to it elicits more general movements, which are retained even after lesions of the motor area.

Frontal Eye Fields

This area lies between the the premotor and prefrontal cortices. It controls voluntary eye movements, mediated by a circuit involving the frontal cortex, superior colliculus, pretectal area, accessory occulomotor nuclei at the junction of the midbrain and diencephalon (Barr & Kiernan, 1988, p. 158), and the three oculomotor control nerves (III, IV, VI). Control of eye movement may be impaired immediately after an accident.

Supplementary Motor Cortex

Motor responses occur with electrical stimulation of this area on the medial surface of the brain, above the cingulate gyrus and rostral to the primary motor area. These include postures, complex patterned movements, and rapid uncoordinated movements (Carpenter & Sutin, 1983, p. 690), vocalization, and visceral responses.

The Prefrontal Cortex

The anterior pole of the brain (anterior to the premotor area) is well developed only in primates (Carpenter & Sutin, 1983, p. 704). It is believed to be associated with the most complex and least routinized aspects of cognitive control, planning, and decision making. These are the most vulnerable to any impairing condition. It is also significant for emotional expression (see Chapter 13 on Cerebral Emotional Deficits, including the Frontal Lobe Syndromes), monitoring behavior (see Problem Solving), orienting response to new stimuli (Lee, Arena, Kimford, Meador, Smith, Loring, & Flanigin, 1988) and anxiety.

Behaviorally discriminable areas include *medial, orbital* (over the eyes), and *dorsolateral convexity.* The basolateral system includes the orbital cortex, insula, anterior temporal lobe, amygdala, and dorsomedial nucleus of the thalamus (Adamovich et al., 1985, pp. 20–23. See also Chapter 13, Cerebral Personality Disorders). It receives projections from the mediodorsal thalamic nucleus and also has a motor function, i.e., the frontal eye fields (see below). It has two-way connections to areas involved with emotion, cognition, and control of the internal environment. The anterior section of the frontal lobe has important connections through the medial limbic system to the reticular activating system.

Inputs to the Prefrontal Cortex

* Association areas outside the primary sensory cortex;
* Projections from the mediodorsal thalamic nucleus, relaying information from autonomic centers to the lateral convexity of the frontal lobes;
* Extensive somatic, auditory, and sensory information (parietal and occipito-temporal association areas);
* Temporal lobe and amygdaloid fibers project to the orbital and medial frontal cortex (Trimble, 1988, p. 92).
* Dorsal frontal cortex links primarily to the hippocampus and parahippocampal gyrus. One circuit is amygdala–thalamus (mediodorsal nucleus)–orbitofrontal cortex–inferior temporal cortex–amygdala.
* The dorsolateral prefrontal cortex is linked by the medial limbic system with the hypothalamus, anterior thalamus, cingulate gyrus, and hippocampus.
* Mediodorsal thalamic projections onto the frontal lobe allow conjunction of motivational and emotional (value-attaching) information to be presented to the cortex of the frontal lobe, which is occupied with behavioral planning in the future.

Output from the Prefrontal Cortex

* The prefrontal cortex has efferents to (but does not receive afferents from) the caudate nucleus, globus pallidus, putamen, and substantia nigra.
* Projections from the olfactory system, septum, amygdala, and other structures of the limbic system also pass caudally directly into the diencephalon. Then, by way of the stria medullaris, less directly the pathway leads also to the midbrain. Finally, the frontal lobes join this downflow through abundant projections into the median forebrain bundle projecting to the midbrain (Livingston, 1985, p. 1284).

Broca's Area

This lies in front of the motor facial area. Damage is associated with difficulties in expressing thoughts in words (Broca's aphasia, apraxia, dysarthria, nonfluent aphasia). The motor apparatus, including larynx, face, and tongue, are intact, but the individual cannot initiate, integrate, and sequence the movements necessary for articulate speech. Probably cognitive deficits participate in this lack of fluency. Buckingham (1981) ably discusses the complexity of this disorder.

Temporal Lobe

The temporal lobe is an integrating center for a great number of functions that have cognitive, emotional and personal significance. Stimulation of various regions (cortex and hippocampus, etc.) creates flashbacks, interpretive illusions, or experiential hallucinations (Penfield & Roberts, 1959, p. 34). See Chapter 6 for a discussion of complex partial seizures and altered states of consciousness. For most people, the left temporal lobe is more important for verbal processing (dominant), although considerable additional verbal meaning is added by the right hemisphere (see Chapter 12 on Communication Deficits).

Cortex

This is a primary area for auditory input, verbal understanding, and processing information and problems that are best coped with sequentially. Temporal gyri, primarily on the left for most individuals who have the usual right-hand dominance, are significant for verbal processing and comprehension and analyzing auditory input. (Note that the right cerebral hemisphere does make an important contribution to verbal processing; see Chapter 3 on Neurobehavioral Principles, and elsewhere, on the limits of lateralization.) The parahippocampal gyrus is adjacent to the hippocampus, and is covered by the entorhinal cortex. This is an evolutionarily old region of cortex, with intimate connections with the olfactory tract. It projects to the hippocampus, and via the fornix to the opposite entorhinal area and hippocampus (see above, and Brodal, 1981, p. 681). Stimulation of the superior temporal gyrus, particularly rostral to the auditory area, provokes sensations of vertigo (Carpenter & Sutin, 1983, p. 683).

Wernicke's Area

The posterior portion of the superior temporal gyrus organizes incoming sounds into a temporal sequence so as to extract linguistic meaning. However, many studies of verbal deficits indicate a widespread anatomical vulnerability, even with the presence of relatively well-defined aphasic deficits, beyond such classical areas as Wernicke's and Broca's (see diagram in Benson, 1985, p. 23, for the "boundaries of the 'language area'").

Hippocampus

The hippocampus (see Figs. 2.12, 2.15, 2.17, and 2.18) is a relay between the cerebral cortex and the hypothalamus. The hippocampus and amygdala are located toward the inner surface of the temporal lobe, near the pole. Hippocampal stimulation can produce psychomotor epilepsy. It is part of the limbic circuit, and

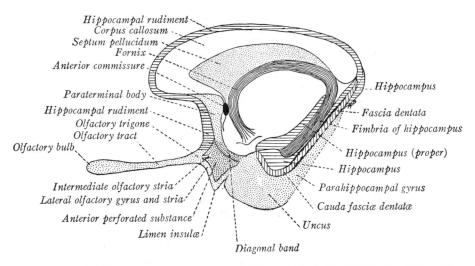

FIGURE 2.17. Rhinencephalon. From Ranson SW and Clark SL (1959), Fig. 237, with permission.

projects to the frontal lobe, cingulate gyrus, hypothalamus, mamillary body, and medial dorsal thalamic nucleus. The pathway from the entorhinal cortex and hippocampal area into the hypothalamus (mammillary bodies) is the *fornix*. Memory problems are particularly affected by bilateral lesions here.

The hippocampus is the principal target for adrenocortical steroids. It is implicated in reduced production of corticosterone (a glucocorticoid steroid) terminating the stress response. Feedback occurs via the hippocampal receptors sensitive to glucocorticoids (Sapolsky, Krey, & McEwen, 1984) to the HPA axis.

Amygdala

The amygdala is at the tip of the temporal lobe, above the inferior horn of the lateral ventricle. It receives noradrenergic afferents from the locus ceruleus and dopaminergic afferents from the ventral tegmental area and substantia nigra of the midbrain, i.e., it has significance for consciousness, muscular output, etc. It projects to the cingulate gyrus and hypothalamus, mamillary body, hypothalamus, and medial dorsal thalamic nucleus to the frontal lobe. The amygdala seems to organize rage reactions (see Chapter 10 on Memory and Chapter 13 on Cerebral Emotional Disorder).

Parietal Lobe

The parietal cortex integrates sensory and motor functions into a sense of personal identity and motives, extrapersonal space, and opportunities for action (Livingston, 1984, p. 1151, citing Mountcastle). Its multiple system representations (e.g., sensory association, limbic, reticular, and motor) provide for convergence between sensations, motivations, states of arousal, and motor potentialities in a given environmental context. Prior to reaching it, sensory signals are processed from unimodal to polymodal signals, and then they receive further processing.

The parietal lobes mediate the orienting response to sensory stimuli in space. The right hemisphere is concerned with both hemispaces, and the left parietal lobe is mainly concerned with stimuli delivered to the right hemispace (Masdeu, 1985a–c).

Somatosensory Cortex (SI)

Although there are are many areas from which electrical potentials can be measured following stimulation of somatic receptors (Livingston, 1985, p. 1148), the postcentral gyrus is considered the principal somesthetic cortical area. It receives sensory input as well as other input from the brainstem and thalamus. It contributes impulses to other sensory centers of the cortex, to sensory relay nuclei providing cortical control of sensory stimulation, and to motor systems in the cortex, basal ganglia, diencephalon, brainstem, cerebellum, and spinal cord.

Sensorimotor Cortex

Certain areas serve both sensory and motor functions. One such area, a somatotopic representation posterior and lateral to the somatosensory cortex, receives input from the primary somesthetic area, and the ventroposterior somatosensory relay nuclei of the thalamus. It receives bilateral stimulation, perhaps contributing to bilaterally coordinated bodily movements.

Sensory Association Cortex

Sensory information is pooled from vision, audition, touch, and olfaction to form a comprehensive image of the body image, the external world, and the person's relationship to it.

Occipital Lobe

Striate Cortex

A somatotopic relationship is maintained between the retina, lateral geniculate body (relay visual nucleus of the thalamus), and cortex. On the medial surface of the occipital lobe, there is a significant landmark, i.e., the *calcarine sulcus*, that divides the lobe into the dorsal cuneus and ventral lingual gyrus. The visual cortex is composed of alternating cortical zones (columnar) that receive ipsilateral input and stimulation from the contralateral cortex (Livingstone, 1985, p. 1080).

The striate cortex is the primary visual area in the occipital lobe, so called because even visually a stripe can be seen within it. The lower quadrants of the visual field project to the superior bank of the calcarine sulcus, and the upper quadrants of the visual field project to the inferior bank of the calcarine sulcus. The representation of the macula (center of retina with greatest sensitivity to detail and color vision) is relatively large at the caudal pole of the calcarine area. Representation of each macula area is unilateral. Each hemisphere receives impulses from the ipsilateral temporal retina and contralateral nasal retina, i.e., the contralateral half of the visual field. Color vision seems to be represented primarily below the sulcus, although it is a physiologically complex process from retina to cortex (Livingston, 1985, p. 1091).

Medial and Interior Landmarks of the Cerebral Cortex

Cingulate Gyrus

This encircles the corpus callosum dorsally, and extends underneath its anterior and posterior extremities. It participates in the limbic circuit.

Insula

A portion of the cerebral cortex that is buried in the lateral fissure. It is observable only when the lateral sulcus is opened (see Opercular Region, below).

Opercular Region

The cortex of the frontal, temporal, and parietal lobes that continues downward into the lateral sulcus (and would be continuous with the insula).

Secondary Olfactory Areas

These areas are part of the limbic circuitry, and are implicated in emotional functioning (Carpenter & Sutin, 1983, pp. 612–621).

Entorhinal Cortex

A region toward the pole of the temporal lobe, on its internal surface, it is part of parahippocampal gyrus. It projects to the hippocampus, and via the uncinate fasciculus (see below) to the anterior insular and frontal cortex.

Pyriform Cortex

The medial surface is at the tip of the temporal lobe. It is an olfactory relay center that projects to behaviorally significant areas, i.e., amygdala and dorsomedial nucleus of the thalamus, and then to the prefrontal cortex.

Nerve Tracts of the Forebrain ("White Matter")

This description is based on Barr and Kiernan (1988, pp. 334–337); Brodal (1981, pp. 841–845), Carpenter and Sutin, (1983, pp. 35–39), and DeGroot and Chusid (1988, p. 1960) (Figs. 2.18 and 2.19).

Projection

Projection neurons or pathways connect different levels of the neuraxis, e.g., corticospinal (from cortex to spine). They include reciprocal connections between the cerebral cortex and the thalamus, brainstem, and spinal cord. Fibers converge toward the brainstem. These fibers form the *internal capsule*, which includes ascending and descending tracts between the cortex, spinal cord and motor nuclei of the brainstem, and to the thalamus.

Corticospinal

Pyramidal tract fibers originate in the motor cortex, premotor cortex, and first sensory area of the parietal lobe. Fibers of the primary motor and premotor areas of the frontal lobe, exercise muscular control, including fine coordination. The pyramidal tract gives off fibers to the basal ganglia, thalamus, red nucleus, reticular formation, pontine nuclei, and inferior olivary complex. These fibers come together in the *internal capsule*, form three-fifths of the *basis pedunculi* of the midbrain, and enter the pons. At the caudal end of the pons the corticospinal tract forms the pyramids of the medulla. Here, 85% of the corticospinal tracts decussate and enter the dorsolateral funiculus of the spinal cord and form the lateral corticospinal tract. The remaining 15% form the ventral (anterior) cortocospinal tract, which descends ipsilaterally in the medial part of the ventral funiculus (Barr & Kiernan, 1988, p. 336) (see Fig. 2.5).

Corticospinal fibers also originate in the first sensory area of the parietal lobe, influencing sensory input. They modulate transmission of data through general sensory pathways.

Corticobulbar Tracts

These tracts end at the motor nuclei of the cranial nerves.

The extrapyramidal tract is multisynaptic, and reaches motor ganglia of the brainstem and reticular formation. It forms the background of fine motion, i.e., posture, automatic movement, and unconscious adjustment of muscular tone. The term "extrapyramidal" refers to abnormal spontaneous motions, but anatomically refers to reticulospinal and vestibular tracts, which do descend into the spinal cord, and, other pathways from corpus striatum, substantia nigra, and subthalamic nucleus, which apparently do not (Barr & Kiernan, 1988, p. 345).

Ascending projection tracts include input from the various nuclei of the thalamus.

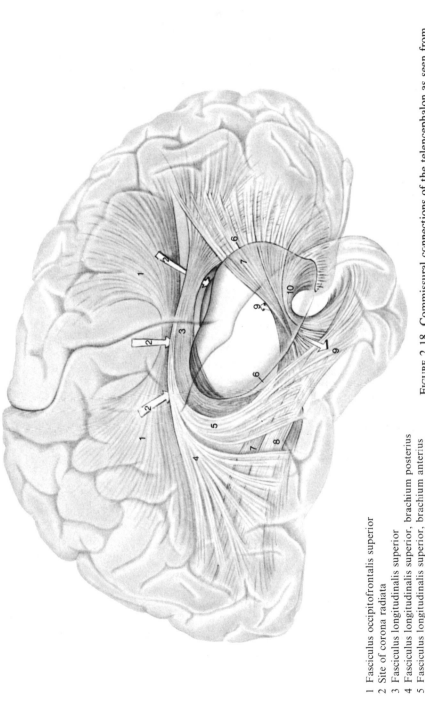

FIGURE 2.18. Commissural connections of the telencephalon as seen from the basal side of the brain. Reproduced, with permission, from Nieuwenhuys R, Voogd J, van Huijzen Chr: *The Human Central Nervous System: A Synopsis and Atlas*, Second Revised Edition. 1984, Springer-Verlag, Berlin, p. 218, fig. 149.

1 Fasciculus occipitofrontalis superior
2 Site of corona radiata
3 Fasciculus longitudinalis superior
4 Fasciculus longitudinalis superior, brachium posterius
5 Fasciculus longitudinalis superior, brachium anterius
6 Outline of insula
7 Fasciculus occipitofrontalis inferior
8 Fasciculus longitudinalis inferior
9 Site of commissura anterior
10 Fasciculus uncinatus

Commissural

These connect fiber paths across the midline, and connect homologous areas, and sometimes different structures, within the cerebral hemispheres. They are located at various levels of the neuraxis. Some pathways connect nonadjacent areas, e.g., via the corpus callosum or anterior commissure, and others connect interacting nuclei (e.g., in the thalamus).

The corpus callosum is a prominent landmark; its anterior edge is called the *genu* and posterior edge the *splenium*. The corpus callosum plays an important role in interhemispheric transfer of information, learned experience, sensory discriminations, sensory experience, and memory. It probably integrates concepts and problem solving by providing different types of information to bear on a task. Transfer across the callosum includes learned discriminations (visual and tactal), sensory experience, and memory. It is believed to play an important inhibiting function as well, e.g., when we alternate between verbal and nonverbal functioning, or during the release represented by nighttime dreaming.

It is easily damaged in traumatic injury. Severing the corpus callosum may not cause gross deficits of cognitive functioning, although on close examination deficits of communication can be detected.

Areas Not Having Callosal Connections

There are no direct commissural connections with the contralateral side for the striate area (visual cortex), the hand, and to a lesser extent the foot region, the somatosensory area, the primary sensorimotor area, and the primary acoustic area (Brodal, 1981, pp. 803, 843). By inference, projection fibers communicate with nearby areas of the cortex (ipsilateral), and then newly formed patterns are transmitted contralaterally.

The anterior commisure is a band of fibers that bifurcates; it connects the olfactory bulb with the contralateral olfactory region, and ipsilateral middle and inferior temporal gyri.

The hippocampal commissure is composed of efferent fiber tracts that are part of the fornix, which originate in the entorhinal cortex and hippocampus. The fibers proceed backward from each hippocampus, arch forward, and join the fibers from the contralateral hippocampus to form the fornix. Some fibers pass to the opposite entorhinal area (anterior medial portion of the temporal lobe) and hippocampus (Brodal, 1981, p. 681). The circuit is continued to the anterior insula and frontal cortex via the uncinate fasciculus (see below). Refer also to Fornix (below) for subsequent portions of this circuit.

The posterior commissure lies rostral to the superior colliculus, where the cerebral aqueduct opens up into the third ventricle. It appears to be involved in eyelid and vertical eye movements (Carpenter & Sutin, 1983, p. 425).

Association Tracts

Association tracts connect gyri, lobes, or widely separated areas within each cerebral hemisphere. Reference to Figs. 2.18 and 2.19 suggests a series of

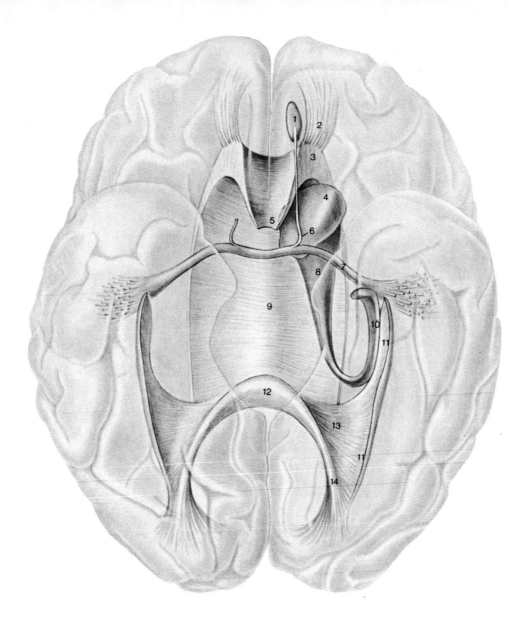

1 Bulbus olfactorius	8 Corpus nuclei caudati
2 Forceps minor	9 Truncus corporis callosi
3 Genu corporis callosi	10 Cauda nuclei caudati
4 Caput nuclei caudati	11 Tapetum
5 Rostrum corporis callosi	12 Splenium corporis callosi
6 Commissura anterior, crus anterius	13 Radiatio corporis callosi
7 Commissura anterior, crus posterius	14 Forceps major

FIGURE 2.19. Long association bunkles of the right cerebral hemisphere in a lateral view. Reproduced, with permission, from Nieuwenhuys R, Voogd J, van Huijzen Chr: *The Human Central Nervous System: A Synopsis and Atlas*, Second Revised Edition. 1984, Springer-Verlag, Berlin, p. 219, fig. 150.

complete circuits pointing to integrated rather than highly localized location of functions (see also, Pansky et al., 1988, pp. 98–99).

Short: Connects adjacent convolutions through the floors of the sulci.
Long: Connects cortical regions in different lobes within the same hemisphere. They are behaviorally significant since they participate in patterns and sequences of complex "higher functions" and due to their length they are vulnerable to many kinds of impact and secondary damage.

Association Tracts on Lateral Aspect of Hemisphere

The inferior longitudinal fasciculus passes from the occipital lobe to the inferior and lateral temporal lobe.

The inferior occipitofrontal fasciculus connects the cortex of the lateral or inferolateral portion of the frontal lobe with the cortex of the occipital lobe and inferior temporal lobe.

The uncinate fasciculus crosses the lateral cerebral fissure, connecting inferior frontal lobe gyri with the uncus and other portions of the temporal lobe. It is significant in verbal processing.

The superior longitudinal fasciculus connects the frontal lobe's superior and middle gyri with the temporal lobe (more posteriorly than the uncinate fasciculus) and with the occipital lobe, passing over the lateral surface of the hemisphere (Ranson & Clark, 1959, pp. 325–326). See also Arcuate Fasciculus.

The arcuate fasciculus starts as a portion of the superior longitudinal fasiculus, which passes over the insula into the temporal lobe.

Occipitofrontal fasciculus radiates from the frontal lobes into the temporal and occipital lobes.

Medial Aspect of the Hemisphere

The cingulum is a band of tissues, within the cingulate gyrus, connecting the anterior perforated substance (which receives some olfactory input) with the parahippocampal gyrus.

The superior occipitofrontal fasciculus is located between the corpus callossum and internal capsule; it connects the occipital and the temporal lobes with the frontal lobes and insula.

The statum calcarium is a sheet of fibers curving around the bottom of the calcarine fissures (which subdivides the visual area), from the cuneus (visual area above calcarine fissure) to the lingual gyrus (medial, inferior portion of the occipital pole).

Fornix

This band of fibers is the main efferent system of the hippocampus, projecting to the mammillary body, and commissural stimulation of the contralateral side (commissure of the fornix). The fornix divides into two bands:

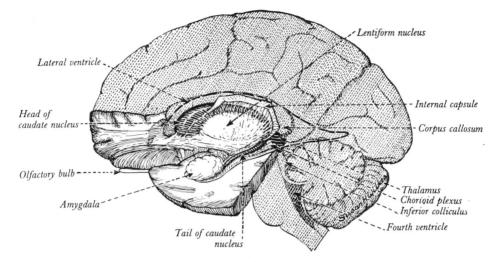

Lentiform nucleus

Lateral ventricle

Head of
caudate nucleus

Internal capsule

Corpus callosum

Olfactory bulb

Amygdala

Thalamus
Choriqid plexus
Inferior colliculus
Fourth ventricle

Tail of caudate
nucleus

FIGURE 2.20. Basal ganglia. From Ranson SW and Clark SL (1959), Fig. 219, with permission.

Posterior commissural fibers traverse the thalamus en route to the mammilary body (hypothalamus), giving off fibers to the thalamus (anterior and intralaminar nuclei).

The anterior band (precommissural fornix fibers) is distributed to the septal nuclei, the hypothalamus, and the midbrain central gray (significant for arousal). From the anterior nucleus of the thalamus, the circuit projects to the cingulate gyrus, via the cingulum fiber tract, and entorhinal cortex, and back to the hippocampus.

Subcortical Structures

These nuclei below the cortex have a variety of cognitive and emotional functions, which are sometimes ignored while exaggerating cortical contributions. Many of these structures are not on the main transmission lines of the neuraxis, but reciprocally exchange impulses with the cortex and nuclei on the main axis. They modify ongoing activity, particularly muscular tone, emotional reactions, and visceral activity.

Basal Ganglia

These nuclei are subcortical structures, including the putamen, globus pallidus, caudate nucleus, claustrum, subthalamic nucleus, substantia nigra (Fig. 2.20). The term striatum (corpus striatum), according to Brodal (1981, p. 211), is practically synonymous with the basal ganglia, including the caudate nucleus, globus pallidus, putamen, and claustrum.

These nuclei, deep within the cerebral hemispheres and brainstem, modulate muscular control, emotional responses, and perhaps memory. Circuits include neocortex to basal ganglia to thalamus back to motor area of neocortex. Basal ganglia are essential for the initiation, control, and cessation of motor activity and posture. They receive input from brainstem motor ganglia, the thalamus, and all regions of the cerebral cortex, project to thalamic nuclei, which project in turn to motor cortical areas. This integrates and transfers information.

Nomenclature of the Basal Ganglia

- *Neostriatum* = striatum = putamen + caudate nucleus
- *Paleostriatum* = pallidum = globus pallidus
- *Lentiform nucleus* = globus pallidus + putamen

Subthalamic nucleus (Diencephalon)

The subthalamic nucleus interconnects with various basal ganglia (globus pallidus and substantia nigra), modulating the activities of the corpus striatum (see basal ganglia nomenclature, above).

Putamen and *globus pallidus* output are modified by impulses from the substantia nigra and subthalamic nuclei. They project via thalamic relays (which receives cerebellar input) to the motor cortex. Integration of information from many sources enhances motor control. Descending influences are via the red nucleus (rubrospinal tract) and the reticular formation (reticulospinal tracts) (Walton, 1985, p. 17).

The caudate nucleus is found in the wall of the lateral ventricle. Its large head protrudes into the anterior horn of the lateral ventricles and is surrounded on the other side by the internal capsule (major fiber paths between cortex and lower centers), the "body" continues on the lateral wall of the ventricle, and the "tail" curves down to enter the temporal lobe terminating near the amygdala.

The red nucleus is a part of the midbrain; it extends from the superior colliculus to the subthalamic region of the diencephalon. It is a way station between the cerebellum and the spinal cord. It reciprocally feeds back to the cerebellum and innervates the brainstem as well. It seems to alternate flexor control during walking with extensor control, by using input from vestibulospinal neurons "to provide appropriate locomotor rhythms" (Carpenter & Sutin, 1983, p. 435). Vestibular function will be discussed in greater detail in Chapter 7 on Sensorimotor Functions.

The substantia nigra is located between the tegmentum and crus pedunculi (descending motor fibers), as they extend from the midbrain to the subthalamic region of the diencephalon. It is a dopamine-producing center, and reduced output is associated with Parkinsonism. It is also a producer of GABA, a significant inhibitory neurotransmitter. It receives input from the caudate nucleus and putamen. Output is to the caudate nucleus and putamen (striatum), thalamus (ventral anterior nucleus), superior colliculus (visual center of the midbrain), and midbrain tegmentum (areas receiving input from the striatum) and feeding back to the substantia nigra.

Limbic System

This is a behaviorally significant group (see Figs. 2.13, 2.15, 2.16, and 2.17) of structures mostly on the inner surface and within the cerebral hemispheres of the brain. It is also known as the "visceral brain," and rhinencephalon (due to the connections with the olfactory system), though it does not process smell per se (see, Barr and Kiernan, 1988, Chapter 18; DeGroot & Chusid, 1988, Chapter 14; Trimble 1988, Chapter 3).

Output to the forebrain suppresses emotional responses to trivial and inconsequential stimuli, i.e., leading to appropriate autonomic and endocrine concomitants of emotions, as well as directing motor responses to external events. Hypothalamic circuits are significant for the emotions, control over the pituitary gland, maintenance of homeostasis, etc. The preoptic region plays a role in gonadal secretions (cyclic in the female and tonic in the male) and the pattern of sexual development early in life, through controlling release of gonadotropic hormones from the anterior hypophysis (pituitary).

Structure

These structures form an anatomical ring and circuit around the base and cortex of the medial surface of the brain (evolutionarily old cerebral cortex), i.e., the anterior lower surface of the temporal lobe (with olfactory connections), nuclei within the medial portion of the temporal lobe (hippocampus and amygdala), medial surface of the temporal lobe including the insula, various nuclei of the forebrain (thalamus, septal nuclei, hypothalamus), midbrain (mammillary bodies), brainstem, dentate gyrus of the hippocampus, amygdaloid body, septal area, hypothalamus, certain nuclei of the thalamus, and pathways that link these structures with the cortex and subcortical structures including the cerebellum.

The limbic system is interposed between the neocortex (sensory processing, integration, and subcortical influences) and the reticular core of the brainstem (autonomic brain function, such as respiration and cardiovascular). It modulates the autonomic nervous system through the hypothalamus, which has a reciprocal relationship with the cortex (Watson et al., 1986). It also has connections "to all brain regions and functions (!)" (Brodal, 1981, p. 690) including viscerally based reactions to internal changes (see below, Visceral Behavior Control System).

Function

1. Preservation of the species and the individual, i.e., motor and visceral responses involved in defense, reproduction, and memory;
2. Emotional experience and expression (feeding, aggression, sex);
3. Integration of environmental information leading to a decision whether to approach or avoid;
4. Processing information leading to communicating feelings such as rage, surprise, fear, alarm, dominance–submission, and mother–infant, male–female interactions (Code, 1987, p. 71);

5. Brainstem mechanisms involved with anger and violence (Chusid, 1985, p. 30; Mark & Ervin, 1970);
6. Subcortical structures within the temporal lobe may trigger epileptic seizures, with a strong emotional component;
7. Encoding recent memories for long-term storage (amygdala and hippocampus);
8. Autonomic functions (cardiovascular and gastrointestinal);
9. Pleasurable reinforcement through input to the septal nuclei;
10. Part of the circuit for drug effects (antipsychotic and narcotics).

Limbic Structures and Behavior

Cingulate gyrus: maternal behavior, play, vocalization;
Hippocampus: memory, anxiety;
Amygdala: fear/anxiety, aggression, sex, mood;
Hypothalamus: eating, drinking, sex, aggression, hormonal control;
Reticular activating system: Arousal, sleep–wake cycle;
Entorhinal cortex: memory, sensory integration;
Ventral striatum: motivation.

These associations have been suggested by Trimble (1988, p. 121).

Septal nuclei: These are cell bodies in the inner wall (septum) separating the lateral ventricles and below the corpus callosum. They are on a circuit to the hippocampus that modulates aggression, anxiety, and dominance, are also part of a pleasure and reward system, and may contribute to memory consolidation.

Cerebellum

The cerebellum contributes to automatic regulation and control of motor functions in space, i.e., *coordination, balance, and kinesthesis* (Carpenter & Sutin, 1983, Chapter 14; Livingston, 1985, p. 1194). It is a servomechanism that accelerates and brakes cortical control over skeletal muscular action, smoothing movements of the body and limb musculature. It collaborates with the vestibular functions (semicircular canal system) to control action in three-dimensional space.

The cerebellum has a cortex, white matter, two lateral lobes, a central section known as the vermis, a transverse section (flocculonodular lobe), and nuclei. Fiber tracts ascend rostrally (superior cerebellar peduncle), caudally (inferior cerebellar peduncle) to the spine, and contralaterally (middle cerebellar peduncle) to the opposite side at the same level in the pons and then descend into the spinal cord.

Cerebellar Input

The cerebellum receives information from all parts of the body, i.e., tension in skeletal muscles, joints, and tendons, and patterns of movements, and from vestibular nuclei of the pons concerning movements of the entire body (vestibular branch of nerve VIII), the spinal column, and the cortex. It has two-way connections with the reticular formation, the extrapyramidal system, and red, vestibular, olivary, and other brainstem nuclei, via superior and middle cerebellar peduncles. These are relayed by nuclei in the brainstem and spinal cord.

Cerebellar Output

Efferent impulses proceed rostrally (superior cerebellar peduncle) and caudally (inferior cerebellar peduncle) (Pansky et al., 1988 p. 115). The vermis and flocculonodular lobe project to the vestibular nuclei. Fibers exiting via the superior cerebellar peduncle decussate at the level of the midbrain and enter the red nucleus. Others proceed caudally to nuclei known to project to the cerebellum, forming a loop.

The Cranial Nerves

All cranial nerves (Figs. 2.10 and 2.11), are bilateral. Many have mixed functions, i.e., their axons originate in multiple nuclei having relatively specialized functions. They exit the brain within the skull, and innervate organs, muscles, and blood vessels within the head and body, serving sensory, motor, and autonomic functions. General references include Barr and Kiernan (1988, Chapter 8). Refer to Wilson-Pauwels et al. (1988), for the most complete summary.

Cranial nerves provide information about adaptive functions and safety. Their integrity is a significant portion of the neurological examination. Deficits help to locate damage within the brain, although somatic damage to the head can be confused for damage to the cranial nerves or their nuclei.

Cranial nerve structure may be summarized as follows (Wilson- Pauwels et al., 1988, pp. x–xi). The olfactory (I) and optic (II) nerves are considered tracts of the brain rather than true nerves; only the peripheral receptor cells (olfactory & retina) are nerve-like, i.e., ganglia outside the brain. Nerves III, IV, and VI, controlling the eyes, function as a group. Voluntary eye movement coordination, which includes input from the frontal eye field, vestibular nuclei, and reticular and superior colliculus, is described in Barr and Kiernan (1988, pp. 125–128).

Motor

The upper motor neuron is in the cerebral cortex, and the lower motor neuron forms the motor group of cranial nerve nuclei in the brainstem. Axons leaving these nuclei form the motor component of cranial nerves.

Sensory

The primary neuron is usually located outside the CNS in sensory ganglia; the secondary neuron is in the dorsal gray matter of the brainstem, with axons crossing the midline to project to the thalamus. Tertiary neurons are in the thalamus and project to the sensory cortex.

Classification of Cranial Nerves

See Livingston (1985, p. 1196).

Somatic efferent: striated muscles of orbit and tongue (III, IV, VI, XII);
Special visceral efferent: striated muscles derived from embryonic gill arches (V, VII, IX, X, XI);
General visceral efferent: smooth muscles and glands (III, VII, IX, X) and preganglionic neurons of the craniosacral autonomic system;
General somatic afferent: sensory nuclei subserving proprioception, touch, temperature, and pain (V, X);
Special somatic afferent: vestibular (balance) and cochlear (hearing) (VIII);
Visceral afferent: taste and other visceral afferents (VII, IX, X).

Details of Individual Cranial Nerves

I. Olfactory

Classification: Special sensory.
Exits brain: It sends fibers through the cribriform plate of the ethmoid bone to the olfactory epithelium.
Nucleus: This is the only sensation in which the cortex is not reached via a thalamic relay station. The nucleus is in the olfactory bulb, which extends under the inferior surface of the anterior pole of the brain. Significant fiber tracts travel via the anterior commissure to the contralateral olfactory bulb, to the uncus and anterior portion of the hippocampal gyrus (anterior temporal lobe), and via the medial olfactory stria to the medial surface of the frontal lobe mediating emotional responses to odors through the limbic system.
Function: Smell.

II. Optic

Exits: It leaves the retina and joins the contralateral nerve at the base of the brain to form the optic chiasma, where it becomes the optic tract. There are branches to the superior colliculus (for oculomotor reflexes) and to the lateral geniculate nucleus of the thalamus (for visual information), and then to the occipital cortex.
Classification: Special sensory.
Nucleus: Lateral geniculate body of the thalamus.
Function: Vision. The temporal halves of each retina (nasal visual field of each eye) project to the ipsilateral cerebral hemisphere. The nasal halves (temporal visual field) cross the optic chiasma and project to the contralateral side. After leaving the lateral geniculate body, the fibers radiate toward the external surface

of the brain, below the cortex, and are vulnerable to temporal lobe lesions, creating diffuse bilateral visual deficits, which become more defined the closer the damage is to the calcarine cortex of the occipital lobe. Each cortex receives input from half of both visual fields, and also through the corpus callosum from the contralateral cortex. The occipital pole receives fibers projected from the center of vision (fovea), while lower retinal fibers are projected to the lateral portion of the optic tract, terminating on the lower bank of the calcarine fissure, and upper retinal fibers project to the superior portion of the calcarine fissure. Portions of the macula project to only one hemisphere. Field deviations can reveal the location of injury, and should be explored by the neurologist, neuroophthalamologist, or neuropsychologist diagnosing the location of brain damage.

III. Oculomotor (Voluntary and Involuntary Eye Movements)

Classification 1: Somatic motor.
   Exits brain: Ventral surface of the brain, between midbrain and pons.
   Nucleus 1: Oculomotor N. in midbrain underneath superior colliculus.
   Function 1: Eye muscles: Superior, medial, and inferior rectus, inferior oblique; levator palpebrae (raises eyelid). Upward, sideward, and downward eye movements. Superior rectus and inferior oblique elevate the eye.
   Classification 2: Visceral motor (parasympathetic).
   Nucleus 2: Edinger–Westphal N. of midbrain.
   Function 2: Pupillary light reflex; accomodation of the eye for near vision (increase of curvature of the lens, pupillary constriction, convergence of the eyes).

IV. Trochlear

Exits brain: Decussates within the brain, leaves via the dorsal surface of the brainstem, travels ventrally around the brainstem, emerging between the pons and the inferior surface of the temporal lobes, underneath the vagus (V) nerve.
   Classification: Somatic motor.
   Nucleus: Trochlear N. of tegmentum (floor) of midbrain.
   Function: Extraocular eye movement, contralateral superior oblique muscle of the eye, rotating and depressing the eyeball.

V. Trigeminal

Exits brain: Motor and sensory roots emerge from the midlateral surface of the pons.
   Classification 1: Branchial motor.
   Nucleus: Masticator (trigeminal motor N. in the pons).
   Function: Muscles of mastication.
   Classification 2: General sensory.

Function: Principle sensory nerve for the head. Sensation from face and scalp, nasal and oral cavities, including tongue and teeth, meninges of anterior and middle cranial fossae, etc.

Nucleus: Sensory nucleus of V is in the pons.

VI. Abducens

This is easily damaged because of its long intracranial trajectory.

Exits brain: Junction of the pons and the pyramid of the medulla.

Nucleus: Abducens N. in the pons, ventral to the fourth ventricle.

Classification: Somatic motor.

Function: Extraocular eye movements, i.e., lateral rectus muscle abducts the eye.

VII. Facial

Exits brain: Emerges from the brainstem, and emerges laterally between pons and medulla, lateral to nerve VI.

Classification 1: General sensory.

Nucleus: Trigeminal N. of the upper medulla.

Function 1: Sensation of concha of external ear and behind ear.

Classification 2: Branchial motor (special visceral efferent).

Nucleus: Pathways originate in the motor cortex, and divide in the midbrain to provide bilateral innervation of the forehead muscles, but contralateral innervation of the remainder of the face. Facial N. of pons.

Function 2: Muscles of facial expression. Innervation of muscles of the forehead (bilateral), and of the face, contralateral.

Classification 3: Visceral motor.

Nucleus: Superior salivatory N of pons.

Function 3: Parasympathetic supply to all glands of the head except skin and parotid.

Classification 4: Special sensory.

Nucleus: Gustatory N. (of N. solitarius). Ascending tracts reach the ipsilateral and contralateral ventral posterior nuclei of the thalami, which then project to the cortical area for taste in the most inferior part of the sensory cortex (postcentral gyrus, extending into the insula).

Function 4: Taste of anterior two-thirds of the tongue.

VIII. Vestibulocochlear

Exits brain: Between junction of pons and medulla, near the cerebellum, but lateral to VI and VII.

Classification: Special sensory.

Auditory branch: Auditory information from the cochlea. Input from each ear does tend to decussate to the opposite auditory cortex, but fibers also project to the ipsilateral cortex. There is bilateral representation of incoming auditory stimulation from the acoustic branch of the vestibulocochlear nerve (VIII). Most auditory processing seems to take place in the contralateral auditory cortex. An excellent diagram of ipsilateral and contralateral connections via the lateral lemniscus and inferior colliculus is found in Livingston (1985, p. 1005). Ascending pathways branch to the contralateral reticular formation, superior olivary complex (providing feedback concerning different timing of events in the two ears), and nuclei of the lateral lemniscus (Livingston, 1985, p. 1006).

Nucleus: Cochlear N. at junction of pons and medulla.

Vestibular branch: Balance information from the semicirculator canals, saccule, and utricle, i.e., movements of the body, changes of position, acceleration and deceleration, and movements of the head and neck. These impulses are of special importance: They create an excitatory influence on the spinal cord, affecting axial and limb muscles; excitatory and inhibitory influences on the spinal cord through relays in the descending reticular activating system; and synapse with neurons that stimulate eye movements (III, IV, and VI) to create vestibuloocular reflexes. These keep the eyes tracking on a moving target when the head or body moves, and contributes to coordination and balance through input to the cerebellum.

Vestibular nuclei: The vestibular ganglion sends branches to the vestibular nuclear complex in the floor of the fourth ventricle (pons) and to the cerebellum.

Ascending tracts are via the medial longitudinal fasciculus to cranial nerves III, IV, and VI.

Descending tracts are via the vestibulospinal tract and descending portion of the medial longitudinal fasciculus.

IX. Glossopharyngeal (Tongue and Pharynx)

Exits brain: Rootlets emerge from the lateral portion of the medulla to form the nerve.

Classification 1: Branchial motor.

Nucleus: N. ambiguous of pons.

Function 1: Stylopharyngeus muscle (elevates pharynx during swallowing and speech).

Classification 2: Visceral motor.

Nucleus: Inferior salivatory N. of medulla.

Function 2: Dry mouth in response to fear; salivation in response to food.

Classification 3: Visceral sensory.

Nucleus: N. Solitarius, which extends from pons into the medulla.

Function 3: Receives information about oxygen pressure from the carotid body, and blood pressure from the carotid sinus, which passes information through the tractus solitarius N. to reticular formation and hypothalamus for reflex responses to control respiration, blood pressure, and cardiac output.

Classification 4: Special sensory.

Nucleus: Gustatory N. of the rostral portion of the N. of the tractus solitarius.

Function 4: Taste sensation of the posterior portion of the tongue. Fibers ascend to the ipsilateral and contralateral ventral posterior N. of the thalami, synapse, and then ascend to the primary sensory cortex of the inferior third of the postcentral gyrus where taste is perceived.

Classification 5: General sensory.

Nucleus: Spinal N. of trigeminal nerve. Secondary neurons decussate, ascend to the ventral posterior N. of the thalamus, and then to the postcentral sensory gyrus (head region).

Function 5: Pain and temperature of the skin of part of the external ear, inner surface of the tympanic membrane, posterior third of the tongue, and upper thalamus.

X. Vagus

Exits brain: Medulla of the brainstem has several rootlets.

Classification 1: Branchial motor (special visceral efferent).

Nucleus: Motor tracts of the motor, premotor, and other cortical areas synapse on motor neurons of the N. ambiguous of the pons.

Function 1: Striated ("voluntary") muscles of the pharynx, tongue, and larynx.

Classification 2: Visceral motor (general visceral efferent).

Nucleus: Dorsal vagus N. of the pons.

Function 2: Smooth muscles and glands of the pharynx, larynx, and thoracic and abdominal viscera.

Classification 3: Visceral sensory (visceral afferent).

Nucleus: Solitarius N. of pons and medulla.

Function 3: Sensations from pharynx, larynx, and viscera.

Classification 4: General sensory (general somatic afferent).

Nucleus: N. of the spinal tract of the trigeminal nerve, projecting to contralateral ventral posterior N. of thalamus, and then to sensory cortex (head region).

Function 4: Skin at back of the ear and external acoustic meatus, external surface of tympanic membrane, the pharynx, and meninges of posterior cranial fossa.

XI. Accessory

Exits brain: Axons ascend from the spinal cord to the medulla, and exit as rootlets.

Classification: Branchial motor (special visceral efferent).

Nucleus: From motor cortex, upper motor neurons decussate in pyramids of medulla; lower motor neurons are located in the accessory N. of medulla and spinal cord (anterior gray column).

Function: Innervate sternomastoid (turns head) and trapezius muscles (maintains position of scapula and shoulder).

XII. Hypoglossal

Exits brain: Rootlets emerge just dorsal to the pyramids of the medulla, to form the nerve trunk.

Classification: Somatic motor (general somatic efferent).

Nucleus: From the motor cortex, via the corticobulbar tract, to the hypoglossal N. of the medulla.

Function: Extrinsic and intrinsic muscles of the tongue.

3
Principles of Neurobehavioral Functioning

Since the purpose of this volume is to consider a wide range of functions in which the brain injured person may be impaired, it is useful to specify some characteristics of the unimpaired, integrated personality.

Adaptation

Definition

Adaptation is the integrated behavior with which an individual or species copes with its environment. Its components are *genetic* (hereditary), *phenotypic* (expression of genes in a particular environment), and *personal style* (how conditioning and other experiences have shaped behavior). A behavioral trait may be adaptive or maladaptive, depending on other traits and the demands of a particular environment. A well-adapted person uses successfully a variety of abilities and strategies, has developed suitable style(s) of problem solving, and has constructive attitudes that seek worthwhile goals. One's mood is generally pleasant, and there are no significant barriers to work, study, social relationships, enjoyment of leisure time, etc. The person avoids large-scale failures such as mental illness or crime. He or she can cope with a variety of demands and changing circumstances, e.g., loss of or changes in significant people, employment, living circumstances, economic conditions, family and community.

Forms of Adaptation

Inability to deal with change and complexity is characteristic of traumatic brain injury. Therefore, it is useful to consider some kinds of normal adaptation, to assess the brain injured person's loss of functioning.

New environment seeking (mobility, i.e., changing jobs, mates, homes, friends, environment);
Autoplastic changes (personality adaptations to the environment);
Alloplastic changes (making alterations in one's external world).

76

Preinjury Self-Destructiveness

Nevertheless, even the unimpaired person is to some extent inefficient and expresses his drives self-destructively. Self-destructiveness is defined as taking actions that are predictably ineffective or damaging (Parker, 1981, Chapter I). The common consequences are poor mental health, ineffective job performance, poor social relationships, crime, mental hospitalization, defective child-rearing, unhappy moods, etc. Consequently, it is axiomatic that a brain injury *reduces the capacity to deal with reality in an already incompletely efficient person.* Impairment is the deviation from a previously more successful level of adaptation (see also Chapter 14 on Adaptability, and Chapter 18 on Recovery).

Personal Integration

A feeling of personal unity and purposefulness is often lost after TBI.

Sense of purpose. An awareness of pleasures to be obtained in the future serves to focus activities and mobilize energy.

Foresight. Discomfort and danger is usually avoided. Discomfort leads to changed goals or behavior.

A clear and positive sense of identity. The unimpaired person has a relatively clear sense of his or her identity, motives, and what is rewarding (Parker, 1983). The person feels sexually and socially attractive.

Adequate Control

Personality factors such as motivation, foresight, and dissatisfaction work together. Inner resources, consistent with a sense of identity, are used to reach reasonable goals. Impulsivity, temper outbursts, inability to learn from experience, etc., do not wreak havoc with plans, and fits of temper do not create danger or antagonize valued associates.

Enjoyment of Life

Activities produce pleasant results; the cooperation of others and their companionship is part of life. The mood is pleasant. One's personal identity is clear and positive (Parker, 1983, Chapter 2).

High Morale

The person feels self-confident that he or she will succeed and meet normal responsibilities. When danger is sensed, it is appropriate, i.e., there is not a disabling belief that the world is overwhelmingly dangerous, or one is excessively vulnerable to damage.

Stress Resistance

Stress resistance may be defined as the ability to continue one's usual activities in the face of events that are dangerous or reduce efficiency. *Brain trauma and its usual accompaniments, somatic injury, anxiety, impairment, and loss of ability to enjoy life, is an example of stress par excellence.*

Personality Characteristics Contributing to Stress Resistance

Coping refers to managing demands (external and emotional) that are experienced as taxing or exceeding the resources of the person. One may discriminate between general techniques for adapting and nonroutine actions dealing with specific events (Lazarus & Folkman, 1984).

Hardiness (Howard, Cunningham & Rechnitzer, 1986; Kobassa, 1979; Kobassa, Maddi & Zola, 1983). The stress-resistant person has a sense of personal control over external events, a deep feeling of commitment and purpose, and flexibility in adapting to change. Kobassa (1979) noted that staying healthy under stress was critically dependent "upon a strong commitment to self, ability to recognize one's distinctive values, goals, and priorities and an appreciation of one's capacity to have purpose and to make decisions."

Stamina (Thomas, 1982) is enhanced by self-esteem, a warm relationship to parents; an open, flexible approach to life; and minimal nervous tension, anxiety, depression, and anger under stress; it is characterized by a lack of morbid, frightening, psychodynamic undertones in response to the Rorschach test. My experience with the Rorschachs of injury victims indicates that such feeling tones are quite characteristic of stressed people, and it is inferred that they contribute to poor morale in facing problems.

Constitution (Adams & Victor, 1985, p. 659). Health and strength contribute to stress resisitiveness. Stable, athletic, tough-fibered individuals take a concussive injury in stride, while the sensitive, nervous complaining types may be so overwhelmed that they cannot expel the incident from their minds.

The will to survive. The dangerous and degrading circumstances offer example of individuals whose desire for self-preservation brought them through when others went under, e.g., concentration camps and prisoner of war camps.

Brain Damage Reduces Adaptive Ability

Impaired Adaptability

Brain damage is more likely to be expressed through reduction of normal functioning than pathognomonic or deviant-pattern symptoms. Reduced ability to function and sudden personality changes alert the professional to inquire about events such as accidents, strokes, illness, or emotional stress, or complaints such as headaches, dizziness, confusion, and loss of balance.

Reduced Reserves

Each brain injury reduces the ceiling of our resources, i.e., reserves necessary to cope with new and difficult situations that one does not have to cope with under current circumstances. A posttrauma drop in adaptive ability may be gradual (e.g., the multiple injuries of a reckless person or professional athlete), or sudden after trauma.

Integration and Complexity

Since the brain functions as an integrated unit, it is an exaggeration to state that a particular brain structure (localization) or side of the brain (lateralization) "does something." Normally, cerebral hemispheres are unified by the commissures of the forebrain (see Chapter 2 on Neuroanatomy), which bringing together bilateral events into a unified experience. Interaction occurs with subcortical structures. While particular information may not be easily available through conscious efforts, behavior is usually unified and coherent.

This proved true (within the limits of the experiment) when two patients were studied who had their corpus callossum, and also anterior, hippocampal, and habenular commissures, etc., severed (Sergent, 1987). This condition is called the "disconnection syndrome" or the unfortunately named "split brain." They were able to make perceptual and other cognitive judgments without conscious awareness, though not as efficiently as under normal circumstances, and illustrate the brain's unified functioning through using subcortical structures.

Neural Processing Is Extended in Space and Time

Complex Functional Units

Long complex pathways, reciprocal connections with other structures, and sequences in processing represent the functional unit. Neural events converge and disperse in space and time.

Various Levels of the Brain Participate in Any Behavior

Individual neurons integrate information from many sources. Its pattern of activity in turn modifies and is modified by other levels, such as those as distant as the cerebral cortex and spinal cord.

Much Behavior is Automatic

Completed circuits and processing at levels lower than the cortex, e.g., visceral functions and sensorimotor adjustment of ongoing activity, occur as a largely unconscious process.

Neural Circuitry Changes Through Life and with Experience

Neuronal activity causes changes of circuitry through life, even though active replacement of neurons after an early age seems not to occur. See Chapter 15 on the effects of stress.

Transmission Is Multiplex

Activity is Processed at Relay Stations

Sensorimotor, higher cognitive functions, and autonomic activities involve integration of pathways from many regions at several integrative centers, followed by transmission to another integrative center. Ultimately, transmission goes via a "final common pathway" to a target organ. Neuronal pathways converge at particular nuclei where activity is modified by facilitatation, inhibition, or information from other centers, and retransmited in both directions and off-neuraxis (Kandel & Schwartz, 1985, p. 220; Livingston, 1985, p. 985; Luria, 1980, p. 110; see Nerve Tracts of the Forebrain in Chapter 2 on Neuro-anatomy).

Complex Tasks Have Parallel Components

Each of the major systems (sensory, motor, motivational, autonomic) is divided into components that function simultaneously. To use *vision* as an example, receptors and nerve centers, movement of eye muscles, and movement of the limbs are all served by different neural groups (Kandal & Schwartz, 1985, p. 220).

Transmission Is Multidirectional

The basic large-scale organizational process of the nervous system is a two-way flow between the cerebral cortex and the periphery, modified by off-axis nuclei (e.g., the cerebellum). Sensory and motor activity transmission in any direction is affected by incoming information from the opposite direction, and information coming in to relay stations (Livingston, 1985, p. 1157). Long lines are further modified by activities of the cerebellum, cranial nerves, and autonomic nervous system (off-axis).

Most Long Pathways Cross at the Midline

Most sensory and motor events are largely controlled by the opposite cerebral hemisphere, with different systems decussating at different levels. Exceptions include bilateral representation by certain cranial nerves, i.e., vision (each eye is represented in both hemispheres, the temporal half of the retina remaining ipsilateral, while the nasal half crosses at the optic chiasm; innervation of the forehead by the facial nerve). Audition and olfaction also have some bilateral representation.

Each Pathway Is Topographically Organized

Pathways are organized according to either the shape of the body (motor, somesthesis) or of the receptor (vision), or characteristics of the stimulus (frequency, for audition). Spatial aspects of transmission retain their position relative to each other from one level to the next (see Somatotopic Localization, Chapter 2 on Neuroanatomy).

Multiple Types of Activities Occur Simultaneously

Processing includes alternation of functioning with other areas, facilitation and inhibition, parallel or sequential transmission, synthesizing, analyzing, modification by information received through monitoring ongoing action and external events, modifying output to match an anticipated outcome, etc.

Systemic and Chemical Factors Are Significant

Sensitivity to Chemical Factors

The neuron is a small scale integrating unit. The nerve cell's threshold of activity is modified by neurotransmitters, neurohormones, neuromodulators, metabolic states, inorganic chemical levels (sodium, potassium, calcium), electrical and magnetic fields, etc.

Systemic Feedback

Feedback from bodily activities and physiological levels creates facilitatation or inhibition. Systemic effects include stamina, health, stress, fatigue, motivation, prior experiences, metabolic status, glandular secretions, status of nutrients, wastes, oxygen, temperature, etc.

Higher Level Functions

"Higher functions" in particular are controlled by the principles of complexity and alternation.

- A child listening to a parent receives both a verbal message (likely left hemisphere predominance) and recognizes the emotional tone (likely right hemisphere predominance).
- Reading requires sequential and verbal processing (likely left hemisphere predomance) and visual organization of the stimulus (predominantly right hemisphere).
- Carrying out a plan involves a mental image (e.g., right parietal predominance, and then monitoring action to effectuate this concept outside the body (frontal lobe predominance).

Motivational Systems

Motivational Level, Affect, Energy, Sex, Expressive Behavior

These nonverbal drives and temperamental qualities represent an interaction of self-awareness, visceral control, arousal, cortical, subcortical, and brainstem activities. The outward expression of feelings, including vocal expression, posture, etc., includes input from both hemispheres.

Emotional Reactions

Assertions have often been made concerning emotional localization that are based on slender evidence in my opinion. It is believed that the right hemisphere processes negative emotions and the left hemisphere processes positive emotions (Heilman, Watson, & Bowers, 1983). The right hemisphere detects the emotional context of speech. With increasing emotional intensity, the right hemisphere's involvment in processing increases (Bryden & Ley, 1983). The right hemisphere may be more effective in processing both negative and positive information due to its superiority in pattern recognition (Sackheim, Putz, Vingiano, Coleman, & McElhiney, 1988).

The Question of Location

It is my position, with respect to higher and complex functions, that concepts such as lateralization and localization reflect vulnerability to impairment more than the actual anatomical area in which functioning actually occurs. Both hemispheres and subcortical structures interact in processing "higher" functions. Brodal (1981, p. 690) said it well: "As research progresses it becomes increasingly difficult to separate functionally different regions of the brain." Further (Brodal, 1981, p. 847), "The classical conception of a clear-cut functional localization cannot be upheld." Some details are offered in Chapter 2 on Neuroanatomy from a behavioral viewpoint. Code (1987) summarizes the joint contribution of both cerebral hemispheres to a variety of functions, particularly verbal. Nevertheless, there are anatomical considerations that affect performance.

Lateralization

Lateralization may be defined as the preponderance of one cerebral hemisphere or the other in processing particular functions. The extent of lateralization varies by function. Complex, "higher functions," e.g., verbal or holistic processing and problem solving, involve widespread participation. Limits on the completeness of lateralization exist between individuals, and for particular functions.

Reciprocal Relationships

Particular functions utilize reciprocal interhemispheric release and inhibition of the opposite hemisphere (probably utilizing the corpus callossum). Cognitive processing involves both cerebral hemispheres. For example, typical right hemisphere "performance" tasks (nonverbal, holistic organization, organization, visual reasoning) are performed with the assistance of left hemisphere predominance functions: verbal signals to the self, reasoning, memory, sequence, planning, storage, and rejection of intervening steps.

Multiple Contributions to Processing

Integrated functioning is commonplace, e.g., manipulating concepts that integrate visual, spatial, bodily image, and auditory information. Emotional reactions are determined in part by a cognitive appraisal, as well as perceiving the mood of others emotional valence (whether pleasant or unpleasant), and overt expression of one's feelings (see Chapter 13, on emotional disturbance).

Different Types of Information Require Different Pathways

Input and retrieval of different types of sensory information (e.g., visual or auditory) or verbal information (dominant hemisphere) versus spatial (nondominant) processing make different anatomical demands (Code, 1987; Eskenazi, Cain, Novelly, & Mattson, 1988; Joseph, 1988).

Localization

Sensory and muscular activities can often be related to specific tracts, mostly those that cross the midline to the opposite (contralateral) side of the body (decussating), connecting receptors with particular areas of the sensory cortex (with exceptions, e.g., vestibular and olfactory senses), and those that electrical stimulation results in fine movements from particular areas of the motor cortex. More complex cognitive, motor and emotional responses, however, are processed by complex circuits.

Anterior–Posterior Specialization

In general, incoming information is processed and integrated in the posterior portion of the brain, and then expressed through the planning and monitoring function of the anterior portion.

Characteristic Right Hemisphere Functions

Bodily image, perception of most aspects of music, comprehension and expression of prosodic, melodic, visual, facial, and verbal stimuli (Bryden & Lay, 1983;

Joseph; 1988), perception, comprehension, and expression of prosodic, melodic, visual, facial and verbal emotion, geometric and visual space, perception of depth, distance, direction, shape, orientation, position, perspective, figure ground, pictorial presentations, colors (Benton, 1985b), bodily orientation in space, the relative position of different parts of the body, conceiving of a situation or problem as a whole (holistic reasoning), creating an image without the use of words, and nonverbal reasoning are considered to be right hemisphere functions.

Characteristic Left Hemisphere Functions

Verbal and Sequential Processing

The left cerebral hemisphere is primary in most individuals, both right and left handed. Right lateralization of cerebral speech is very rare in right handers, but is more frequent in left handers, though the exact proportions are not known (Rey, Dellatolas, Bancaud, & Talairach, 1988). Refer to Code (1987) and Joseph (1988) for right hemisphere contribution to verbal processing. The left hemisphere is considered to organize and categorize information through linguistic coding and temporal units. It also creates sequential control of movements (limbs, articulation, etc.).

Functions Interacting with Lateralization

Handedness

The proportion of left handers is stated to be 10% of the general population with an overrepresentation among mental retardates, epileptics, the reading disabled, and alcoholics. Degree of left handedness exists on a range from strong to weak, including mixed handedness. There is inconclusive evidence that left handers have less distinct lateralization of language functions (Code, 1987 asserts that there are left handers with bilateral representation for language), and bilateral lateralization of verbal functions can interfere with right hemisphere functions such as spatial abilities (Filskov & Catanese, 1986). The overwhelming majority of right handed individuals (between 88–96% of the population according to Code, 1987, p. 17) have left hemisphere specialization for language, as well as most lefthanders. There are exceptions to this rule: 4% of right handers were determined to have right hemisphere specialization for speech (using the sodium amytal technique of Wada to anesthetize one cerebral hemisphere); 15% of left handers have right hemisphere specialization.

Age

Degree of lateralization and relative maturity of a particular mental function may vary with age. There can be individual differences for a particular function. See also Chapter 19 on Children's Brain Damage, for the significance of change of handedness.

Sex

The degree of lateralization is somewhat less in females than males for verbal, spatial, and hearing tasks (Crockett, Clark, & Klonoff, 1981). Such differences were not confirmed by Bornstein (1984), using as a criterion left hemisphere injury causing reduction of Verbal IQ, and right hemisphere injury reducing Performance IQ. Code (1980, pp. 13–14) suggests that sex differences may be related to different approaches to a task. In my own study of TBI (usually diffuse), no significant deficits by sex were detected for Full Scale, Verbal, or Performance IQs, for factor scores (Verbal; Perceptual Organization; Freedom from Distractibility/Numerical/Memory). Significant differences were detected for different nonverbal tasks: men were higher in Block design, and women in Digit Symbol. Brain-damaged women were more effective with the Stroop Color Identification task and Color Word task (suppress the incorrect printed color name used to print a different color) (Stroop Color and Word Test, Golden, Stoelting, 1978).

Complex Interactions

Several parameters may interact in the process of lateralization. Even for a bilaterally represented sense such as olfaction, females made more consistent judgments than males, and right handers had greater differences in internostril judgment than left handers (Gilbert, Greenberg, & Beauchamp, 1989).

Conclusion Concerning the Brain and Adaptation

Successful living requires the integrated functioning of complex, interdependent, and sometimes antagonistic systems. Safety and achievement, comfort and stress, excitement and avoiding boredom are difficult to reconcile. Consequently, damage to the very organ of adaptation, the brain, is especially impairing, particularly when it is accompanied by physical trauma, anxiety, loss of self-esteem, pain, illness, loss of mobility, etc.

The complexity of the brain, i.e., its interconnectedness and multiplication of ongoing functioning processing for any task, helps in understanding why even small amounts of damage can impair many types of performance.

4
Trauma and Brain Damage

Brain trauma is a process with multiple variables, including type of injury, intensity of injury, pathological reactions to the injury that may increase over a period of time, and finally processes of healing and adaptation. This chapter will give primary consideration to impact injuries, and then to the pathophysiological conditions that may occur after any type of TBI.

After serious *initial* injury, e.g., at the moment of the accident (e.g., impact and/or inertial forces), pathological processes occur, that create permanent *secondary* damage (see below). Trauma physically disrupts cells, and ischemia causes metabolic derangement. Later histopathological consequences cause increased neuropsychological impairment in survivors. The center of the lesion is devitalized, and the surrounding margin of tissue is compromised by edema and inflammation. The devitalized center becomes contracted and scarred. At the periphery of the lesion the pathological changes are largely reversible so that much of the function returns (Towbin, 1987) (see Chapter 3 on Neurobehavioral Consequences, i.e., "Soft Signs").

Concerning the question of recovery of function of nerve tissue that is damaged, but not killed: damaged (killed) brain cells are not regenerated after trauma (Kelly, 1985). However, there are inherent (and external) biochemical factors that enhance recovery. With animals, the fact that sequential lesions seem less impairing than the same damage incurred at once also implies some recovery of function (Hass & Hawkins, 1978; Stein, 1988). The hypothesis is offered that during the process of recovery the locus of functions shifts (Stein, 1988).

However, clinical observation suggests that brain damage actually reduces judgment and makes the individual more vulnerable to errors and thus repeated injury. The reduced ceiling of ability is likely to be detected with confrontation with complex tasks (see Chapters 5 and 21 on Overview and Assessment).

Mechanically Induced Trauma

The major sources of initial brain trauma are direct impact, shaking, and penetration. Mechanical forces progressively penetrate the brain, affect cell membranes and structure, and ultimately lead to multiple, impairing secondary effects

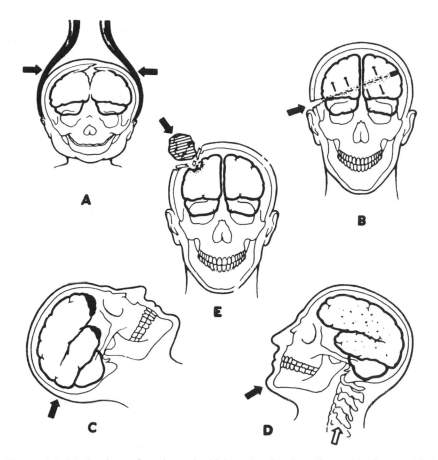

FIGURE 4.1. Mechanisms of craniocerebral injury. (A) Cranium distorted by forceps (birth injury). (B) Gunshot wound of the brain. (C) Falls (also traffic accidents). (D) Blows on the chin ("punch drunk"). (E) Injury to skull and brain by falling objects. From Courville, CB: *Pathology of the Central Nervous System*, Part 4. 1937. Pacific, Mountain View (now Pacific Press, Boise), Fig. 34–1, with permission.

(Graham et al., 1989). We are now learning about chemical reactions that affect the neuron's ability to "communicate, store, retrieve, and integrate information" (Jenkins, Lyeth, & Hayes, 1989). The chief processes responsible for TBI are diffuse axonal injury (DAI), a primary result, and brain ischemia, a secondary process (Langfitt & Zimmerman, 1985) (Fig. 4.1).

A common term for impact is *cerebral concussion*, described as a usually reversible traumatic paralysis of nervous function. *Since it is doubtful that many injuries causing temporary loss of awareness, or altered awareness, are totally lacking in sequellae, this term should be discarded as significantly misleading.*

Primary and secondary processes are influenced by physical principles and the structure of the brain within the protecting yet confining skull and meninges.

Axonal disruption is considered to be the basic pathology of minor brain injuries and is associated with loss of consciousness and traumatic amnesia. The final outcome, however, will depend on the presence and nature of secondary pathophysiological processes. Diffuse damage occurs to cortical, subcortical, and vascular structures (Alves & Jane, 1985). A comprehensive discussion of traumatic brain and spinal cord damage is found in Becker and Povlishock (1985) and Cooper (1987d).

Although injury is often not medically verified, the soft brain may be torn, internally separated, stretched, or cut when a jolt occurs. This is likely to be followed by the posttraumatic concussion syndrome (e.g., dizziness, amnesia, headaches, unconsciousness, confusion). Diffuse damage to white matter (conducting fibers) is characteristic of impact injuries. Brain stem injury, characterized by loss of consciousness, seems always accompanied by other abnormalities (Adams, Mitchell, Graham, & Doyle, 1977).

Trauma and Key Aspects of Head Anatomy

The Brain Is Tethered to the Spinal Column by Its Brainstem

The foramen magnum is a large circular window through which the central nervous system exits the skull. When impetus is transmitted to the body, for example, in a fall or automobile accident, the head continues to move, perhaps to the front or rear, or to the side in an angular direction. It accelerates forward as far as the neck will permit, and then swings back. Rotation of the cerebral hemispheres around the relatively fixed brainstem, at the midbrain–subthalamic level, is believed to create the maximal shearing stress (Adams & Victor, 1989, p. 697). This is part of the mechanism of "whiplash." The rapid to and fro motion, at a high rate of speed, stretches and tears brain tissue, and brings the brain into contact with the inner surface of the skull. If the head is at an angle to the body when the motion in one direction stops, then rapid lateral motions (swirling) occur, which can impact the inferior surface of the brain against the bottom of the skull, i.e., scraping it to cause lacerations.

The Skull Consists of Flat and Sharp Surfaces

Sharp surfaces intrude between or are adjacent to brain areas. These include the frontal crest and crista galli (separating the frontal lobes). They are the anterior support for the dura mater (falx cerebri). When the brain hits a flat surface, the result may be a contusion or bruise.

Location of TBI

When the brain rotates on one of the sharp surfaces of the inside of the skull, scratches are called lacerations. This occurs characteristically to the frontal and temporal lobes (see diagrams in Adams & Victor, 1989, Chapter 35, for various types and locations of TBI). The frontal lobes (inferior orbital; polar surfaces), upper mesencephalon, and medial–inferior surface of the temporal lobes are particularly susceptible to damage (Stuss & Benson, 1986, p. 46).

The brainstem is very vulnerable to twisting, pressure within the skull, etc., due to its location at the exit of the brain from the skull and continuation as the spinal cord. Damage here contributes to mortality of traumatic head injury. Injury above the corticospinal decussation can cause contralateral paralysis of the limbs.

The Dura Mater Makes the Brain Vulnerable to Impact Trauma

The dura mater is a dense and inelastic membrane. Its structure and strength create a hazard when the brain is pressed against it. The following forces press the brain against the sharp edges of the dura mater, causing lacerations and other damage:

1. *Momentum* of the brain caused by acceleration or deceleration forces parts of the brain into contact with the dura mater, which may cut or bruise it. A common injury is a cut to the corpus callossum, which connects the two cerebral hemispheres.
2. *Brain swelling*, i.e., edema, is increased fluid volume. This causes the brain to be cut as it herniates through the dura, causing structural distortions as some portions move and others are stretched or pushed against hard surfaces.

Trauma

A lesion directly underlying the skull where the blow was struck is called a *coup*. Damage to the opposite side is a *contracoup*, and occurs primarily at the frontal and temporal poles (Cooper, 1987b). Coup lesions are produced by deformation of the bone, with transient brain compression. The most significant lesions occur distant from the impact, i.e., when the head is free to move or is suddenly decelerated. Energy is transmitted from the skull through the brain, which may move as it receives it.

At impact, or with acceleration and deceleration, the brain is impelled forward to make violent contact with the skull, shearing forces separate structures of the brain, there is pressure against the base of the skull, pulling on the brain stem, and turning of the entire brain around the brainstem causes impaired circulation and injury, or movement of the brain against sharp edges of the external covering of the brain, described as leather-like, i.e., the dura mater.

Trauma Usually Creates Diffuse Brain Damage

Focal brain injuries are those in which a lesion large enough to be visualized with the naked eye has occurred, e.g., contusions, subdural hematoma, epidural hematoma, and intracerebral hematoma (Fig. 4.2). These lesions lead to brain shift, herniation, and brainstem compression.

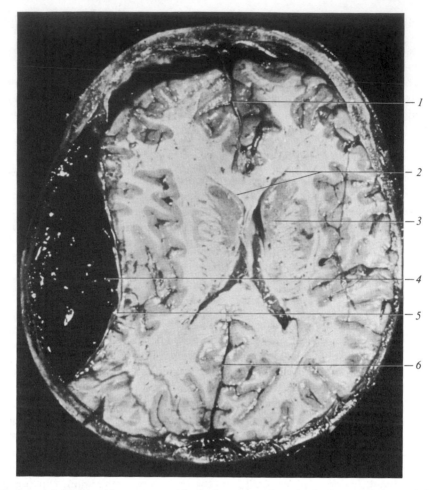

FIGURE 4.2. Epidural hematoma with displacement of cerebral parts. (1) Falx cerebri, lateropositioned. (2) Cornua frontalia ventriculi laterales, lateropositioned. (3) Caput nuclei caudati. (4) Epidural bleeding. (5) Dura mater pushed off from the side wall of the skull. (6) Fissura longitudinalis. From Samii M and Brihaye J: Traumatology of the Skull Base: Anatomy, Clinical and Radiological Diagnosis, Operative Treatment. (First International Congress of the Skull Base Group). 1983, Springer-Verlag, Berlin, Fig. 1, with permission.

Diffuse brain injuries are associated with widespread disruption of neurological function, and are not usually associated with macroscopically visible brain lesions. They are the consequence of a shaking effect caused by inertia, rapid acceleration and deceleration, and, in particular, rotational acceleration (Gennerelli, 1987a) (Fig. 4.3).

Traumatic brain injuries create typically diffuse brain damage, i.e., both cerebral hemispheres, brainstem, and the cerebellum may be damaged. Impact, secondary damage, or toxicity transmitted through the cerebrum causes exten-

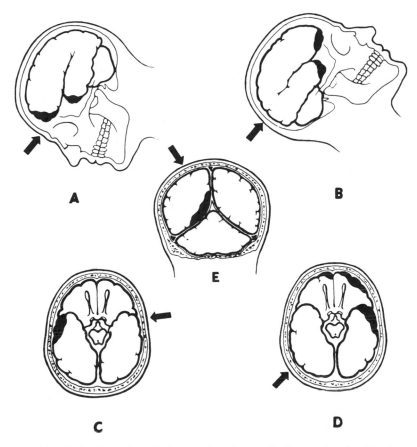

FIGURE 4.3. Mechanisms of cerebral contusion. Arrows indicate point of application and direction of force; black areas indicate location of contusion. (A) Frontotemporal contusion consequent to frontal injury. (B) Frontotemporal contusion following occipital injury. (C) Contusion of temporal lobe due to contralateral injury. (D) Frontotemporal contusion due to injury to opposite temporooccipital region. (E) Diffuse mesial temporooccipital contusion due to blow on verte. From Courville, CB: *Pathology of the Central Nervous System*, Part 4. 1937. Pacific, Mountain View (now Pacific Press, Boise), Fig. 34–3, with permission.

sive damage to association tracts and commissures (see Fig. 2.18), providing the anatomical basis for diffuse brain injury, and frequently produces paradoxical results. Although lateralized damage may be documented through imaging techniques, there are no lateralized deficits. Both cerebral hemispheres, the brainstem, and the cerebellum may be damaged. When symptoms of focalized brain damage occur, it is usually but one aspect of the overall neural pathology. Dysfunctioning results from varied pathophysiology and destruction of tissue. When focalized brain damage is detected after trauma, generalized disfunctions may accompany it.

Primary Injury

Injury caused directly by the initial insult has been categorized as focal concussion (reversible or irreversible trauma to a restricted, usually cortical region), cerebral concussion (diffuse symmetrical pattern of functional disruption), primary brain lesion (visible structural disruption that may not agree with actual site of concussion), and skull fracture (Alves & Janes, 1985, citing Ommaya and Gennarelli).

Neuronal Damage

During traumatic injury, neurons are separated at the synapse, or there may be damage or destruction of the axon, or damage to the neuron itself. Death of CNS neurons is not followed by regeneration. Neuronal or axonal damage causes dysfunctioning of postsynaptic cells.

Transneuronal Degeneration

This refers to death of neurons, beyond the synapse, which a neuron ordinarily stimulates, when the stimulating neuron dies. This lethality may cross more than one synapse, and proceed in an anterograde or retrograde direction. It is concluded that "neurons are dependent on one another for survival. This illustrates the widespread changes brought about by damage confined to a small part of the brain" (Kelly, 1985). See diaschisis, below.

Mechanical Forces

Nerve disruption is distributed according to physical laws (Thibault and Gennarelli, 1985). When an impact injury occurs, there are usual sequelae: loss of muscle tone causing the patient to drop to the ground motionless, with loss of consciousness, reflexes, and respiration. Respiration soon returns. Later the patient becomes restless, begins to regain consciousness, with irritability, apathy, and confusion, and is occasionally uncontrollable and abusive. Autonomic dysfunctioning is common (nausea, vomiting, hypothermia, and alterations of pulse and blood pressure). They may act purposefully, but not recall what happened (Strub & Black, 1988, p. 318).

The brain movement may result from impact within the skull due to a violent blow against the skull, or because the the skull hits a hard object, e.g., from a fall or the dashboard of a car. The brain may swing within the skull and hit the other side of the skull, penetrating the cerebrospinal fluid and causing a contusion, or various internal injuries. Alternatively, the head spins forward, or around, when restrained by a seat belt. When the skull has stopped, the brain keeps moving and becomes contused by the area of contact.

Impact Loading or Contact

An object strikes the head or the head strikes an object. If the object is broad, flat, and slow moving, energy puts the head in motion. If the object is rapid and small, it dissipates its effect through shock waves and skull perforation, and heat.

Impulsive Loading

The head is set into motion without direct impact to the skull. Force or change of speed is applied to the torso, neck, or face (Thibault and Gennarelli, 1985), but not directly to the head. Inertia causes the tethered neck and head to swing forward due to inertia. Whiplash is an example, i.e., the head moves rapidly, and then is restrained by its own structure, and bounces back.

Acceleration

Movement is imparted to the skull, e.g., by a blow or falling object. This may be followed by deceleration as the head's movement is restrained by a stationary object or the neck.

Translational

The blow comes from the side, or the head hits on the side. The force is called translational, and movement is in a horizontal plane.

Deceleration

A car stops suddenly, and the head and/or torso move forward.

Rotational (*Angular*)

The brain rotates around the long axis. The skull rotates because its attachment to the neck permits movement only in an arc.

1. Rotation of the brain around the brainstem may cause compression of fibers, cells, and blood vessels, apparently *leading to coma or other lapses of consciousness*.
2. Swirling brain movements laterally across the orbital, and petrous ridges, and the sphenoid wings cause *lacerations*, most frequently in *parts of the frontal and temporal lobes*.
3. Diffuse brain damage occurs because of shearing and tensile forces. The damage is known as diffuse axonal injury (DAI).

Destructive Intracranial Forces

Cavitation

The uneven distribution of force may cause the brain tissue to separate temporarily, perhaps causing contusions and focal intracerebral hematomas (Thibault & Gennarelli, 1985).

Pressure Waves

In acceleration type injuries (head pushed forward by an object), pressure is transmitted from the point of injury. As the brain rebounds from contrecoup, there is a reduced, or perhaps even negative pressure, which may add to the shearing destruction and impact. Axial compression can contribute to head and neck injuries (Cytowic et al., 1988) and produce coup and contracoup injuries (Stuss & Benson, 1986, p. 47).

Shear

Shear is movement of part of the brain at a different speed or angle than surrounding tissues. Different planes or areas of different strength slide past each other. This causes stretching of fibers, which may not function again, or be slow to recover. It contributes to diffuse brain damage, minor in each area, but clinically significant in overall effect on consciousness and ability to function normally.

Strain or Tension

Strain or tension is to pull, draw, or stretch tight beyond legitimate limits. The brain cannot move forward since it is tethered to the spinal cord beyond the skull. This type of injury requires electron microscopy to detect, not being detectable by MRI or CT (Barth, Gideon, Sciara, Hulsey, and Anchor, 1986).

Torsion

This is defined as the stress caused when one end of an object is twisted in one direction and the other end is held motionless or twisted in the opposite direction.

Typical Contact Injuries

Skull Deformation

Skull deformation is compression of bone caused by a blow to the head, the fixed head being more vulnerable than the freely moving head. Depending on the velocity of the impacting force, there may be depressed fracture, linear fracture, or skull deformation.

Increased Intrathoracic Pressure

A blow from a steering wheel is transmitted to the intracranial and orbital compartments (Cytowic et al., 1988). Increased intracranial and arterial pressure is associated with breakdown of the blood–brain barrier, followed by edema of the brainstem and white matter (Tornheim 1985).

Primary Brain Damage

Lacerations

Lacerations are actual tears in the cortical surface, i.e., visible breach in the brain substance.

Contusions

Contusions (Adams, Graham and Gennarelli, 1985; Graham, Adams & Gennarelli, 1987; Walton, 1985, p. 226) are focal damage to the surface of the brain and white matter, with extravasation of blood, but without rupture of the pia-arachnoid membrane. The brain appears red from the damaged tissues, which leak blood. There are local areas of swelling and capillary hemorrhage resembling bruises. It is a diffuse state characterized by nerve–cell and axonal damage, multiple punctate hemorrhages, and edema.

Contusions are caused by impact, rotation, and depression of the skull, and typically occur at the frontal and temporal poles. They are associated with impact of short duration (short pulse), e.g., blows and falls. The sites can be independent of the locus of impact, usually, frontopolar, orbitofrontal, anterotemporal, or lateral temporal, specifically at the frontal and temporal poles, and on the inferior surfaces of the frontal and temporal lobes where brain tissue comes in contact with bony protuberances in the base of the skull. Gliding contusions of the cortex and white matter occur on the superior surfaces of the cerebral hemispheres, when the medial parts of the temporal lobes are impacted against the dura mater, and the cerebellum against the foramen magnum at the time of injury.

More severe contusions tend to be associated with a fractured skull. They are less severe in patients with diffuse axonal injury. They may be more severe at the point of impact than diametrically opposite (contrecoup). This is illustrated by the fact that patients who received frontal injuries had more severe contusions in the frontal lobes.

Diffuse Axonal Injury (DAI)

DAI has been defined as traumatic coma lasting more than 6 hours. Mechanically it has been described as a combination of abrupt deceleration followed by abrupt cranial acceleration resulting in sudden angular motion of one cerebral hemisphere in relation to the other. Shear injuries are characterized by small focal hemorrhages and cerebral swelling (Weiner & Eisenberg, 1985). DAI is damage to the white matter or tracts connecting groups of cells, with temporary or permanent loss of function, but without mass lesions or ischemia (Gennerelli, 1987). Axonal injury can occur with even simple concussion (Langfitt & Zimmerman, 1985). DAI may be responsible for disability following minor head injury.

It is associated with focal lesions of the corpus callosum, and of one or both quadrants of the rostral brainstem, usually involving the superior cerebellar peduncle or peduncles, and the dorsolateral brainstem. It is associated particularly with motor vehicle accidents. With increasing severity there is mechanical disruption of fibers potentially including both hemispheres and extending as far caudally as the brainstem. Damage may occur in isolation or with tissue tears (small hemorrhages). Severe DAI can be present with few or no CT abnormalities. It may not manifest itself in the focal neurological examination or EEG, CT scan, etc.

DAI occurs at the moment of impact, including falls from a height. It is more common in road traffic, than in falls and assaults. Motor vehicle accidents have a long pulse (duration of deceleration) and tend to be associated with diffuse axonal injury. It is not secondary to hypoxia, brain swelling, or intracranial pressure. *DAI is highly impairing, but tends not to be associated with skull fracture, contusions, hematomas, cerebral swelling and displacement, and it will not be detected up by the usual neurological techniques.*

Sensorimotor and cognitive consequences may ensue. Deficits of cognitive functioning are related to the extent of DAI, and are considered the most commonly encountered cause of a vegetative state or severe disability after head injury. Less severe failures of recovery of intellectual function after minor head injures may be related to milder degrees of diffuse axonal injury.

More Severe White Matter Damage

With severe impact, there is damage to the corpus callosum, fornix, brainstem (ascending and descending tracts), cerebellum, etc. (Adams et al., 1977). Such impact damage can occur in the absence of high intracranial pressure, and in the absence of hypoxic brain damage.

Whiplash

Intensive acceleration/deceleration accidents, *without direct head contact with any object* (whiplash), can cause fatal or impairing neuropsychological deficits. Examples include automobile accidents and a trip followed by a fall. The brain is subjected to acceleration then deceleration, or rotation, due to a trip and fall, or being in a vehicle struck by another vehicle, and then deceleration when the skull is restrained by the neck. The brain's impetus brings it into contact with flat or rough internal surfaces of the brain, or it rotates around the brain stem.

Injuries include subdural hemorrhage, retinal damage, neurotransmitter deregulation, vocal cord paralysis, hearing loss and vertigo, and dissociated amnesia similar to transient global amnesia, neck injuries, nasal fracture, vocal cord paralysis, and headaches (Cytowic et al., 1988).

Whiplash is described as causing major debilitation (Yarnell & Rossie, 1988). One and a half years later, no member of a group of 16 patients had returned to the previous level of occupational function. Although standard neurological tests revealed only occasional deficits, neuropsychological examination revealed impairment in vigilance, selective attention, memory, mental stamina, and cognitive flexibility. There were features of posttraumatic stress disorder, hypochondriasis, depersonalization, phobias, apathy and blunted affect, depression and suicidal ideas, anhedonia, and alienation. One patient developed a florid paranoid psychosis. Additional symptoms included distractibility, loss of drive and initiation, increased irritability, and decreased frustration tolerance.

Neuronal Changes

Release of cytotoxic substances secondarily released due to disruption of cell membranes (Bakay & Wood, 1985). Changes in electrolytes (calcium and potassium) result in hyperexcitability or electrical silence depending on the degree of membrane disruption.

Damage to Neurons

Even with minor trauma, axonal swellings (retraction balls) occur over a period of 12 hours (Povlishock, 1985). I have inferred that an examination of the patient immediately after injury might not reveal behavioral problems present half a day later. Moreover, Povlishock asserts that posttrauma morbidity, in minor head injury, without evidence of neurological abnormality, is related to axonal damage. Adams et al. (1977) believe that milder and transient forms of cerebral dysfunction are due to transient failure of conduction of nerve fibers, rather than focal damage. At the point of contact, blood vessels may be torn, causing extracerebral hematoma, i.e., epidural or subdural. Enzymes bound to the membranes and neurotransmitter receptors are altered by the mechanical disruption.

Neurotransmitter Changes *(Rosner, 1985)*

Many of the systemic responses described below are related to catecholamine release (described as a "storm"). The level of neurotransmitter release is related to injury severity [norepinephrine (NE), epinephrine (E), dopamine]. Acetylcholine (ACH) and opiates are also involved. Within seconds after trauma NE can increase 10,000%, and E 40,000–50,000%. After 1 hour, there have been measurements of E at six times and NE at two times baseline. After 500 seconds peripherally circulating opiates are secreted (the source is not definitely known). Opiates may serve activating and inhibitory functions.

There is evidence that motor deficits can occur due to agonist-receptor interactions, in the absence of neuronal injury (Jenkins et al., 1989). That vestibulomotor deficits were treatable in rats is used as evidence for neuronal receptor damage.

Skull Fractures

Skull fracture implies a blow containing considerable energy. A depressed skull fracture occurs when an object with relatively large amounts of energy makes contact with the skull over a small area, depressing the bone at the point of contact. Typically the head is struck by an object (club, bat, golf ball, etc.). The fracture may be closed or open, i.e., laceration of the scull, which can lead to infection (see also missile injuries, below).

There may be no signs of symptoms of CNS injury, or these may occur in the absence of skull fracture. Although skull X rays are routinely administered in the ER, and are generally negative, diffuse brain damage usually exists in the presence of an uninjured skull and absence of hematomas large enough to appear on an X ray. Subdural hematomas, an indicator of severe trauma, can occur twice as often without skull fractures as with them (Cooper, 1988a).

Depressed

A depressed fracture of the skull can create focal damage due to underlying contusions, but rarely causes loss of consciousness.

Penetrating, or Missile, Injuries

A rapidly moving small object causes skull perforation and shock waves. Gunshot and other penetrating objects typically embed the brain with fragments of scalp tissue, hair, bone, and metal (Weiner & Eisenberg, 1985). Air is compressed in front of the bullet so that it has an explosive effect on entering the tissue, causing damage for a considerable distance around the missile tract. The missle is slowed by friction with the brain tissue and converts mechanical energy into heat. This causes considerable local damage but little rotational injury. The missile is deflected by the bone and dura, rotates, and may break into fragments. The velocity of military weapons, now used by criminals, is supposed to be greater than that of weapons usually available to civilians with different patterns of damage (Graham et al., 1987; Thibault & Gennarelli, 1985; Stuss and Benson, 1986, p. 46).

A bullet of low velocity may represent a penetrating missile injury, i.e., it enters the cranial cavity but does not leave it. The brain damage may be focal with no LOC, or there can be ricochet creating multiple destructive tracts with fragments of bone, soft tissue, and clothing, and danger of cerebral abscess or meningitis.

Perforating

The missile leaves the head. Although there may be no LOC, brain damage is severe because of shock waves, extravasation of blood, alterations to the permeability of the blood–brain barrier, and hypoxia.

Basal Skull Fractures

When the base of the skull is broken, causing rupture of the dura mater, a fistula is created that exposes the cerebrospinal fluid (CSF) (see Pathological Consequences, below).

Skull Fracture of Frontal Bone and/or Sinus

Hitting the head, commonly in automobile accidents, may create a bony depression over the frontal sinus (forehead), or damage to the protruding bones of the nose. This creates a hazard of infection from a fistula in the posterior wall of the frontal sinus. Cosmetic repair may be necessary.

Pathological Consequences of Skull Fractures

Rhinorrhea and Otorrhea

Rhinorrhea and Otorrhea are leakage of cerebrospinal fluid from the nose (fracture of the frontal bone, with tearing of the dura mater, and arachnoid membrane) or from the ear (fracture of petrous bone, dura mater, and arachnoid membrane torn, and perforated tympanic membrane), respectively. These conditions indicate an opening through which the CSF is exposed to bacteria. They are sometimes misattributed to a cold.

Infection

When the dura is penetrated (rhinorrhea, otorrhea, entry of foreign material through the skull and meninges), bacteria accompany the weapon, broken skin, bone fragments, etc. into the brain.

Osteomyelitis

Osteomyelitis is associated with compound or depressed fractures of the skull, rhinorrhea, otorrhea, and scalp lacerations. It requires prophylactic antibiotic therapy and meticulous aseptic technique for dressings.

Pneumocephalus

The presence of air within the cerebral ventricles has the same implications as a CSF fistula.

Early Posttraumatic Seizures and Coma

Early Posttraumatic Seizures

These may occur immediately after impact. Early posttraumatic epilepsy contributes to brain swelling. Of patients 1–2% have seizures within the first 24 hours, and 5% with nonpenetrating head injuries have seizures in the first week. Generalized seizures adversely affect CNS homeostasis by increasing oxygen consumption (leading to oxygen desaturation of the blood) and intracranial pressure (Guss, 1985). Seizures are discussed at greater length in Chapter 6 (Consciousness) and Chapter 19 (Childrens' Brain Damage).

Loss of Consciousness (LOC)

Transmission of energy through the brain substance to the brainstem results in a disturbance of consciousness (dizziness to coma). The extreme case is brain death (Korein, 1978). There is experimental animal evidence that maximal loss of responsiveness compatible with life is associated with bilateral mesencephalic lesions in the rostral reticular formation between the superior portion of the inferior colliculus and inferior portion of the medial geniculate body (Hass & Hawkins, 1978). During coma, there is a reduction in the electrical activity of the reticular core, while leaving conduction relatively intact in the sensory (lemniscal) pathways and cortex (Rosner, 1985). LOC indicates brain damage resulting from impact through the brain substance, probably as far as the brain stem, or rotation of the brain around the brain stem. It is believed that primary damage to the brainstem does not occur in isolation (Graham et al,. 1987), i.e., it is inferred that LOC accompanies generalized brain damage.

Diffuse brain damage has been related to coma. Some injuries, e.g., penetrating missile wounds, may not cause initial loss of consciousness until pathological processes or hemorrhage cause unconsciousness. Unconsciousness may be caused by damage to both cerebral hemispheres, or by dysfunction of the diencephalon–brainstem (mass lesions such as hematoma or compression) (Gennarelli, 1987).

Duration of coma has a significant bearing on recovery. Extended coma is associated with a vegetative state, i.e., a condition of wakefulness without awareness (Levy, Knill–Jones, & Plum, 1978). Most survivors never attain an independent existence, and if they do they are severely disabled.

For individuals with relatively short coma, perhaps even lasting weeks, the correlation between length of coma and outcome seems low. There are many individuals with gross disability with short periods of coma, and some individuals in extended coma may achieve surprisingly high levels of recovery, particularly if social support and rehabilitation services are prompt and superior. Nevertheless, they have significant neuropsychological residuals. In any event, the definition of "recovery" varies with the orientation of the researcher, and the victim might not always agree with the assessment.

Lucid Interval

A lucid interval is determined by whether a patient talked between the time of injury and death (Graham et al., 1989). Absence of an immediate loss of consciousness, or when a patient is unconscious and then regains consciousness, is associated with hemorrhage. This may occur after severe injury even a week later. Another example offered is a child who has fallen or suffered a blow to the head, and is only momentarily unconscious (Adams & Victor, 1989, pp. 704– 707).

Brain Trauma Without Loss of Consciousness

Significant brain damage may occur without loss of consciousness, e,g., penetrating head injuries, or where there is no transmission of injury to the brainstem.

False reports of no brain damage are often made because of the observation that there has been "no loss of consciousness."

Many significant injuries occur without loss of consciousness (e.g., football and boxing, and perhaps minor household blows and falls), although the victims may experience confusion, lethargy, or amnesia. The blow has disrupted normal functioning, and it can be considered a concussion. Activities that are overlearned can be continued, although the victim is in anterograde amnesia, and outsiders lack awareness that the individual has been concussed (Strub & Black, 1988, 315–318).

Somatic Injury

Neck and body

Neurological Effects

Injury to the neck may affect decussating tracts. Whether proprioception or temperature and touch will be affected ipsilaterally or contralaterally depends on the sensation involved and the level of crossing the midline (see Chapter 2 on Neuroanatomy).

Impaired Immunological System

Trauma effects the various immune systems, which are correlated with susceptibility to infection and other causes of mortality. Of head injury patients 40% die because of extracranial causes, mostly infection (Gadisseux, 1985).

Pain

Neural Effects of Pain

Pain (see also headache, below; Chapter 15 on Stress) pathways (spinothalamic) send branches to the reticular system (affecting alertness), and to the limbic system (hypothalamus and forebrain), thus contributing to the emotional component of chronic pain (Hendler, 1981a, p. 192). Descending pathways may suppress the conscious experience of pain, particularly during intense emotional stress (Barr & Kiernan, 1983, p. 280).

Radiculopathy

Radiculopathy refers to irritation and compression of the sensory roots entering the spinal cord, in this case, often consequent to mechanical trauma. It can be experienced as pain in the extremities, bodily axis, paresthesias, and weakness.

Headaches

Although headaches are often attributed to emotional causes, they are one of the most common after-effects of traumatic brain injury (Adams & Victor, 1985,

Chapter 9; Cytowic et al., 1988; Herskowitz & Rosman, 1982, Chapter 11). Although pain is a sign of damage to soft tissue of the head, its intensity can be related to inability to express feelings, depression, secondary gain, etc. (see Chapter 15 on Stress). Persistent headaches can disrupt a patient's life (Rimel et al., 1982).

Areas of the Head Vulnerable to Trauma

The face and scalp are richly supplied with pain receptors to protect the contents of the skull. Nasal and oral passages, the eye and ear, are delicate and sensitive. Other head structures that are affected by trauma are the intracranial arteries and veins, cranial nerves, muscles that go into spasm, meninges, and contents of the skull, which react to increased intracranial pressure, skin, subcutaneous tissue, scalp and skull, muscles, arteries, periosteum of the skull, eye and orbit, ears and mastoid sinuses, nasal cavity and sinuses, teeth and oropharynx, intracranial venous sinuses, dura at the base of the brain, and arteries within the dura mater and pia-arachnoid,

Direct Result of Injury and Tissue Damage

Long lasting trauma in the form of headaches can occur after application of force directly to the skull, and the effects of inertia swinging and shaking the soft external and internal tissues of the torso, head, and neck, before and after impact. The mechanisms include traction, dilatation, distention, or displacement of intracranial arteries, extracranial arteries, intracranial veins of the dura, compression, traction or inflammation of sensory cranial and spinal nerves, voluntary or involuntary spasm or inflammation of cranial and cervical muscles, meningeal irritation, raised intracranial pressure, hemorrhage, and migraine. Speed (1982) attributes the physiological process of chronic posttraumatic headache to muscle contraction, vasodilation (including migraine), scar formation in the scalp, and injuries to neck structures. He asserts that 30% of head injured patients will develop this condition. Headache is associated with prolonged cerebral circulation time (Lishman, 1987, p. 170).

Pain Receptors

The head is supplied by these cranial nerves: trigeminal (cranial nerve V), facial (V), glossopharyngeal (IX), and vagus (X), and the first three cervical nerves (C1–3).

Damage Outside the Skull

Damage to upper cervical nerve roots (radiculopathy) may be experienced as headaches (Spindler & Reischer, 1982). A detailed description of the interrelationship between the spinal column, muscles, connective tissue, and the head is offered by Zohn (1982). He stresses the complexity of balance and movement, and the formation of pain–provoking trigger points, after trauma, which contribute to headaches. The mechanism may be radiculitis, or damaged soft tissues in the muscle. Trigger points outside the head may be experienced as headaches. In addition, there may be nerve entrapment by muscular spasm, fibrositis, and other soft-tissue damage.

Headaches can result from direct or indirect trauma to the neck, a fall on an outstretched hand, or an extended fall (Reichmeister, 1982) (see also TMJ syndrome, below). Disorder of cervical muscle tone occurs with damage below the occiput. Mechanical strain of the cervical spine is associated with ANS dysfunction (Cytowic et al., 1988).

Confusion as to the damaged area may arise from the fact that damage within the skull (above and below the tentorium cerebelli) can be referred to different areas of the skull and neck.

Temporomandibular Joint Syndrome (TMJ)

TMJ (Gelb and Siegel, 1980, Chapter 2) occurs when the jaw joints are forced out of alignment, for example, by a blow. However, spasms of the muscles that operate the jaw are considered of greater etiological significance by Pincus and Tucker (1985, p. 295). When the head is not in the proper position, it does not rest comfortably on the neck and shoulders. The consequences are headaches, muscle tension, spasm, and trigger points, jaw clicking and other noises, earaches, pains in various parts of the head, various somatic symptoms, etc. TMJ is subject to misinterpretation since the victim may not relate it to the injury.

Secondary Processes

Brain injury may be considered to be a process. The initial impact or other deficit (e.g., neurotoxin, infection, anoxia), perhaps an apparently "trivial" head injury, can set into motion a sequence of events leading to secondary brain damage (see below) with a neuropsychological impairment or fatal outcome or permanent and severe injury (Graham et al., 1987). Accompanying somatic injury and pathology further impair recovery, add to emotional stress, and can result in permanent illness or even mortality. Excellent general sources are Becker and Povlishock (1985) and Cooper (1987c).

Walker (1978), in a study of the brains of people maintained on a respirator, observed that the secondary reactions seemed more significant than the primary pathological lesion. Lesions, inflammation, and necrosis were observed in the spinal cord, brainstem, cerebellum, diencephalon, and cortex. The medulla bore the brunt of brainstem lesions, due to displacement and compression by the cerebellum. The changing status of the injury is illustrated by the finding that "late MRI (magnetic resonance imaging) lesions in severely head injured children have little anatomical relationship with earlier defects seen on computed tomography" (McCullough comment, in Levin et al., 1989).

Secondary brain damage may cause general brain damage. For example, a depressed skull fracture can cause immediate impact damage, followed by bleeding, pressure on nearby parts of the brain, restriction of blood flow in other parts of the brain, accompanied by swelling, in turn forcing the brain against internal edges of the skull and dura mater. Metabolic changes cause destruction of cell membranes, causing further edema and reduced blood flow.

Loss of Autonomic Self Regulation

Brain functioning requires optimal physiological conditions, and is itself the controlling organ. Damage to the brainstem is associated with impairment of cerebral blood flow and cerebral oxidative metabolism (Hass & Hawkins, 1978). Brain damage also impairs the ability to combat more general systemic effects accompanying somatic injuries.

Acute injury results in autonomic stimulation of the cardiac and respiratory centers, which can increase cardiac output, central blood volume (hyperemia), oxygen delivery, and intracranial hypertension. Vascular dimensions change according to the need for oxygen and glucose (Muizellaar & Obrist, 1985). In some patients with severe head injury, the intensity of the hyperdynamic state exceeds other types of trauma (Perkin, 1985). Metabolic autoregulation is disturbed directly by head trauma, or functions inadequately, when seizures or increased metabolism are superimposed on other disturbances such as increased intracranial pressure.

Systemic Responses to Brain Injury

These ensue from the neurotransmitter storm (see above) and somatic injury:

- *Vascular* (Bakay & Wood, 1985; Bruce, 1985; Kishore & Hall 1987; Miner, 1985; Rosner, 1985): Trauma, infection, hypoxia, and any condition elevating intracranial pressure result in changes in cerebral blood flow and its control mechanisms. Blood clotting abnormalities lead to rapid death, or delayed and recurrent hematomas. ECG changes are present in 90% of head injured patients. After anoxia and ischemia, acidic metabolites produce vasodilation, and thus ischemia. Increased serum norepinephrine levels create hypertension, hypotension, bradycardia (reduced heart rate), apnea, pupillary dilation, myocardial necrosis, and arterial spasm (hypotension and cardiovascular collapse).
- *Shock:* When head injuries are complicated by severe injuries to the trunk and extremities.
- *Hypermetabolism and hypercatabolism* (Clifton, Robertson, & Grossman, 1985; Gadisseaux, 1985; Miner, 1985; Nillson & Pontin, 1985): After head trauma there is a hypermetabolic nutritional state, to meet the needs of damaged organs, i.e., increased resting energy expenditure and caloric needs. Hypercatabolism refers to abnormally high urinary nitrogen excretion and negative nitrogen and protein balance. These are related to the severity of the injury.

There are alterations in glucose, fat, and protein metabolism. The HPA plays an important, though not the only role in the hypermetabolic response. This is mediated by glucagon, the catacholamines epinephrine and norepinephrine, and glucocorticoids (e.g., cortisol, stimulated by ACTH release). Hypermetabolism persists during the duration of coma. There is a markedly increased energy requirement varying with the severity of trauma. Intravascular volume must sustain oxygen delivery and cardiac output. Caloric and oxygen requirements are greatly increased. Body temperature and pathological posturing also increase metabolic expenditure. There is increased oxygen consumption, which may be impaired by vascular spasm, which causes reduced cerebral blood flow and oxygen availablity, resulting in energy depletion and anoxia.

- *Pulmonary* (Beckman, 1985): Respiratory distress resulting from a shift of blood to the pulmonary circulation results in pulmonary edema, one of the most striking effects of brain injury. Fat emboli may be involved.
- *Hyperthermia:* Results from shock stemming from injury to the hypothalamus or brainstem, local or general infection, or marked dehydration.
- *Enhanced bone formation:* Although loss of calcium from the skeleton during immobilization is well known, hypercalcemia can occur in the presence of metabolic derangements of organic mental syndromes. This increases obtundation and also aspiration and pneumonia (Seliger, Cosman, Abrams, & Lindsay, 1989. Traumatic lesions of the brain, accompanied by long coma, is associated with new bone formation around large joints. Such patients appear to have an abnormally high release of GH to thyrotropin–releasing factor (Szabon & Groswasser, 1989).
- *Dysphagia:* Many seriously head injured individuals have problems swallowing, resulting in aspiration, malnutrition, poor wound healing. These lead to increased medical problems and prolong hospitalization (Field & Weiss, 1989).

Traumatic Encephalopathy

Changed Neurological Functioning

Diaschisis (Long Distance Effect)

Neuronal death and dysfunctioning cause disturbed functioning at distant sites to which connnections were interrupted. Thus, disturbed function is far more widespread than that implied by a focal injury, contributing to the difficulty in "localizing" or "lateralizing" a given function. Areas distant from the lesion will tend to recover more than damaged ones, but their functioning probably will offer subtle impairment due to loss of adequate input (see transneuronal degeneration, below).

Metabolic

Neuronal activation may be disturbed due to pathological changes (e.g., metabolic) or loss of tissue. Healing may take 1–3 weeks if proper connections are restored; otherwise the cells atrophy (chromatolysis) or degenerate totally (Kelly, 1985).

Denervation Supersensitivity

Removal of presynaptic input, i.e., deafferentiation due to destruction or injury of stimulating neurons, increases sensitivity to the remaining neurotransmitter. The mechanism is an increase in the number of receptors on the target cell after an axon is cut (Schwartzkroin & Fuchs, 1989).

Neuronal Sprouting

Branches of neurons from nearby undamaged areas invade damaged or degenerated areas. Afferent inputs fill the receptor sites left by degenerating ascending and descending trasts. This has been demonstrated both in the brain (hippocampus) and spinal cord. The damaged area is served by neurons that ordinarily serve a different function, and it may be presumed that the newly established connections are not identical with the preinjury patterns. When the spinal cord is severed, regenerating axons are prevented from reaching their target sites by the barrier caused by scarring, i.e., growth of glial cells (Livingston, 1985, p, 1172–3; Schwartzkroin & Fuchs, 1989).

Posttraumatic Epilepsy

Seizures may occur immediately on injury or years later. The more severe the injury, the greater the possibility of seizures. The incidence of late posttraumatic epilepsy is related to the severity of the injury, an amnestic period of more than 24 hours, an intracranial hematoma, depressed skull fracture, or penetrating injury (Dacey & Dikmen, 1987). EEG studies are useful to determine the likelihood and control of seizures.

Seizures can cause pathological cellular effects, with potential neuropsychological consequences (Bolter, 1986), including exaggerated metabolic demands, ischemia secondary to anoxia, hypoglycemia, hypotension, hyperthermia, and acidosis.

Long Term Neurotransmitter Effects

There are a variety of neurotransmitter effects that contribute to impairment. At the time of injury, increased secretion of catecholamine and opiate–like materials appears to have a permanent effect on brain organization and behavior. These substances cause immediate activation and inhibition, with a variety of long–lasting cognitive and emotional effects (see Chapter 15 on Stress). In addition, damage to neurons and axons prevents neurotransmitters from being transported to synapses where they will stimulate the next sequence in a pathway (diaschisis).

Neuronal and Transneuronal Degeneration

Degenerative changes take place in the damaged neurone and beyond the synapse in both directions: anterograde (affected cell is ordinarily stimulated by the injured neuron) or retrograde (affected cell makes synapses on the injured neuron) (Kelly, 1985). Damage to the axon interferes with transport of nutrients and neurotransmitters and by–products toward the next synapse (anterograde) and also back to the cell body (retrograde). Retrograde death of a neuron can occur after the axon is severed. Transneuronal degeneration occurs when there is the death beyond the synapse of other neurons not directly damaged, i.e., anterograde (the course of the impulse) or retrograde (neurons stimulating the damaged neuron). Transneuronal degeneration can affect functioning at considerable distances (diaschisis, see above) since it may cross more than one synapse, i.e., involve the death of two or more consecutive impulses in a pathway (Kelly, 1985; Schwartz, 1985).

Damage to Hypothalamus and the Attached Pituitary Gland

The pituitary gland is vulnerable to trauma involving change of momentum to the brain relative to the skull, or direct blows, since it is attached to a stalk at the base of the brain (infundibulum) and actually located within of the skull at the base of the brain (sella turcica). The pituitary stalk can be torn at the time of head injury. Thus, when the brain moves, this stalk, and/or its attachment within the hypothalamus may be torn, stretched, or rotated. Head trauma and child abuse are clearly stated to be etiologic considerations for hypopituitarism (Findling & Tyrell, 1986). Cooper (1987a) asserts that most of the damaged to the hypothalamus and pituitary gland is secondary to raised intracranial pressure, brain shift, and distortion of the brain. When the brain moves, this stalk, and/or its attachment within the hypothalamus, may be torn, stretched or rotated. The integrity of hypothalamic releasing factors, and of anterior and posterior pituitary secretion, is jeopardized by damage to the infundibulum (stalk of the pituitary) or to local circulation connecting the brain with the pituitary gland. (See Chapters 8 and 19 on visceral control centers and children's brain damage).

Some endocrine deficits include *hypopituitarism* which is attributed to head trauma and child abuse (Findling & Tyrell, 1986) (developmental problems are discussed further in Chapter 19 of Childrens Brain Damage) and *diabetes insipidus*, which is attributed to mechanical disturbance to the pituitary or hypothalamus (Ramsey, 1986).

Cranial Nerve Damage

Cranial nerve damage occurs in 10% of head injuries (Cartlidge & Shaw, 1981, p. 81). Sensory and motor deficits occur due to damage to the sensory organs, nerve pathways leading to the brain (inside and outside the skull), and nerve centers and pathways within the brain. The symptoms include disturbed vision, hearing, eye movements, balance, anosmia, facial pain and paralysis, and hampered movements in the tongue, pharynx, and upper limbs, trapezius muscle of the back, and oculomotor movements (Cartlidge & Shaw, 1981; Rouit & Murali, 1988; Wilson-Pauwels et al., 1988) for a detailed description of the anatomy and function of the cranial nerves).

Damage to sensory and motor functions can be diagnostic as to the location of the head injury. The damage may be to the nerves directly, to surrounding bone and tissues as they exit the brain, or to sensory and motor nuclei in the brainstem. The reader is referred to the discussion of cranial nerve functions in Chapter 2 on neuroanatomy, and to neuropsychological deficits in Chapter 7 on Integrated Sensorimotor Functions.

Intracranial Pathology

Increased Catecholamines

Circulating levels are related to the severity of the injury, and abnormally high levels may last for weeks. Elevated levels of norepinephrine cause a variety of metabolic effects, including vasoconstriction (hampering distribution of oxygen, nutrients, and removal of wastes) and reduced CSF formation (same effects) (Bakay & Wood, 1985; Miner, 1985).

Cerebrospinal Fluid (CSF) Dysfunctions

Head injury, e.g., basilar skull fracture with infection, can disturb CSF absorption leading to elevation in intracranial pressure (Bakay & Wood, 1985). Vasoconstriction caused by elevated catecholamines in the CSF, and drugs administered to head injured patients, can interfere with CSF production. Loss of calcium from the CSF to brain cells causes a variety of intrabrain cell dysfunctions and lesions indistinguishable from impact injury.

Increased Intracranial Pressure and Edema (Brain Swelling)

Edema is defined as an increase of cerebral tissue water causing an increase of tissue volume, and is associated with impaired absorption of cerebrospinal fluid (CSF), obstruction to its flow due to disruption of the lining of the capillaries of changes in the blood–brain barrier (McComb, 1985; Pacyna, 1985) or chemical changes of the affected tissue (Unterberg & Baethmann, 1985). It is caused by a variety of conditions including trauma, toxic effects, and hemorrhage (Langfitt & Zimmerman, 1985). Disturbance of CSF pressure control leads to brain herniation and death (Marmarou and Tabaddor, 1987).

Swelling of the brain takes place adjacent to contusions (Graham et al., 1987; Langfitt & Zimmerman, 1985) or intracerebral hematoma. After evacuation of a mass lesion (hematoma), when the skull is opened during surgery, edema pushes brain tissue through various compartments within the brain, or outside the skull, causing considerable damage. Cerebellar herniation isolates the spinal cord.

Some damage is due to disruption of the tissue and damage to the blood–brain barrier of small vessels due to shear strains, with electrolytes leaking into brain tissue. By–products of cell injury may be carried in the edema fluid, affecting the microenvironment of the brain, traversing the extracellular space of the white matter, and affecting distant locations. Many neurotoxic substances (mediator compounds) are released that enter the brain through the broken blood–brain barrier, causing further edema, and carrying neurotoxins such as glutamic acid to distant sites (Tornheim, 1985; Unterberg & Baethmann, 1985).

Increases in the blood volume (hyperemia) and edema (addition of fluid to the brain substance) are separate conditions (Clasen & Penn, 1987). Increased intracranial pressure occurs when there is interference with circulation within the brain, or increased mass, e.g., hematoma, edema, or impaired circulation of the cerebrospinal fluid. The latter condition can lead to hydrocephalus, i.e., increased retention of fluid in the ventricles. This places pressure on the tissue, and can result in permanent brain damage.

Behavioral signs of brain swelling include changes in consciousness, headache, restlessness, etc., which suggests intracranial bleeding.

Effect of Alcohol at the Time of Trauma

Severe acute alcohol intoxication results in abnormal permeability of the blood-brain barrier and cerebral edema (Bakay et al., 1980, p. 357). Alcohol might interfere with the ability to diagnose even mild brain injury and could interfere with normal recovery (Kraus & Arzemanian, 1989). It is not conclusive that alcohol affects outcome, i.e., different reports indicate higher or lower mortality in different series of patients. Nevertheless, for severely brain injured individuals, positive blood-alcohol concentration was correlated with a longer duration of hospital stay, and chronic alcoholics had a higher mortality rate than contrasting groups. Moreover, there may be a synergistic effect between severe brain injury and intoxication to prevent the patient's homeostatic injury response (Kraus, Morgenstern, Fife, Conroy, and Nourijah, 1989). Drinking at the time of injury has a greater negative effect on outcome than habitual drinking per se; the effects vary from measure to measure, and may have an additive effect with post-traumatic amnesia.

Brain Shift

The mass of the brain may be shifted from its symmetrical position around the midline. This process can also can compress the brainstem (or other areas (causing death or unconsciousness).

Herniation and Brainstem Compression

This is forcing of the brain outside of its normal compartments (e.g., meninges or foramen magnum), due to factors such as brain swelling, hematoma, or increased intracranial pressure that increases in size. There can be obliteration of the cortical sulci and ventricles, ultimately herniating under the falx cerebri displacing the lateral and third ventricles across the midline (Weiner & Eisenberg, 1985; see dura mater in Chapter 2). Ultimately the midbrain and spaces of the brainstem (cisterns) are obliterated. Herniation through the tentorium can cause blockage of the foramen magnum by cerebellar tissue. A mass lesion, brain swelling, or increased intracranial pressure can compress the brainstem and cause herniation outside the foramen magnum. Initially there is loss of consciousness, and ultimately death due to loss of visceral functions. Intracerebral hematoma can put pressure on the brainstem, injuring it, with poor outcome. Brodal (1981, p. 694) observes that a mass lesion (a tumor) can push the brainstem to the other side, compressing the contralateral cerebral peduncle against the tentorium (dura mater) above the decussation, resulting in paresis on the side of the lesion!

Hydrocephalus

This is defined as an accumulation of CSF, due to lack of absorption, or mechanical obstruction. It may lead to ventricular enlargement (McComb), implying loss of tissue and/or stretching or compression.

Hypoxic Brain Damage

The brain is extremely susceptible to deficits of oxygen since it consumes 20% of the entire body's oxygen supply although composing only 2% of body weight and receiving 17% of cardiac output (Barr & Kiernan, 1983, p. 359). Hypoxia has a high incidence, and occurs soon after injury (Langfitt & Zimmerman, 1985), with various pathological processes contributing to it. It is associated with high intracranial pressure, and arterial spasm. Therefore, it can occur in the absence of an intracranial mass lesion. Damage is found more frequently in the hippocampus and basal ganglia than in the cerebral cortex and cerebellum. After the initial impact, there is usually a general paralysis of nervous function characterized by loss of muscle tone, causing the patient to lose muscular control, perhaps drop to the ground motionless, with loss of respiration. Arterial spasm can occur soon after an injury. Also, high intracranial pressure may cause ischemia (local anemia due to mechanical obstruction of the blood supply). Hypoxia is a frequent finding in patients who remain vegetative or severely disabled after a head injury. It occurs in half of brain injured patients studied (Marshall & Marshall, 1985).

Metabolic Derangements

Trauma or ischemia creates chemical changes, edema, reduced blood flow, and breakdown of membranes leading to complex inorganic and organic reactions. Some cells are sacrificed that would linger and consume oxygen and metabolic substrates better utilized by the remaining cells (Young (1987).

Ischemia

Ischemia is local anemia due to mechanical obstruction of the blood supply, e.g., large mass lesions, or intracranial hypertension. Ischemia subsequent to trauma increases the likelihood of neuronal death. Much of the neuronal dysfunction results from aberrant information flow. There is a "sublethal excitotoxic process" after mild trauma that is brought to a lethal level by subsequently developing ischemia (Jenkins et al., 1989).

Hemorrhage or Hematomas

This is caused by escape of blood from the vessels due to shearing (varied speeds of acceleration and deceleration of tissues), or alterations in the blood–brain barrier (Povlishock, 1985). The arteries and veins of the skull, meninges, and within the brain may be torn or penetrated.

Hematomas are localized masses of extravasated blood, relatively contained within a space, and usually clotted. As space occupying lesions, they interfere with circulation (oxygen, nutrients, removal of wastes), resulting in anoxia, displacement of brain tissue against the sharp edges of the dura mater, or internal and sharp edges of the skull. Sufficient internal pressure can push brain tissue out of the skull through the foramen magnum (exit of spinal column).

The meninges are landmarks describing location of the bleeding.

- *Subarachnoid:* Next to the brain. It is relatively common in patients who have been unconscious for at least 1 hour.
- *Epidural:* Bleeding between the dura mater and the skull, relatively distant from the brain surface, following traumatic rupture of the middle meningeal artery or vein. It is considered to have a somewhat less damaging effect than blood applied directly to the brain surface, e.g., subdural. There may be a transient loss of consciousness. After a lucid interval lasting a day or more, increased intracranial pressure will cause loss of consciousness and further brain damage.
- *Subdural:* Bleeding into the space between the dura mater and arachnoid membrane, which may originate from a subdural vein rupture. Mortality and morbidity are greater than in epidural hematoma (Cooper, 1987b). The patient may have little initial impairment of consciousness, since this condition may be delayed in onset. Weeks or months after a trivial accident, the symptoms of a subdural hematoma may occur, presenting as a stroke or dementing process (Teasdale & Mendelow, 1984). Chronic subdural hemorrhage or hematoma requires operative relief since the hematoma increases in size. Eventually, the hematoma, which is encased in a membrane, increases intracranial pressure.
- *Petechial:* Minute hemorrhage, on the surface of brain and also the internal surfaces of the brainstem, seems to be caused by acceleration/deceleration impulses characteristic of road traffic accidents. They are often found in fatal injuries (Langfitt & Zimmerman, 1985). Personality changes may appear weeks or months after the precipitating injury. The outcome is worse than epidural hematoma or diffuse brain damage (Rimel et al., 1982).
- *Intracerebral hemorrhage:* Subcortical hematoma or small multiple areas. The incidence is increased in patients with a posttraumatic amnesia of more than 24 hours, an intracranial hematoma, a depressed skull fracture, or a penetrating injury (Dacey & Dikmen, 1987). Seizures are discussed at greater length in Chapter 6 (Consciousness) and Chapter 19 (Childrens' Brain Damage).
- *Delayed traumatic intracerebral hematomas (DTICH):* These are secondary insults that occur hours and days after impact. They occur chiefly in the frontal

and temporal lobes, and may be caused by weakness due to trauma, increased intravascular pressure, and hypoxia leading to vascular dilatation; they finally result in rupture of the injured vessels (Cooper, 1985).

Effectiveness of Neurological Diagnostic Procedures

Much of the damage associated with trauma may not be detectable by a focal neurological examination, imaging techniques, or X ray. Adams, Mitchell, Graham, and Doyle (1977) state that a head–injured patient, without a fractured skull or even a blemish, may sustain severe and irreversible damage due to rapidly developing brainstem damage secondary to a high intracranial pressure and herniation of the brain.

Skull X Rays

Skull radiographs are of little use in making the diagnosis of chronic subdural hematoma, since a fracture is found less than 10% of the time (Cooper, 1987b). The presence of a fracture on a skull X ray does not indicate the severity of injury or predict outcome, and is probably unnecessary most of the time (Weiner & Eisenberg, 1985).

Isotope Brain Scans

The accuracy of isotope brain scans in detecting chronic subdural hematoma ranges from 50–100% (Cooper 1987b) (see PET scan).

CT Scan

It is effective in detecting subdural hematomas, but can misdiagnosis a lesion when the hematoma is isodense with relation to the brain subtance (Cooper, 1987b). It is not effective in detecting cytotoxic edema, a major contributor to severe brain swelling accompanying acute subdural hematoma. It detects DAI only when there is relatively gross hemorrhagic destruction of white matter in the corpus callosum and occasionally in the brainstem (Langfitt & Zimmerman, 1985).

Nuclear Magnetic Resonance (NMR)

It is useful in differentiating kind of hematomas, in particular, isodense ones (same density as brain) in contrast to contusions, hematomas, and their extent. It is better than CT for ischemia, cysts, and edema, which create hypodense conditions (Langfitt & Zimmerman, 1985). Changes may be seen immediately after TBI and then disappear.

Conclusion

The brain is extremely vulnerable to a variety of mechanical, physiological, and pathological processes. Their effects are not always documentable through routine medical procedures, but the practitioner should be alert to behavioral deficits that can reasonably be attributed to traumatic brain injury.

5
Overview: Neurobehavioral Consequences of Brain Damage

The Effect of Trauma on Integrated Functioning

Some generalizations concerning the effect of brain trauma on behavior will be considered, followed by a taxonomy of specific dysfunctions and deficits.

Trauma Usually Creates Diffuse Brain Damage

Narrowly defined dysfunctioning after neural trauma is infrequent since it is more characteristic for complex circuitry to be damaged by trauma. Symptoms are sometimes classified as follows:

Focal: localized because associated with damage to a relatively small, or well-differentiated area;

Diffuse axonal injury: axonal and cell damage spread out over the central nervous system, without gross pathology as a large hematoma, though smaller damage may be visualized;

Lateralized: defects are confined to one side of the body, usually associated with damage on the opposite side of the brain;

Generalized: widespread damage with many symptoms.

Diffuse damage is more characteristic of traumatic brain injury (TBI) than focal lesions. Occasionally focal symptoms occur with generalized brain damage (e.g., visual scotoma in Chapter 7 on Sensorimotor Functions), but they are but one aspect of the overall neural pathology.

Limited Correlation Between Location and Dysfunction

Focal Injuries

Focal brain damage often results in more narrowly defined deficits than diffuse brain damage. It is primarily associated with direct impact, e.g., a fall (frontal and temporal lobes), depressed skull fractures, and penetrating missile injuries.

Damage to the left cerebral hemisphere is more likely to result in focalized disturbances than damage to the right hemisphere, where more generalized damage is required (Davidson, 1980).

However, a focal lesion need not result in a narrow range of dysfunctions. This follows from the brain's complex circuitry and multiple contributions to a given function. Moreover, damage to one part of the brain is rarely localized, i.e., adjacent nerve tracts are cut, pressure extends to other regions, etc.

Complex Circuits May Be Damaged

Focal lesions may result in a wide range of dysfunctions, due to interference with complex circuits, interference with nearby circuits due to secondary pathological processes such as edema, increased intracranial pressure, hematoma, etc., and diaschisis ("long-distance effects"). Damage to an identified area or link could result in dysfunctioning whose "basis" may be at a different portion of the nervous system.

The Damage Cannot Be Accurately Localized

Common injuries such as impact, neurotoxins, as well as secondary effects of severe injuries lead to generalized brain damage. For example, DAI is associated with high-acceleration injuries, e.g., motor vehicle accidents. Multiple damage to the central, autonomic, or peripheral nervous systems and/or the soma can coexist. Unpredictability of symptoms may be conditioned also by a long-distance effect (diaschisis). Damage affects input to certain centers and output to others, and impairs nearby long lines (see Chapter 4 on Trauma and Brain Damage). Dysfunctioning of a distant region may result. Paradoxical neuroimaging studies have been observed, i.e., lateralized damage without focalized or lateralized deficits.

Functioning May Be Bilateral

Thus, bilateral transmission pathways permit some retention of functions that would be detected only with careful examination. Functioning may be retained despite unilateral damage. Examples include vision and audition (see the diagram in Livingston, 1985, p. 1005).

Complex Functions May Be Subserved by a Circumscribed Area

Combined somatosensory and motor cortex (Brodal, 1981, p. 847), unity representation of sensory and motor mechanisms in lower centers (Livingston, 1985, p, 1157), speed of processing, and accuracy of perception can be impaired by damage to a circuit integrating multiple sensory channels (Luria, 1980, pp. 42– 51).

Some Functions Are Sensitive to Lesions Anywhere in the Cortex

Examples include reaction time, detection of hidden figures, and language performance (Woods, 1987).

Somatic Damage Contributes to Neurological Dysfunction

- *Damage to joints, bones and muscles* leads to deficits of strength, sensation, pain, and/or loss of range of motion. Ipsilateral deficit is caused directly by damage to muscles, peripheral nerves, bones, etc., or neural tracts below the point where sensory and/or muscular pathways decussate (Menkes, 1985, p. 489).
- *Gross systemic effects* such as poor stamina, poor morale, poor health, pain, continued stress, anxiety, fatigue, etc., contribute to impaired neuropsychological performance.

Lateralization of Symptom Varies with Level of Damage

Expression of sensory and muscular deficits depends on whether the level of the nervous system that is damaged is above or below decussation. One must assess whether trauma has occurred to nerve pathways outside the central nervous system, the spinal cord, the particular level of the medulla, midbrain, or cerebrum. The pattern of impairment is a helpful tool in localizing. For example, the degree of similarity of shape of a bilateral visual scotoma will vary with the closeness of the lesion to the occipital cortex (Bajendas & Kline, 1987, pp. 11–12). A left-sided muscular weakness has a different significance according to whether or not there are also symptoms of right parietal lobe damage. A variety of evaluation procedures may be needed to gain a broad enough picture to make a judgment (see Chapter 7 on Sensorimotor Functions).

Damage Does Not Reveal the Function of a Part

When a neural structure is absent or damaged, it reveals what the rest of the nervous system can do without it (Livingston, 1985, p. 1179)! As Trimble (1988a, p. 153) states, "any destruction of brain leads to both the effects of that lesion in that area and the continued, but now different, action of the rest of the brain. *Moreover, post injury functioning reflects the interaction of pathological processes (from damaged but somewhat functional tissue) interacting with the integrated functioning of the remaining tissue.*"

The Significance of "Soft Signs"

Although small lesions may be "clinically silent," they can cause lesser symptoms, i.e., "soft signs." Loss of function "within normal limits" does not consider the "subtle loss of versatility and acumen previously possessed prior to the cerebral damage" (Towbin, 1985).

Overview of Neuropsychological Symptoms

1. *Varied conditions effect the quality of recovery* (see Chapter 18 on Recovery):

    - The locus and degree of primary and secondary pathophysiological damage;

- Different impairments may improve at different rates;
- Rapidity of rehabilitation;
- The age of the victim;
- Demands of the environment for performance.

2. *Traumatic brain injury is expressed in different ways*

Deficits of variable breadth: Symptoms may be *narrow* (e.g., particular sensory problems) or broad (comprehension problems with aphasia). Within the context of retained general ability, specific dysfunctions can occur: anomia, i.e., inability to remember the names of people and objects, loss of memory for recent events, acalculia, inability to concentrate, reduced psychomotor speed or speed of mental processing, etc.

Deficits from the baseline: For outpatient assessment, the most characteristic deficit is reduction of performance from an estimated baseline. The actual level of performance may be within the normal range, emphasizing the impor tance of making an estimate of preinjury performance, or obtaining test or work samples of it (see Chapter 21 on Assessment).

Pathognomonic symptoms: Characteristic responses to psychological tests found primarily after brain damage are quite rare. Examples include *perseveration* (repetition of a previously given response) and some kinds of perceptual–spatial errors in copying geometric figures (e.g., inverted angles, rotations).

Release of normal neurological inhibition: Functions that are normally inhibited become expressed, e.g., the rage dyscontrol syndrome (Mark & Ervin, 1970, Chapter 9). Somatic release symptoms are discussed in Chapters 8 and 15 on Neurophysiological Dysfunctions and Stress.

3. *Immediate neuropsychological symptoms predict subsequent deficit*
Neuropsychological symptoms at the time of injury (loss of consciousness, confusion, loss of memory, feeling dazed) are almost always associated with subsequent neuropsychological deficits (cognitive and emotional).

4. *The cognitive effects of trauma are complex*
Diffuse brain injury and secondary pathological processes interact with the extensive location for processing creates a variety of symptoms. Damage to areas that integrate different senses, e.g., hearing and vision, can reduce speed of information processing, misperceptions, etc.

5. *A particular symptom can result from different anatomical damage*
Anomia (inability to remember names of objects) illustrates the complexity of localization (Kirshner, Casey, Kelly, & Webb, 1987). Different locations of anatomical damage caused different kinds of errors. With impaired visual input, perceptual (visual) errors led to misnaming. The stimulus was inadequately conveyed to verbal processing areas, leading to ineffective identification. Left cerebral damage led to verbal and/or communications problems, i.e., relatively few visually related errors compared to semantic ones.

7. *The neuropsychological effects of brain damage are cumulative*
Slight impairment may indicate reduced efficiency and lessened reserves against further injury. Each TBI reduces judgment, and perhaps coordination,

contributing to increased likelihood of dangerous incidents. Small cumulative injuries may permit some degree of recovery compared to a single major injury (see Chapter 4 on Trauma and Brain Damage). This research finding, based on excisions of rat cortex, might have little relevance for human victims of TBI.

8. *Emotional distress following brain damage seems almost universal*

When a previously well-adapted individual suffers illness or injury, the consequences include an interaction of actual emotional disorder caused by damage to the brain directly, reaction to reduced competence, a feeling of reduced attractiveness, depression and disturbed self-esteem, and/or withdrawal (see Chapter 15 on Stress).

9. *Reduced Competence*

Even if a person seems only slightly impaired, efficiency is likely to be reduced (memory and communications problems, inability to concentrate, bad judgment, inflexibility, poor self-control, etc.). The victim is less able to devise strategies to cope with necessities, and make life pleasant and constructive.

10. *Communications problems prevent description of dysfunctioning*

Aphasia is most common immediately posttrauma. Subsequently, superficially communications seem normal, i.e., the person can respond to simple, but nonprobing questions, but close scrutiny reveals deficits in understanding and communicating ideas, memory, etc. Close inquiry will reveal an inability to self-describe well.

11. *The nature of the damage depends on the age of the individual*

- *Young individuals* lose the ability to learn and develop, but have less stored information to lose (see Chapter 19 on Children's Brain Damage).
- *Older individuals* also lose the ability to learn, but can function with stored information. If memory is intact, they may continue with routine vocational skills and other habits, though with less flexibility.

The same injury occurring at different ages may have different effects, depending on the degree to which the impaired area of the brain has become specialized. For example, the degree of left hemisphere specialization for verbal ability ("age-aphasia" interaction, Code, 1987, p. 16) increases, while the likelihood of posterior cerebrovascular lesions also increases.

12. *Exceptions occur to expected localization/dysfunction effects*

Not all localized lesions create predicted patterns. A 13-year-old girl was examined who 3 years before suffered a left-sided generalized hematoma and cerebral contusion. Contrary to the expected pattern of reduced Verbal IQ, her WISC–R Verbal IQ was 103, Performance IQ 86, and Full Scale IQ 94. Neither intrasubtest scatter nor V–P score reached statistical significance (Kaufman, 1979, Chapter 6).

13. *Reserves are lessened against further injury*

The neuropsychological effects of brain damage are cumulative. With brain damage, the person's judgment and coordination might become somewhat more deficient, and the likelihood of further dangerous incidents increases.

14. *The significance of impairment varies with environmental demands*

Impairment is expressed as a function of the patient's competence and adaptive demands of his environment. The same damage may be more or less impairing according to what is expected of the TBI victim. An intelligent person, in a relatively unskilled job, may have no call for high level performance.

15. *There is no totally accurate criterion of prognosis*

Some measures used for prediction of outcome include the length of coma, length of posttraumatic amnesia, and the Glasgow Coma Scale. Recovery depends on many conditions (for example, see Item 1, above). Although severity of damage is associated with length of posttraumatic coma, the correlation is not high (long coma may be followed by relatively good recovery, depending on factors such as rehabilitation efforts).

16. *Brain damage differentially affects the processing of tasks that are old and new ontogenetically and phylogenetically*

Two general principles apply:

- *New and unfamiliar tasks* are more effected by TBI than overlearned and familiar ones.
- *Phylogenetically new functions* are more vulnerable to brain damage than older ones. Indeed, when archaic support systems (circulation and breathing, for example) are destroyed (medullary damage) so is life! The least overlearned and routineized behaviors are likely to be impaired after damage to the newest portion of the CNS, i.e., the prefrontal cortex (Bilder & Goldberg, 1987).

Taxonomy of Neuropsychological Systems and Deficits

A taxonomy is proposed to systematize symptoms occurring after brain damage. An overview of the range of potential deficits was developed, proposing the concept of neuropsychological systems.

Definition of a System

A "system" refers to components of behavior that are unified in terms of ability to adapt, and subtended by an identifiable pattern of neural activities. The symptoms included in each system are consistent with studies in neurology, neuropsychology, and clinical experience (including hundreds of persons referred to the author for neuropsychological evaluation after personal injury and emotional trauma, social security disability, and workers' compensation claims, with ages from age 2 until pregeriatric).

Utility of the Taxonomy

Rehabilitation planning
Assessing damage for forensic purposes

Planning a comprehensive examination
Assessing the completeness of available information
Identifying the need for referrals to other experts
Conveying information to victims, family, schools, psychotherapists, courts, etc.

Overview of Systems

Each of the following is described in a later chapter:

Chapter   6: Consciousness, Orientation, Attention, and Arousal
Chapter   7: Integrated Sensorimotor Functions and Body Image
Chapter   8: Neurophysiological, Humoral, and Visceral Functions
Chapter   9: Intellectual Functioning
Chapter 10: Memory: Short- and Long-Term
Chapter 11: Efficiency and Control
Chapter 12: Communications Problems—Aphasia
Chapter 13: Cerebral Personality Disorders and Frontal Lobe Syndromes
Chapter 14: Adaptability, Independence, and Daily Functioning
Chapter 15: Anxiety, Stress, and Psychodynamic Reactions

Neuropsychological developmental problems of children are given separate consideration in Chapter 19, as an additional dysfunctioning, in addition to the systems referred to above.

Brain damage/stress checklist items correspond to each system in the taxonomy (see Intake Procedures).

6
Consciousness, Orientation, Attention, and Arousal

Overview

Adaptive action requires awareness, optimal level of arousal, and useful focusing on inner and outer stimuli. As information is processed at higher levels of the neuraxis, it becomes integrated with other increasingly diverse information, and becomes transformed to new cognitive forms. Automatic acts become minimized and choice and evaluation are increased (Davidson, 1980). Sensations are given meaning and perhaps receive a sense of familiarity. Ultimately diverse functions are integrated, e.g., verbal and emotional awareness, consciousness and unconsciousness, and verbal and rational thought with movement of the body in space (Ornstein, 1977, pp. 16–39).

Definition of the System

This system controls self-awareness, alertness to the environment, selection of new or ongoing events for continued appraisal, and possible danger, determining relevance for prior plans or other interest, bodily needs, curiosity, etc. Distractibility is overcome to focus attention, and new events are selected for attention. Control is exerted over the general level of activity.

Neuropsychological Dysfunctioning

Altered consciousness is one of the most characteristic after-effects of brain damage. Altered states of consciousness impair ability to receive and understand information from the environment and one's body. Information processing at the poles of sensory overload or unconsciousness is inefficient or nonexistent. The level of inefficiency from common environmental distractions is higher. Brain dysfunctioning can change the level of somatic functioning (arousal). Bodily functions are experienced as distressing. Physical activity is poorly controlled.

Primary Neural System

Level of consciousness depends on the reticular activating system, ascending and descending, and cerebral cortex. As noted in Chapter 2 on Neuroanatomy, lemniscal and cerebellar systems stimulate the reticular activating system (RAS). Cortical activity or stimulation alone does not necessarily lead to any conscious experience (Libet, 1987), but is dependent on the integrity of the *ascending reticular activating system*. Concentration and alertness are very vulnerable to damage to widely scattered areas of the brain, creating deficits from poor alertness to coma. The following statements concerning deficits of attention associated with different areas of the brain are consistent with the assertions made above concerning a diffuse vulnerability of any complex function to trauma.

Altered consciousness has been variously attributed to lesions that are in the left hemisphere, bilateral, diencephalon, hypothalamus, midbrain reticular formation, and pons. Slowly developing lesions, i.e., destruction of the area between the rostral midbrain and posterior diencephalon, is always followed by deep coma, from which the patient is unarousable. Walton (1985) states that lesions or dysfunctions of the reticular system produce stupor or coma when they are bilateral, are located between the lower third of the pons and the posterior diencephalon, and are either of acute onset or large in extent. Unconsciousness is related to the rapidity with which lesions develop. Hemorrhage produces sudden unconsciousness and coma. Tumors and slow hemorrhoraging may not disturb consciousness for a considerable period of time (Carpenter & Sutin, 1983, p. 443).

Attention involves several control processes and neural centers (Pribram, 1980). Associated functions include the *orienting response* [bodily movements and neural processes that optimize information reception, and reduce distraction (amygdala)], *readiness to respond* (basal ganglia), and *"effort,"* coordinating the response to input and readiness (hippocampus). Selective attention implies that other signals are prevented from reaching consciousness and being processed, and also that prior stimuli are disengaged permitting the focus of attention to be changed (Posner, 1988). Both of these functions are impaired in TBI. The amount of attention directed toward an effort increases the responsivity and selectivity of the neurons that process it. The amount of effort needed to perform a perceptual task affects how the information is processed (Spitzer, Desimone, & Moran, 1988). I infer that part of the attentional deficits of TBI victims evolves from deficient motivation and/or the extra effort required by impairment.

Focusing attention has been attributed to a wide variety of areas. These are reported here to illustrate its complexity, as well as for the interested reader: the right parietal lobe (Farah, Wong, Monheit, & Morrow, 1989), the temporal–parietal junction, and projections to the posterior superior temporal gyrus from the visual cortex and inferior parietal lobe. Global information is more efficiently processed in the right hemisphere and local information in the left (Lamb, Robertson, & Knight, 1989); the midprefrontal, anterior cingulate, and superior posterior parietal cortices are used for goal-directed behavior, and the midprefrontal and hippocampal cortices, and possibly the orbitofrontal and temporal cortices are used for stimuli that are not currently salient but are emotionally charged, in memory, or being extinguished (Cohen, Semple, Gross, Holcomb, Dowling, & Nordahl, 1988). Deficits of attention are related to lesions at the junction of the midbrain and pons (locus ceruleus) and to dysfunction of mesencephalic dopaminergic neurons, a site of injury in severe closed head injury (Adamovich, Henderson, and Auerbach, 1985, p. 26). Interrupted projections to cerebral and cerebellar hemispheres interfere with general attention, causing "global neglect" (Livingston, 1984, p. 1152). Neglect of unilateral information has been attributed to the right parietal lobe, midbrain, and thalamus (Posner, 1988).

Orientation has autonomic components that are facilitory (related to the dorsolateral frontal system) and inhibitory (orbitofrontal limbic neural network) (Lee et al., 1988).

Sleep is regulated by more rostral portions of the ARAS, the basal forebrain, and other areas. Sleep problems may occur after thalamic lesions, indicating a sleep–inducing function.

Symptoms Related to Different Dimensions of Consciousness

Activation

Because of ambiguity in the literature, I will refer to levels of consciousness as related to "activation." It is a function mediated by the asacending reticular activating system (ARAS), which, by desyncronizing the cerebral cortex, contributes to awareness, consciousness, attention, etc. Lesions result in inability to be awakened, to maintain wakefulness, and follow stimuli or commands.

Syndromes Associated with Loss of Consciousness (LOC)

Stupor

Mental and physical activity, and responsiveness are minimal.

Coma

The patient appears to be asleep, and is insensitive to all stimuli.

Brain Death

The brain is irreversibly damaged and ceases to function, but pulmonary and cardiac functions are artificially maintained (Korein, 1978).

Pseudocoma, or "Locked in" State

Patients are unresponsive but not unconscious (catatonia, abulia). They are awake and alert, mute, and able to communicate only by eye blinks or movements. Lesions of the ventral pons, sparing the brainstem reticular formation, but interrupting motor pathways, result in the "locked in" syndrome, i.e., tetraplegic but awake, alert, and suffering from insomnia (Kales & Kales, 1984, p. 115). This is caused by head trauma, frontal lobe disease, lesions of the pons, or a drug effect. Drug treatment that increases the dopamine content of the basal ganglia and substantia nigra seems effective by enhancing modulation of motor pathways to the entire body (Rao & Costa, 1989).

Akinetic Mutism, or "Vegetative" State

Bilateral corticospinal tract damage ("Pyramidal") leaves only autonomic functions intact. In contrast to the "locked in state" an examiner will have the impression that he cannot arouse the patient's attention and interest (Masdeu, 1985b). After severe trauma, there can be a period of complete unresponsiveness, followed by sleep–wake cycles. The wakefulness is without awareness, communication, or complex behavior.

Posttraumatic Confusion and Posttraumatic Amnesia

As a person leaves a coma, a period of poor memory may occur. Posttraumatic amnesia (PTA) is the length of time between the injury and return of ongoing memory. It includes the period between an accident, in which a patient was in coma, and/or any period of confusion or occasional incidence of poor memory, until relatively continuous memory becomes available. The patient may appear to be quite clear mentally, but in retrospect will be unable to remember anything that occurs. Their reports may be merely repetitions of what they have been told, or confabulations in an attempt to reconstruct the accident and its consequences. I have examined some professionals who have resumed work in the condition of PTA, and only later became aware of their total lack of memory for this period.

During recovery from coma, there is an unclear consciousness with an inability to store memories and/or islands of memory. This lends confusion to the attempt to measure the length of PTA. The confusional state (alterations in the content of consciousness) usually results from extensive subcortical and cortical dysfunction (Strub & Black, 1985, p. 16). Other symptoms include disorientation, incapacity to think with customary speed, clarity, and coherence (Adams & Victor, 1985, p. 301; Bond, 1984), and uncontrolled behavior, such as agitation, wandering, combativeness, and restlessness. The patient may be aware of his surroundings, but unable to register memories (Levin, Benton, & Grossman, 1982, pp. 73–79).

Although the length of amnesia has been considered to be a reliable index of the severity of the concussive injury, the correlation between length of PTA and outcome is not high (Tabbador, Mattis, & Zazula, 1984). Its components, e.g., coma, retrograde and anterograde amnesia, and disorientation, may have different courses of recovery. Unconsciousness can exist from a time before the injury occurred (retrograde amnesia) until the victim can form consecutive memories after the accident (anterograde amnesia). One study showed no correlation between length of coma and ability to withstand distraction (Kewman, Yanus, and Kirsch, 1988).

It is also important to realize that many individuals with significant neuropsychological impairment have had only brief loss of memory or confusion, without total loss of consciousness. On awakening, the person can think strangely, have patches of memory, or be confused for a considerable length of time.

Confusion

Inability to orient oneself can exist over an extended period. One victim stated: "I'm confused. I don't know if its all in my head or if it really happened. I can't understand why I can't dust myself off and start over again."

Seizures and Related Dysfunctioning

Posttraumatic Seizures

Seizures may occur early (at the time of the impact) or late (more than 1 week later) (Kennedy & Freeman, 1986). Mild seizure activity can create intermittent interruption of consciousness. Anticonvulsant medication can impair attention and psychomotor functions, and create false positive lateralizing signs (Hartlage & Telzrow, 1986, p. 147).

Apart from immediate seizures within the first week, the overall incidence after closed head injury is around 5%. Infection of the brain and its meninges may lead to acute seizures, or scarring with later seizures. Hematomas and depressed skull fractures increase the likelihood. Of patients who will have seizures more than half will have them the first year, and one-fifth will have them 4 years after injury, with reduced likelihood of remission (Lishman, 1987, p. 5).

Some patients with penetrating brain wounds received in the Vietnam war remained at risk for epilepsy even 10–15 years later, although they were 95% certain of avoiding epilepsy if they were seizure free for 3 years. Subsequent head injury, other encephalopathy, and alcohol or drug abuse played an important role in occurrence, particularly in the late–onset group. It was concluded that most head–injured patients can be 95% certain of remaining seizure free if they have been seizure free for 3 years after injury (Weiss, Salazar, Vance, Grafman, & Jabbari, 1986).

Classification of seizures (Adams & Victor, 1989, p. 250; Strub & Black, 1988, pp. 392–393):

1. *Generalized* (bilaterally symmetrical, without local onset). This is a convulsion. A variety of movements or different feelings in the body precede it, which when remembered as a sign of an impending seizure is called an *aura*. One patient described his aura: "I'm trying to control myself mentally. When I get the seizures I fight with it. Sometimes I can control it. The aura is dizziness, headaches, floating feelings, double vision, sleepiness."

2. *Tonic–Clonic* (grand mal)

- *Tonic phase:* The whole musculature is seized by a spasm. There are movements of the mouth, eyes, legs, and arms, the tongue may be bitten,

the respiratory muscles are contracted (preventing breathing), and the bladder is emptied.
- *Clonic phase:* Increasingly violent muscular contractions of the entire body, with rapid pulse, bloody froth from the bitten tongue, sweating, occasional periorbital hemorrhages, and loss of breathing (refer to Chapter 7 on Sensorimotor Functions).

3. *Absence* (petit mal). There is a sudden disruption of consciousness that is brief, and little motor activity. Even the patients may not be aware of them and they appear to be a moment of absentmindedness. Simple types involve LOC alone. Complex ones also include brief tonic, clonic, or automatic movements.

4. Other less common seizure types.

4a. *Partial (focal)* beginning locally.

- Without loss of consciousness but with motor, sensory, autonomic, or psychic symptoms.
- Complex with impaired consciousness, although it may begin as a simple partial seizure, with a variety of cognitive, affective, sensory, and motor symptoms, sometimes called "temporal lobe" or "psychomotor."
- Partial, simple or complex, with secondary generalization.

4b. *Unilateral* (with or without impaired consciousness and with a variety of muscular convulsions).

- Partial seizures secondarily generalized.

4c. *Unclassified,* e.g., pseudoseizures (nonepileptic, sometimes associated with syncope, migraine, ischemic attacks, hypoglycemia, and sleep disorders, Trimble, 1988, p. 296).

4d. *Temporal lobe focal attacks* ("psychomotor attacks"; automatisms; complex partial seizures) are the type of seizure most commonly observed in psychiatric practice. They are characterized by a wide variety of altered states of consciousness (hallucinations, illusions, déjà vu, dreamy states, and depersonalization), depression, fear or elation, old memories, and disturbance of thought, behavior, affect, and consciousness. This is usually attributed to epileptic centers in the temporal lobe, but similar symptoms can occur due to a focus in the frontal lobe (Adams & Victor, 1985, pp. 236–237). Elaborate actions can be carried out, with motor control and sensory reception preserved, but there is complete amnesia for what occurred (Brodal, 1981, p. 696).

Altered States of Consciousness

These are associated with other forms of neurological damage besides seizures. Changes in the activation level (circuits between the brainstem and cortex) interfere with normal processing of cognitive and bodily functioning (see Adams & Victor, 1985, pp. 255–257; Levy et al., 1978; Posner, 1978).

Symptoms include disorientation, clouding of consciousness, depersonalization, derealization, seizures, impaired ability to receive and understand information from the world and one's body, and altered alertness (excitement, drowsiness, sleep, coma).

This is how one man described his experience after his car was struck from the rear. After a period of unconsciousness, whose length he does not know, "I felt like a robot. I saw things but I couldn't do anything about it. I felt like I was paralyzed. I wanted to go home."

Clinical Examples of Altered Consciousness

Case 5. A man whose automobile when stopped was struck in the rear by another car: He sometimes has seizures. After an aura he was choking, and had an urge to vomit, urinate, and defecate. He threw up on a rug, and urinated in the bathroom. He describes his experiences as follows: "Things take a long time. I slide in and out" (of consciousness). He lacks self–direction, and needs it from others. "I need bite size pieces," i.e., a flow of directions. He is too sensitive to noise since he cannot filter it out. On a trip to take care of family responsibilities, he describes himself in a state of bliss. "It was very quiet . . . In broad daylight, or at any moment, I can have an intrusive, disturbing recollection of the accident. I initially felt frightened and out of control. I felt like somebody else changed the channel I was viewing. The picture or smell or touch changes."

Case 6. An adolescent who came out of a long coma: "It's like a dream. It's scary to have thoughts about the accident." He thinks he blacks out when this happens.

Case 7. A woman who hit her nose against the dashboard in a moderately high speed crash: She has had dizzy spells. She was told it would go away in 6 months. She attempted secretarial work, but did not succeed because of poor handwriting, because she could not take messages. She also fears panic attacks and becoming disoriented. She asserts that she has a weakened immune system. She could not find her way back to the office from the main lobby. "I am afraid to go inside a building on my own. Without warning, the room spins violently around. It's very violent and I must be on the ground. I'm terrified of what could happen on the street. I could be killed. When I'm on the ground I am nauseous. It takes a while to go away. The room is spinning. Its like a ping-pong ball going back and forth in my head."

"I was speaking on the phone to someone who asked me what show I had seen, when everything went black. It was as though I was in a movie theatre and the lights went out. I couldn't see. It was very shocking and terrifying." She does not know what happened, and is uncertain if the other person was there when she came to. "I go into the next room to do something and I completely forget what it was. I sit down and 10 minutes later it comes back."

Attention is the process of selecting new or ongoing events for continued appraisal, and signaling their importance to the sensory muscular system and general awareness (see also Chapter 11 on Efficiency and Control). It may be narrowly focused, generalized, or vague. Attention focuses on tasks that are relevant for survival, well–being, or curiosity. These can be internal bodily events, external events, or ego operations (thoughts, feelings, complex movements, and memories, including ideas, past events, and self-concept; Pattison & Kahan, 1986).

Sensory information can be received, and acted on, without apparent verbal contribution, under *conditions of sensory deficit* (visual field loss), i.e., "blindsight" (Ellis & Young, 1988, pp. 66–70; Pribram, 1980), *separation of the hemispheres* (cutting of the corpus callosum and anterior commissure).

Attention can be split so that two stimuli are attended to simultaneously. Sometimes attention is shifted from self-awareness to environmental awareness, from one modality to another (e.g., visual to auditory) or one visual field to the contralateral one (Farah et al., 1989), or from more to less inclusive aspects of a hierarchy (Lamb et al., 1989).

The significance of attention for memory was noted by Penfield (1959, pp. 74–75): "Conscious attention adds something to brain-action that would otherwise leave no record . . . Permanent facilitation of a patterned sequence . . . is established only when there is a focusing of attention on the phenomenon that corresponds to it in consciousness." A less salient stimulus may represent extinction, or placement in memory of inhibited or painful events (Cohen et al., 1988).

Problems of Attention

Hyperalertness

This is a stress–related experience, probably a consequence of multiple physiological reactions accompanying fear and injury.

Inattention, Confusion, and Clouding

Dizziness, confusion, disorientation, or coma may be momentary or last for extended periods. The patient does not take into account all elements of the situation, and does not think with customary speed and clarity.

Distractibility

Slowness of central processing time may reflect difficulty in screening out irrelevant information (Levin, 1985). Distractions impair auditory comprehension in all individuals, but particularly in brain damaged victims. This effect must be separated from memory and comprehension problems, as well as impaired attention (Kewman, et al., 1988).

Reduced Concentration

Reduced capacity to maintain attention over a period of time (concentration) is very characteristic of brain damage. People complain that after a short period, perhaps

5 minutes, they cannot continue what they have started due to an inability to reject irrelevant input and to focus on a problem or situation. Insufficient information is obtained, and the person drifts further away before anything significant is accomplished. Concentration problems may be momentary or last for extended periods.

Arousal

This refers to levels of behavioral output and "levels of awareness" (Kandel & Schwartz, 1985, p. 560). Awareness is related to level of arousal, i.e., unclear, distorted, or fluctuating awareness of internal and external events. Whether arousal describes a level of activity or awareness is controversial. Kandel and Schwartz (1985, p. 609) describe it as a state of awareness whereas Strub and Black (1985, p. 16) assert that it refers to energy and not awareness.

Arousal is a general state of available energy, a physiological preparatory state, or activity, that influences or energizes different behavioral systems simultaneously (Jennings, 1986). It is characterized by a low threshold for, or exaggerated release of muscular or autonomic activity. Arousal level is affected by somatic activities and moods such as anxiety and it increases after stress. Organ systems affected are those controlled by the autonomic nervous system, and also muscular reactions (see Chapter 15 on Stress).

Altered Arousal

Kandel and Schwartz (1985, p. 609) assert that arousal "varies from states of excitement . . . to drowsiness, sleep, and coma." There may be many arousal states since autonomic activities can be high during drowsiness, and intercorrelations of measures of physiological arousal are low. Insomnia can also be related to a high state of arousal associated with anxiety or depression.

High arousal, i.e., heightened muscular and visceral responsiveness, occurs at times of heightened receptivity to danger and other environmental conditions. It is characterized by a low threshold for, or exaggerated release of muscular or autonomic activity.

Reduced arousal, even mild underarousal (or overarousal), results in apathy, poor motivation, and irritability (Filley, Cranberg, Alexander, & Hart 1987). The patient may be unable to initiate behavior, reacting primarily to external direction, or may not be reactive at all. He may seem lazy or unmotivated (Lezak, 1983, p. 81).

Orientation

Characteristic functions include perception of oneself in a context as time, place, or person, ability to locate oneself in space and find one's way around, awareness of the location and relationship of different parts of one's own body, and a sense of left and right.

Disorientation

The person is unsure of time, place, or person, creating difficulties in orienting oneself in space with regard to distance and objects. The victim gets lost, experiences a changed sense of time, deficits in left–right identification, mis-identifies familiar people and attending staff, experiences perplexity and dis-orientation, and is bewildered what to do.

One man must carry a compass to find his way around the city. An adolescent, who had a skull fracture and repeated seizures, described his disorientation as follows: "I woke up, got out of bed, looked in the mirror, saw a bump the size of a baseball, but it didn't mean anything to me. From that day on I felt different." He returned to school in another area and thought that he was in the city in which he had been injured.

Strange Experiences

A patient may be in a state of full consciousness, but experience gross dis-tortions of reality: confusion, hallucinogenic, psychotic-like experiences, delu-sions, illusions, perhaps due to lesions (Walton, 1985, pp. 640–641) or seizures (Pritchard, 1983).

7
Integrated Sensorimotor Functions and Body Image

Overview

The content of this chapter overlaps most with the traditional focal neurological examination. The integrity of senses and motor apparatus is significant for safety, the ability to earn a living or study, to ambulate, and to enjoy one's life. The emphasis here will be on the kinds of deficits that are observed in outpatient practice, i.e., after the person has presumably recovered sufficiently to go home, in the case of the severely injured person, or soft signs of dysfunctioning after so-called minor head injury. Many details in Chapter 2 on Neuroanatomy were specifically included to aid in understanding sensorimotor dysfunctioning. Some procedures that the reader can utilize in performing a sensorimotor examination are detailed in Chapter 21 on Assessment.

Definition of the System

This system maintains consciousness through input to the ascending reticular activating system. It also receives stimuli, analyzes and encodes them for use and later retrieval, and integrates them with motor functions at all levels of the nervous system (reflexive and purposful). Muscular activity orients receptors to receive significant stimuli. Purposeful movements may require complex, serial motions, performed in order, that require ongoing modification according to the relative position of the person's body, joints, and a stationary or moving target. Stimulation from the periphery creates the body image.

Neuropsychological Dysfunctioning

Particular symptoms may be attributed to different levels of damage, because of decussations and the complexity of the nervous system. *Contralateral* dysfunctioning is attributable to damage above the decussation. Examples include inability to detect stimulation on one side of the visual field (e.g., visual neglect), and loss of sensation, strength, or muscular control. Other deficits include impairment of sensory receptors and central processing (loss of hearing, sight, vestibular functions, smell, over- or undersensitivity to stimuli such as light or sound, etc.); impairment of integrated sensorimotor functions such as co-ordination, balance, and kinesthesis, resulting in paralysis, tremor, and poor gross and fine muscular control; and complex patterns. Damage to the central nervous system can create a disturbed bodily image (defective right–left orientation, and/or incomplete, disproportionate, asymmetrical, or undetailed self-perception).

Primary Neural System

The sensory and motor systems are an integrated unit, including the cerebral cortex (motor, visual, auditory, somesthetic cortex, olfactory cortex), basal ganglia, cerebellum, thalamus, ascending and descending tracts of the spinal cord, and brainstem, cranial nerves, and sensory neurons of the autonomic nervous system. Lower centers project to the ascending and descending reticular activating systems enhancing cortical arousal and muscular tone, respectively.

Sensorimotor Integration

Integrated Functioning

Rapidly changing environmental conditions require convergence of diverse control systems on the pathway required for action, followed by modification of performance to match some inner or external criterion of success. A motor response integrates meaning, memory, and feelings, visceral support, and input from the internal and external world. As stimuli are detected inside and outside the body, they are encoded, modulated by ganglia at intermediate levels between the receptor and the cerebrum, where they interact with ongoing neural activity. Then responses are selected for transmission according to relevance, and information is extracted and compared from cortical, subcortical, and contralateral sources (Livingston, 1985, p. 1081).

The Motor Response

Muscular action must take into consideration movement by the person and the object. Vision, hearing, somesthesis, and vestibular function are thoroughly integrated. Their interacting nuclei are in the brainstem, and they also exchange with the cerebral cortex, basal ganglia, cerebellum, and spinal cord. The actual activity is often a program, or complex series of commands, originating somewhere else than in the motor cortex (see comment about Cerebellum, below). Sequential release of these instructions starts movements. However, it is possible to inhibit the program momentarily by cortical stimulation. The decision "go" or "no go" is believed to take place between the diencephalon and brainstem (Livingston, 1985, pp. 1263, 1269). When inhibition is completed, action resumes under feedback control from some internal monitoring system (Day et al., 1989).

The final pathway (though not necessarily organization) of motor impulses originates from the contralateral motor areas of the cortex. They are integrated with, and modified by, motor, sensory, and autonomic input at cortical and lower centers, before and during transmission to the cranial nerves and spinal cord. Manipulation is a decision developing in the cerebrum, after interplay between limbic, diencephalic, and frontal systems. This is executed through the motor cortex via pyramidal and extrapyramidal pathways, modified by stimuli from the external and postural receptors, nuclei in the pons, reticular formation and inferior olive, and cerebellum.

In addition to relatively direct corticospinal circuits, the cerebellum (anterior lobe) maintains a representation of bodily performance that enables it to modify ongoing activities, and then feed back to the motor cortex. A practiced movement sequence is organized before the onset, so that it will be executed in one smooth unit (Inhoff, Diener, Rafa, and Ivry, 1989). Although skill acquisition for athletics and music may be based upon adaptation of "low level" sensory and muscular circuits (Livingston, 1985, pp. 1036–1037), these circuits are certainly rapid and integrate complex information!

Consider a batter facing a pitcher who takes a stance at the plate, follows the ball with his eyes, feels the weight of the bat as he swings it slightly back and forth, senses the position of muscles, bones, and body position with his kinesthetic and vestibular (balance) receptors, then swings the bat to some anticipated position when he sees the pitcher bring his arm around, modifying the motion with the trajectory of the ball traveling around 90 miles/hour.

Multiple Processing of Sensory Input

Integration with other sensory modalities (intermodal)
Output to motor units where they immediately affect further action
Output to motor units to orient stimulus receptors
Transmission to the cortex for the finest analysis of detail
Routed to the RAS to maintain consciousness and level of motor response
Routed into limbic and association areas for meaning
Channeled back to receptor to modulate ongoing stimulation.

Assessing Deficits

Deficits may be considered from the viewpoint of their adaptive significance, e.g., loss of psychomotor speed and strength, or what they contribute to localization. From the viewpoint of rehabilitation the first task is to establish the level of impairment, e.g., when a carpenter or mechanic, or other manual worker, whether skilled or unskilled, can no longer perform at the previous level.

Localization is sometimes difficult to establish since a symptom might be referrable to cranial nerve damage, to the spinal cord, peripheral nerves, cranial nerves, receptors, nerve tracts, nuclei in the brainstem, thalamus, cortex, cerebellum, or to a body, head or neck injury. Further information concerning localization is obtainable from Brazis, Masdeu, and Biller (1985) and for cranial nerves specifically from Wilson-Pauwels et al. (1988).

Central Sensory Deficits

Sensory Agnosias

Perception in any modality is a complex process. One may use as an example recognition of a visually presented object. Stimuli are built up into small units and then into a shape, and finally a multiple process occurs in which the object is compared to stored knowledge, and also elicits processes of recognition and associations (Riddoch & Humphreys, 1987). Also involved are visual memory for that type of object, and retrieval of verbal information, e.g., its name. Additional symptoms include inability to recognize environmental, musical, and emotional components of communication (Joseph, 1988).

Perceptual Disturbances

These have been classified by Benton (1985b) as *visual perceptual* (agnosia, or inability to recognize information coming from a particular sensory modality; visual analysis and synthesis; facial recognition, impaired color recognition); *visuospatial* (defective localization of points in space, defective judgment of direction and distance, defective topographical orientation, unilateral visual neglect), and *visuoconstructive* (defective assembling performance, and defective graphomotor performance). There is a substantial trend for this type of deficit to be associated with posterior, right cerebral lesions, but it is not confined to this location, and is found certainly with diffuse damage.

* *Hemiattention and neglect*—not receiving information from the side opposite the lesion, not attributable to sensory or motor defects. It is observed in the somesthetic, auditory, and visual modalities (Heilman, Watson, & Valenstein, 1985).

  An example of neglect is restricted peripheral visual fields, which are often overlooked in neurological and ophthalmological examinations. A head injury victim bumped into walls and open filing cabinets (visual "neglect"). This symptom (inaccurately attributed to alcoholism) was caused by a right parietal lobe hematoma that eliminated his left visual field. Another man hit his head falling out of a hospital bed: "I misjudge turns and I'll hit the side of the wall. I miss steps going up and down. I've fallen many times. I've tripped over a hose right in front of me."

* *Anosognosia,* i.e., unawareness of the sensory impairment independent of severe disturbance of intellect (Damasio & Van Hoesen, 1985). Examples include *visual* (color, space, faces), *auditory,* and *tactile* (form recognition, fingers, body parts), as well as loss of ability to identify a finger (which may be specific or related to a sensory loss) (Benson & Geschwind, 1985).

• *Paresthesias:* Changed sensation associated with neurological damage.
• *Astereognosis:* Inability to recognize an object through touch.
• *Loss of cross-modal sensory integration:* Inability to recognize the equivalence of stimuli offered in different sensory modalities.

Significant adaptive functions require simultaneous processing from several sensory channels, and then further processing in the form of memory, associations, familiarity, significance, and ultimately into a general concept or plan that is stored or executed.

A child learning to read requires association between what the teacher or parent says (auditory channel) while organizing visual information and associating to it. The entire task includes (at least) cross-modal sensory integration, verbal reasoning and labeling, retrieval of information from long-term memory storage as words, self-instruction and storage of portions of a solution in verbal terms, and recodification of problem solutions into motor expression (written or oral).

Suppression or extinction is a deficit of complex sensory analysis: When there are two stimuli simultaneously occurring bilaterally, one of them may be suppressed, i.e., not detected. This can be demonstrated with vision (peripheral stimulation) and somesthesis (simultaneous stimulation of cheek and hand). See Heilman et al. (1985) for further explanation and anatomical loci.

Cranial Nerve Sensory Deficits

Cranial nerve dysfunction may indicate damage close to the periphery (e.g., eyes and ears), pathways in the tissues and skull, pathways between the brain and skull, or to nuclei and pathways within the brain itself. Lack of deficit of cranial nerve function does not mean that no neuropsychological impairment exists. For details of cranial nerve deficits see Rouit and Murali (1987) and Wilson-Pauwels et al. (1988).

Odor

Permanent anosmia can result from even trivial injuries to the brain. Anosmia, that can be unilateral or bilateral, can be due to shearing cranial fractures, that sever fibers of the olfactory nerve (I), skull fracture, rhinorrhea between the olfactory bulb and the receptor surface of the nose, bleeding, edema, and ischemia. There is anatomical evidence that permanent posttraumatic anosmia results from inability of the olfactory epithelium to regenerate axons through the cribriform plate after they have been torn by shearing forces creating movement (Jafek, Eller, Esses, & Moran, 1989).

Of patients with severe head injury 60% were found to be anosmic. Of the 40% who could detect odors, half were unable to identify the stimulus, suggesting a more central type of damage (Costanzo, Heywood, & Young, 1987). Difficulties in identifying odors sometimes appear to be due to an inability to associate names to stimulus, rather than loss of sensitivity itself. Inability to recognize odors may result from focal and diffuse injury to the orbitofrontal and temporal regions (Levin, High, & Eisenberg, 1985), or loss of the anterior the pole of the temporal lobe (unilateral lobectomy, including two-thirds of the hippocampus and the entire amygdala) (Eskanazi et al., 1988).

The fifth cranial nerve (trigeminal) makes a considerable contribution to smell, interacting with the olfactory nerve (I) at central levels (Alarie et al., 1987; Bouvet, Delaleu, & Holley, 1987). Head injuries considerably raise the threshold for sensory irritants (e.g., ammonia) detected by the trigeminal nerve (V) (Alarie et al., 1987).

Temporal lobe seizures may cause olfactory hallucinations (Brodal, 1981, pp. 694–696).

Vision

Trauma can create somatic damage interfering with vision, and can occur in the retina, optic nerve, optic tract, thalamus, or optic radiation leading to the calcarine cortex of the occipital lobe. Lesions create specific patterns of blindspots depending on their location. The pattern of visual deficits will depend on the location and extent of injury to the eye and visual pathways. Since the visual pathways extend from the anterior to the posterior portion of the cerebrum, careful examination offers a rich opportunity to obtain information concerning the location of lesions (Bajandas & Kline, 1987, offer many examples with extensive diagrams; standard neurological texts).

Field Defects

Particular patterns of visual scotomata are associated with rather specific areas of the visual pathways. Field defects after trauma may occur at any point in the visual pathways, from retinal tears and posterior vitrious detachment (Cytowic et al., 1988), to occipital lobe damage. Charts are presented to show that field deficits may become less apparent with time, though eventually show some mild constriction. I am in complete accord with these authors' implied criticism of many ophthamologists who, after receiving a referral from a neurologist or other specialist in head injury, conduct a conventional eye examination and conclude that nothing is wrong. I sometimes conduct a careful visual field study with a revolving perimeter, to the limit of peripheral vision on all sides, for both eyes. If there is evidence for restricted fields, than a referral is made for automated visual fields *specifying that these must be performed to the periphery.*

Field deficits may be associated with relatively localized injuries occurring after cerebrovascular accidents, tumors, etc. Right hemisphere deficits include hemiattention or neglect, prosopagnosia.

• *Quadrantopsia:* A fraction of one or both visual fields (e.g., a quadrant, unilateral or bilateral). The closer the damage is to the occipital cortex, the more "congruous" or similar the bilateral field deficits become. Otherwise, they are homonymous, but dissimilar.

- *Hemianopsia:* Loss of one-half the visual field of one or both eyes.
  Heteronymous hemianopsia: Loss of different fields for each eye.
  Homonymous hemianopsia: Loss of the same visual field in each eye. Homonymous hemianopsia may cause individuals to bump into objects on the side of the field defect (neglect, see example below), and represents a hazard in driving. Lesions of the optic chiasma cause bitemporal deficits due to damage of the centrally located fibers (receiving information from the sides of the head), which decussate at that location.
- *Scotoma:* Loss of vision in a particular areas of the visual field.

Vestibular

Output from the superior colliculus orients eyes, head, and body for further sensory input. It participates in a feedback circuit, i e , receiving axon branches from the retina, feeding into the midbrain reticular formation, which activates the thalamus, and subsequently the entire forebrain, including the visual (striate) cortex. It interacts with vestibuloocular stimuli to maintain balance and orientation of the eyes on a target while the target and/or head is moving.

The vestibuloocular reflex stabilizes a visual image on the retina during head movement, e.g., when the head moves in one direction the eyes compensate through movements in the opposite direction. Input includes antigravity muscles, somatosensory stimulation (perception of motion), visual and vestibular systems, and their cortical areas (Farber & Zoltan, 1989).

Symptoms

Somatic injury, e.g., a blow to the head, may damage the canals of the inner ear, and/or their pathways, resulting in one of the most common signs of head injury, i.e., dizziness and vertigo (sensation of movement).

Deficits in these functions point to brainstem damage: poor arousal, attention, and level of awareness, poor integration of postural reflexes, abnormal muscle tone, and poor balance and equilibrium.

It was estimated that half of patients recover by the end of 6 months, but dizziness can persist for as long as 2 years after head injury, with evidence of labyrinthine damage (Cartlidge & Shaw, 1981, Chapter X, "Dizziness," which includes a description of medical procedures for studying it). A screening test for vestibuloocular deficit is inability to follow a moving finger that rotates around the visual field creating a sense of dizziness.

Case 8. A woman in the front seat of a car with her fiance, who was driving recklessly on a slippery road: "I was concerned because he was skidding. Just before the accident, when I realized we were going to crash, I had this feeling of peace and afterward euphoria. I was ecstatically happy I wasn't dead." She has had dizzy spells. She was told it would go away in 6 months. She has attempted secretarial work, but did not succeed because poor handwriting prevented her from taking messages, she had panic attacks, and was disoriented. She could not find her way back to the office from the main lobby. "I am afraid to go inside a building on my own. Without warning, the room spins violently around (vertigo). It's very violent and I must be on the ground. I'm terrified of what could happen on the street. I could be killed. When I'm on the ground I am nauseous. It takes a while to go away. The room is spinning. It's like a ping-pong ball going back and forth in my head." She asserts that she has a weakened immune system.

"I was speaking on the phone to someone. She asked me what show I had seen. All of a sudden, everything went black. It was as though I was in a movie theatre and the lights went out. I couldn't see. It was very shocking and quite terrifying." She doesn't know what happened. She is uncertain if the other person was there when she came to. "I go into the next room to do something and I completely forget what I was to do. I sit down and 10 minutes later it comes back."

Audition

Bone Conduction

Sound vibrations transmitted through the skull to the cochlea. It is tested by applying tuning forks to the top of head and/or behind the ears. Bone conduction sensitivity, in the absence of air conduction, indicates that the auditory branch of nerve VIII is intact, although there may be a mechanical interference with the usual transmission through the eardrum.

Air Conduction

Sound is transmitted through the tympanic membrane and bones of the inner ear to the cochlea.

Complaints about difficulties in hearing, and/or measured deficits, particularly if unilateral, should be referred for audiological examination.

Spinal Level Sensory Deficits

Pain, Temperature, Light Touch

Damage to the spinothalamic tracts of the spinal cord at the point of damage, or within one or two levels lower or higher, will hamper ipsilateral sensation, whereas damage to tracts at higher levels will interfere with contralateral sensation.

Radiculitis; Radiculopathy

The dorsal and ventral radicles (rootlets) combine as they leave the spinal cord to form the dorsal or ventral root itself. Trauma or injury to the spine can create pain or other sensory deficits at the periphery, or muscular weakness.

Proprioception (Kinesthesis)

There are many influences on motor neurons (see Chapter 2 on Neuroanatomy, descending motor pathways) making them vulnerable to trauma at distant points or over long connecting circuits. Impairment causes loss of skilled movements. Brainstem damage can affect bodily coordination in a variety of ways: (1) reflexive motor responses based on positional stimuli occur both within the spinal cord, and via brainstem reticular formation and reentry into the spinal cord; and (2) vestibular information influences posture and locomotion, converging with proprioceptive information (Livingston, 1985, p. 1250).

Muscular Symptoms

Adams and Victor (1985, pp. 35–36) point out that motor functions can be disturbed by damage or disease to motor cells of the spinal cord and cranial nerves, motor cells of the cerebral cortex, brainstem nuclei, subcortical systems (basal ganglia and cerebellum), and premotor and other areas of the cortex. Deficits of strength and sensation can be caused by peripheral neural damage, or damage to joints, bones, and muscles (weakness, pain, and/or loss of range of motion). Damage to the basal ganglia can result in varied disorders of movement (Walton, 1985, pp. 322–324).

Terminology

See Adams and Victor (1989), Carpenter and Sutin (1983, p. 489), Lawson (1988, p. 275).

* *Akathasia:* Motor restlessness, inability to sit still and constant fidgeting.
* *Akinesia:* Decrease of spontaneous movements.
* *Ataxia:* A loss of muscular coordination, most usually in gait. It can be due to cerebellar dysfunction (including input from frontal lobes), posterior (sensory) columns of the spinal cord, or to peripheral nerve disease.
* *Athetosis:* Disturbance of posture and motor control resulting in involuntary movements described as writhing, i.e., inability to sustain fingers, tongue, or any part of the body in one position. Flexion and extension may alternate with each other, and face and limbs can be involved.
* *Chorea:* Involuntary arrhythmic movements that are forcible, rapid, and jerky.
* *Clonus:* Involuntary rhythmic muscular contractions occurring at a frequency of 5–7 times/second, in response to an abruptly applied and sustained stretch stimulus.
* *Dyskinesia:* Involuntary repetitive and stereotyped movements.
* *Dystonia:* Muscular rigidity limiting the range of motion.
* *Fasciculation:* Visible twitching within a muscle at irregular intervals, involving several muscular units. It is not a reliable diagnostic sign of neurological damage, occurring in normal muscles. It is a spontaneous, local contraction of muscles innervated by a single motor nerve element.

- *Fibrillation:* Random contraction of denervated, individual muscle fibers, involuntary and invisible, from spontaneous activation of single muscle cells or fibers.
- *Hemiballismus:* Uncontrolled movement, limited to one side of the body, with rotation and flinging of the limbs. Involuntary sudden movement of great force and rapidity.
- *Hemiparesis:* Slight paralysis, affecting one side only.
- *Hemiplegia:* Paralysis of one side of the body.
- *Hypotonia:* Muscles are flabby and tire easily.
- *Parkinsonian syndrome:* Rigidity, tremor, postural alterations, masklike facial expression, shuffling gait.
- *Rigidity:* Resistance to passive stretching of the muscles. Resistance to stretch remains constant (see spasticity).
- *Spasticity:* When a spastic muscle is stretched, more and more motor units respond, resistance mounts, and then suddenly ceases (see rigidity).
- *Tonic:* A form of seizure, in which the entire musculature, including breathing apparatus, is seized in a spasm.
- *Tremor:* Involuntary shaking caused by rhythmic, alternating contraction of opposing muscle groups. An action tremor occurs with the arms outstretched or through the entire range of motion. Intention tremor is not present at rest. It involves the muscles at the base of the limb, and is transmitted mechanically to the extremities. It increases towards the end of motion as the limb approaches a target. Rest tremor is present in the absence of voluntary movement.

Classification of Motor Deficits by Site of Lesion

See Chapter 2 on Neuroanatomy for definitions.

Upper Motor Neuron

Muscles are affected only in groups (Adams & Victor, 1989, p. 47; DeGroot & Chusid, 1988, pp. 45–49). With damage, voluntary movements are absent or weak. Rather than atrophy, there is spasticity with weakness. The stretch reflexes are not inhibited by descending pathways; tendon jerks are exaggerated; plantar reflex is abnormal (Babinski sign); other superficial reflexes are suppressed or absent: abdominal, cremasteric. Nerve conduction studies are normal.

Substantia nigra: Parkinson's disease; the lesions confined to the primary motor area cause a flaccid paralysis appropriate to the position of the destroyed cortex. When only small cortical areas are damaged recovery occurs with functions taken over by the adjacent areas. Symptoms frequently seen include unilateral loss of strength, paralysis, and insensitivity.

Lower Motor Neuron

Individual muscles may be affected:

1. Muscle tonus is reduced or absent, i.e., flaccid paralysis.
2. Tendon-jerk reflexes are weak or absent.

3. Muscles atrophy progressively, i.e., there is loss of muscle mass, due to inactivity, but tone and reflex activity are increased due to release.
4. Nerve conduction potentials are abnormal.

Cerebellum

Cerebellar damage results in "decomposition of movement," i.e., serial movements are "decomposed into independent sequential constituents that are executed with errors of force, amplitude, and timing." This can occur during the planning or execution of the movements (Inhoff et al., 1989). Dysfunctions appear as ataxia, hypotonia, and intention tremor. Errors occur in the rate, range, force, and direction of willed movements. There is rigidity, tremor of the distal muscles and poverty of movement, dyskinesias (chorea, athetosis, dystonia musculorum deformans), and ataxia of gait (see also Biller & Brazis, 1985; Brazis et al., 1985).

Cranial Nerve Level

Extraocular Movements

Damage to the frontal eye fields causes deviation of the eyes toward the side of the damage. There is an inability to converge the eyes on an approaching target and an inability to track smoothly vertically and/or horizontally. Accurate visual pursuit requires that the object remain on the fovea of the eye. As the object moves, there has to be inhibition of the vestibular ocular reflex, as well as smooth pursuit of the eye muscles, and vergence movements (convergence and divergence). Parietal lesions and damage to the cerebellum result in impaired pursuit in the direction of the impaired side. This topic is discussed in detail by Masdeu (1985c).

Intraocular Movements

Loss of pupillary constriction to bright lights.

Loss of Gag Reflex

Damage to the glossopharyngeal nerve (IX).

Tongue Deviation

Upper motor lesions deviate to the opposite side; *lower motor lesions* deviate to the same side, due to flaccid paralysis. This can be observed when the tongue protrudes.

Spinal

Visceral

Spinal cord injuries result in visceral overreactivity below the level of transection. Bladder and rectal stimulation may cause hypertension, headaches, flushing, and pilomotor activity, which are recognized by the patient as signs that the bladder or rectum needs evacuation. There is lack of temperature control below the transection. If output from T6 to S3 is preserved the person may be fertile or potent. Fertility may remain in the absence of potency or ejaculation.

Loss of Speed and Strength

Reaction time in head-injured patients is reduced. With increasing degrees of injury, these factors achieve more importance: complexity of the task, ability to screen out distractions, and speed of information processing. Even 1 year after an injury reaction time reduction is detectible (Levin, 1985). Related symptoms include lethargy, neurasthenia (fatigue, weakness, pains, etc.), and slowness in repetitive and directed movements.

Grip Strength

The frontal lobes (premotor, supplementary motor areas) play an important role in skilled motor activities. For hand grip, males are usually 40% stronger than females. One quarter of normal subjects are reported to have a stronger left hand (for further discussion, see Chapter 21, Assessment).

Distortions of the Bodily Image (Body Schema)

Impaired body image: impaired conceptualization of one's own body or other's bodies; inability to identify body parts, phantom limbs, and left–right dysfunction (Schilder, 1950).

Body image is created by sensory input from the somesthetic information from the surface of the body, proprioceptive stimuli from joints and muscles, emotional conditioning (Parker, 1983), visceral and vestibular stimulation, moods, appetites, satisfaction of internal motives, etc. The parietal lobe contributes to orientation in space and to awareness of bodily sensation (Chapter 2, Neuroanatomy and Organization). Neglect of sensory stimulation coming from the limbs, or one side of the body, can be attributable to right parietal damage (somesthetic dysfunctioning). It is likely to be accompanied by inappropriate euphoria or indifference; they may fail to perceive left-sided stimuli, and may dress, wash, or groom only the right side of the body, or misperceive the side that is being stimulated, etc. (Joseph, 1988). Further deficits of body image include feeling of bodily asymmetry (accompanying unilateral sensory or motor deficits), loss of the detailed awareness of one's body, and imbalance (accompanies seizures or vestibular dysfunctions).

Integrated Sensorimotor Deficits

Coordination

Deficits in coordination involve clumsiness and loss of coordination, subcortical tremor, primitive reflexes, hyperreflexia and hyporeflexia, ataxia, primitive grasp, chorea, inability to control the strength, pacing, and coordination of planned small and large movements, and tremor. Injury to the cerebellum results in reduced muscular tone and incoordination, without loss of kinesthetic sense, since these impulses do not enter consciousness (Carpenter & Sutin, 1983, p. 279).

The examiner will be interested in control on drawing tasks; improvising procedures such as the speed and care in which 10 beads are strung on a shoelace in a defined task, e.g., 60 seconds, and formal and informal tests of tapping speed or other psychomotor coordination.

Oculomotor

Deficits of eye movements indicate possible damage to the skull, eye, muscles of the eye, cranial nerves III, IV, and VI, pathways and nuclei within the midbrain, and also deficits of function of and integration with the vestibular branch of nerve VIII.

The following definitions of eye movements are offered by Bajandas and Kline (1987, p. 43), and Livingston, (1985, pp. 1042–1043):

- *Saccades* bring images of objects onto the fovea.
- *Nystagmus* is movement of the eye during high angular acceleration, with relatively slow components in the direction opposite to that of the acceleration, and quick movements in the direction of acceleration. The purpose is to direct the fovea toward the oncoming visual scene during rotation.
- *Smooth pursuit* holds the images of the world steady during sustained head rotation.
- *Vestibular and orientation:* The intact person holds images steady on the retina during brief head rotation. The vestibular stimultion resulting in nystagmic eye movements may cause movements of the head or body opposite to that of the direction of rotation, with increased tone in extensor muscles on the side of the direction of movement and flexion away from the direction of movement, with the direction reversed following deceleration. This is used in vestibular testing with the Barany chair.

    A useful procedure is to ask the person to track a rotating finger, with one's head steady. A high proportion of individuals who suffer vertigo complain of dizziness during this procedure (15 seconds or less).
- *Vergence* moves the eyes in opposite direction to movement so that images of an object are placed on both foveae.

Kinesthesis and Proprioception

Individuals with cerebellar and brainstem damage will not coordinate proprioceptive stimulation from the medial lemniscus with cerebellar nuclei. Consequently they are clumsy and do not orient their body in space, and tend to bump into things.

Clinical Examples of Sensorimotor Examination

Case 9: Middle-Aged Man

This section of a comprehensive neuropsychological examination integrates clinical and sensorimotor observations to illustrate these points:

1. Observation of the ability to follow instructions and emotional qualities.
2. A man who had suffered dementia was unable to assess his own condition. His Full Scale IQ was 48, with an estimated baseline of 83.

Reason for Referral

To examine after-effects of an accident in which he was knocked down by a car.

Medical Records

1. Sufficient impact to infer very severe neurological injury (maxilla, frontal bone, orbital bone).
2. Further brain damage secondary to the initial injury: meningitis (which would involve large areas of the cortex and other portions of the brain) caused by infections due to the tear in the dura mater; hydrocephalus would cause expansion of the ventricles, damaging brain tissue by pressure and interfering with circulation (nutrients, oxygen, disposal of wastes, etc).

While the focal neurological examination was normal, this is not a measure of emotional or higher mental functions, and certainly not verbal or problem-solving ability.

Clinical Impression

Mr. X appeared to be of average height and slender for his age. He was a black man, accompanied by his nephew (translator), who arrived 1/2 hour late. He did not bring a sandwich despite instructions. He was neat, clean, and informally dressed. There was a scar visible when his hair was parted.

Social quality: Cooperative, and related adequately.
Alertness: He was goal-directed, followed directions, but was unable to learn certain simple tasks (digit symbol, i.e., associating a number with a mark). He could not perform so simple a task as tapping into consecutive rows of boxes without stopping because he forgot the instructions. He could not follow instructions to alternate each foot. Asked to rotate his arms, he did not understand the instructions.
Problem-solving style: He performed so poorly at even the simplest level of many assigned tasks, that it was not meaningful to ask whether he used immature or well-developed approaches to tasks.
Reaction to event: Minimized deficits, anxiety, and any complaints, i.e., he had no insight into his impairment.

Emotional behavior: He was motivated to do well, when he could perform. When he did not get the idea or could not begin, e.g., in creating images for the Rorschach Inkblot Test, he was resentful at being pressed.

Morale: Where he could perform, he did what he could without anticipating difficulties.

Communication: Total lack of ability to speak English, although he has lived in the United States for several years, and seeming inability to discuss any deficits from his injury.

Coordination problems: No gross problems observed.

Physiological/stamina: He was able to perform the examination without needing extra breaks. The exam was broken into 1-1/2 and 3-3/4 hour segments.

Neuropsychological implication: The examination is a suitable sample of his performance. Evidence for impairment includes inability to learn, dull affect, inability to describe sequelae of the accident, inability to perform simple tasks, inability to follow instructions for motor activities, and inability to learn new tasks.

Sensorimotor Functions

Preferred hand: right.

Grip strength (Smedley hand dynamometer, average of three trials measured in kg):

	kg	Dev. age
Right hand	27.7	13
Left hand	34.7	15

Using appropriate sex standards, and taking into account his age, stature, and occupation, *there is not only a general loss of strength, but in particular a relatively high loss of right hand strength.*

Psychomotor speed (Parker Test of Bilateral Directed Tapping, Experimental): The task is to tap with each hand into rows of 1/2 inch boxes. His speed was approximately 15% of the average for available norms for his age (an unpublished procedure), which is far below the normal range. The ratio between preferred and nonpreferred hand speed was +14%, which is normal, but meaningless in view of the speed deficit. *Evidence for loss of psychomotor speed.*

Oculomotor movements: Eye tracking in the vertical and horizontal planes was jerky and poor. His eyes did not converge for an approaching target. He was able to track a stationary target when he moved his head.

Visual fields by confrontation: No evidence for deficit.

Visual double simultaneous stimulation: No evidence for deficit.

Somesthetic sensation (finger identification; double simultaneous stimulation-cheek-hand): No evidence for deficit.

Stereognosis (identification of objects by touch): He was asked to identify four different coins, with each hand, with eyes closed. He made three of four misidentifications with each hand. The examiner is not certain as to the precise meaning, since it may reflect to some extent unfamiliarity with the coins (although he recognized them in advance).

Hearing (using tuning forks of 128, 256, 512, 1024, and 2048 cps, measured at the skull vertex, and both ears, for air and bone conduction): At each frequency, a different ear was reported as less sensitive. The meaning is obscure.

Vibration (128 cps at elbow and knee): His results were somewhat variable, but in balance there is no reliable evidence for a deficit.

Odor (pocket smell test): Not examined.

Balance and vestibuloocular functioning: Toe-heel walking was unsteady. Standing on toes was unsteady. Evidence for deficit of balance. He was able to regard a rotating target without feeling dizzy, indicating some sparing of vestibular-ocular functioning.

Gait: No evidence for deficit.

Coordination and motor control—gross/fine: (tapping performance, special movements, handwriting, various drawing tasks, digit symbol writing, bead stringing): He was able to string 10 beads on a shoelace in 78 seconds, an informal test of gross coordination whose results seemed to show very slow gross psychomotor coordination. Indeed, he seemed tremulous. He missed many boxes with either hand, while tapping. Toe–heel tapping was clumsy with the right foot.

Kinesthesis (see procedure, below): His ability to locate an object in space from nonvisual sensory clues was marginal.

Neuropsychological Implications

Although the neurological examination was normal, there was evidence for loss of psychomotor speed, strength (particularly on the preferred right side), control, ability to alternate movements, sensory deficits of recognition and object identification by touch, etc. Moreover, there was actually evidence for brainstem damage, consistent with the impact and concussion, i.e., the oculomotor deficits, balance and vestibuloocular functioning, kinesthesis, etc. In addition there were marginal deficits of vibration and hearing, whose origin might be the inability to concentrate and/or understand the examiner, or neurological damage. Thus, *massive brain damage (impact, meningitis, hydrocephalus) contributed to generalized cognitive and sensory motor deficits, although the patient expressed no complaints* (see Chapter 16, Expressive Deficits).

Case 10: A Child of 9 Years 9 Months

Reason for Referral

To explore neuropsychological status after he was struck by a truck. His IQ was in the average range, although he was in a special education class. John was a stocky, overweight boy, who otherwise appeared healthy. Scarring was only intermittently visible. Some abstracts from direct observation: *Problem-solving style:* He used preplanning, a mature style, for easy items, and trial-and-error for items of midrange difficulty. His approach is not goal-oriented, i.e., he was asked to make a design with blocks from a model, which he covered with his hands so he could not see it. *Coordination problems:* This was clearly observable, i.e., he found it hard to assemble the block design and jig-saw like Object Assembly designs precisely.

Sensorimotor Functions

Preferred hand: right.

Psychomotor speed (Parker Test of Bilateral Directed Tapping, Experimental): There are no precise norms available for his age, but his speed was consistent with a group of children his age known to be impaired. There was a ratio of approximately +55% between preferred and non-preferred hand which suggests a loss of speed of control for the left hand.

Grip strength (Smedley Hand dynamometer, average of three trials, measured in kg):

	kg	Dev. age
Right hand	13.7	8
Left hand	11.5	7

Using appropriate age and sex norms, there is a deficit for left hand strength consistent with reduced left hand psychomotor speed.

Hearing (see above case): There seemed to be a loss of auditory sensitivity at 128 cps, and for left ear sensitivity at 2028 cps.

Odor (pocket smell test): two of three standard stimuli were detected. He misidentified so familiar an odor as "smoke" as "dill pickle."

Visual fields by confrontation: No evidence for deficit.

Oculomotor function: There were jerky eye movements when tracking a moving target in the verbal and horizontal plains. When a target was rotated in front of his eyes, his eye movements were uneven (i.e., they did not go all the way around, or would stay in one position). Accommodation to light was adequate.

Double simultaneous visual stimulation: No evidence for deficit.

Somesthetic sensation: (finger identification; double simultaneous stimulation-cheek-hand: No evidence for deficit.

Vibration: No evidence for deficit.

Stereognosis (coin identification): Of 16 identifications of 4 coins, twice with each hand, he made 1 right hand and 3 left hand errors.

Balance and vestibuloocular functions: It was hard for him to balance himself on his left leg. Toe–heel walking was insecure. Standing on his toes was insecure. He could not skip. He could stand with his eyes closed without swaying. Evidence for deficit of balance.

Coordination and muscular control—(Gross/Fine) (tapping performance, special movements, handwriting, various drawing tasks, digit symbol writing, bead stringing): He was asked to string 10 beads on a shoelace, and he was stopped at 61 seconds, after stringing the 12th. Asked why he did 12, he stated that "I forgot. I didn't forget, but you know, I didn't want to count 'em, to hurry up and do 'em." In this informal test of coordination, speed, and planning, his approach was inefficient, i.e., he lifted the string and beads off the table. He also found it hard to follow instructions for muscular action (to move his head up or down; toe–heel tapping, alternating feet). His mother stated that "He has problems with his feet, always dropping things. He spills milk, picks up a cup with the tip of his hands so he can't get a grip." His tapping in a speeded situation was poorly controlled for both hands, even taking his age into consideration. He rotated his arms asymmetrically. There was possible hand tremor. His ability to make a thumb to finger circle was marginal. His smile was symmetrical, he could control forehead muscles. He could shrug his shoulders appropriately. He does not hold his body symmetrically.

Kinesthesis (with eyes closed instructed to touch his nose, his knee, the examiner's finger in space, then back to own nose.): His ability to locate an object in space from nonvisual sensory clues was poor.

Neuropsychological Implications

There is evidence for left hand deficits of psychomotor strength, speed, and identification of objects. Kinesthesis and balance problems probably contribute to poor muscular control. There are deficits of gait, posture, and limb movements. The pattern is consistent with right cerebral deficits (primary for left-sided motor control and reception of sensation), and for possible cerebellar and/or brainstem deficits (balance and kinesthesis).

This case illustrates the complexity of localization. Using significant left hand deficits of strength and psychomotor speed as a reference point (potentially right cerebral hemisphere), his performance on the Wechsler Intelligence Scale for Children-Revised was paradoxical. With a Full Scale IQ of 92, and insignificant deviation in favor of Performance Scale (96) over Verbal Scale (90), there was a modestly higher Perceptual-Organizational Factor mean of 10.4 than Verbal Factor mean of 8.8. This would suggest relatively retained right hemisphere functioning in a right handed child. The lowest Factor score was Freedom from Distractibility (7.0), which is consistent with his problems of following instructions.

8
Neurophysiological, Humoral, and Visceral Functions

Overview

This system integrates neural and visceral organ systems used for normal activities, for survival in times of acute or chronic stress (danger, deprivation, environmental extremes, and disease) and daily rhythms. It controls energy output and metabolism, contributes to sensitivity of detection of sensory stimuli, and affects moods and overt emotional responses. The pineal gland and other tissues transduce environmental information (e.g., light, heat, and magnetism) into signals that modulate neuroendocrine mechanisms. Neurohormones, neuromodulators, and neuroimmune responses affect endocrine glands, central nervous system activities, and peripheral tissues.

The brain is considered to be an endocrine organ because of the variety of neuroendocrines it secretes having local and distant targets (Reiser & Reiser, 1985). There is no longer a distinction between hormones, which are products of endocrine glands transported by blood to exert their action at distant sites, and brain substances, which modulate neurotransmission when released into a synapse, or are transported via extracellular space or the blood to more distant sites.

Neuropsychological Dysfunctioning

Damage to limbic and other central areas, the pituitary stalk, and spinal pathways, and long–lasting reactions to stress reactions cause a variety of somatic disorders: developmental problems, sexual dysfunction, impaired ability to resist disease, increased or decreased endocrine and visceral functioning, loss of bowel and bladder control, and hyperarousal, i.e., exaggerated motor and autonomic functions (heart, bladder, colon, sweating). Posttraumatic stress conditions increase somatic functioning in ways characteristic of anxiety (urination, heart rate, sweating) or reduce the general level of functioning. Brain damage also contributes directly to anxiety and depression.

Neural Systems

Anatomy

The older regions of the cortex, limbic system, hypothalamus, and medulla are expressed via the autonomic nervous system, spinal pathways. and medulla (cranial division of SNS). Physiological mechanisms (and arousal) are integrated through the cerebral cortex, subcortical ganglia such as the amygdala, nuclei in the hypothalamus and brainstem, and a reticulum of poorly organized cells around the cerebral aqueduct. As one ascends the nervous system, visceral expression varies from reflexes in the brainstem to more integrated visceral patterns at the hypothalamic and limbic levels, and particularly at the limbic level, visceral functions integrated with emotional experience and expression (Livingston, 1985, p. 1221). In addition to the hypothalamic–pituitary axis (HPA), the reader should review the autonomic nervous system (see Chapter 2 on Neuroanatomy).

Hypothalamic Neurohormones

Among the neurohormones manufactured by the hypothalamus, which have behavioral as well as physiological functions, are thyrotropin-releasing hormone (TRH), luteinizing hormone-releasing hormone (LHRH), somatostatin, also known as growth hormone-releasing inhibiting hormone (GH-RIH), corticotropin-releasing factor (CRF—significant for stress), and growth hormone- releasing factor (GRF). Hormones produced along the HPA (CRF, ACTH, and corticosterone) have regulatory roles with the immune system (see below).

Endogenous Opiates and the Amygdala

Endogenous opioids regulate various behaviors, and may create retrograde amnesia (Flood, Cherkin, & Morley 1987). Opiate-containing fibers running from the amygdala to the sensory systems serve a gate-keeping function by releasing opiates in response to emotional states generated in the thalamus. This influences what is perceived and learned, i.e., retention of emotionally charged events (Mishkin & Appenzeller, 1987).

Hypothalamic–Pituitary Axis

Pituitary Gland (Hypophysis)

The pituitary stalk and blood vessels pass through the dura mater. The blood supply of the anterior and posterior pituitary lobes is described by Findling and Tyrrell (1986). There is a retrograde blood flow between the pituitary and hypothalamus providing feedback between pituitary hormones and their neuro-endocrine control. Since the pituitary gland is connected to the base of the brain by a stalk, and sits in a cavity within the base of the skull (sella turcica), its stalk is susceptible to damage by movement caused by trauma, and to local tumors.

The pituitary has two embryologically and histologically separate components, with different functions.

The posterior pituitary (neurohypophysis) is embryologically an outpouching of the third ventricle, i.e., neural tissue formed as a downgrowth of the hypothalamus. Thus, it is an integral portion of the nervous system. It receives two hormones by axoplasmic transport from the supraoptic and paraventricular nuclei of the hypothalamus: and *vasopressin* (antidiuretic hormone, which controls blood volume via urine release). These are secreted into the bloodstream.

It secretes *oxytocin* (initiating contraction of the uterus and milk ejection) and *vasopressin* (antidiuretic hormone [ADH], which affects urine flow, water balance, and blood volume via urine release).

The anterior pituitary (adenohypophysis) is nonneuronal, i.e., it forms during the embryological period as an outpouching at 4–5 weeks of fetal age of the pharynx (Findling & Tyrrell, 1986; Ganong; 1986). It is somatic tissue, while the posterior pituitary is neural tissue. Secretion is controlled by releasing hormones (neurohormones) secreted into the hypophyseal portal circulation that stimulate secretory peptide hormones of the anterior pituitary.

The anterior pituitary (AP) is controlled by two neuronal circuits, and also by negative feedback from hormonal levels secreted by target glands. Feedback to the hypothalamus by adrenal cortical steroids (following stress) is shared by the limbic system and brainstem (Plotsky, 1987).

One circuit begins with the supraoptic and paraventricular nuclei of the hypothalamus, with pathways that lead to the neurohypophysis (posterior pituitary gland). Substances released there are transported by the portal blood supply to the anterior pituitary. Another circuit leads to the median eminence (at the base of the hypothalamus), which bypasses the neurohypophysis and secretes different neurohormones into the blood supply of the AP. The median eminence also is connected to the neurohypophysis via the hypothalamic–neurohypophysial tract (Pelletier, 1988).

The AP is stimulated by CRH to secrete ACTH, which in turn stimulates the adrenal cortex to secrete cortisol and androgens. Related peptides (POMC-precursor of ACTH) modulate nervous system functioning, i.e., motivation, attention, concentration, arousal, aggression, social behavior, grooming behavior, developmental processes, nerve cell regeneration, sexual behavior, pain, addiction, mood, learning and memory processes, food intake, temperature regulation, and maternal behavior (De Wied & De Kloet, 1987), and also sensory processing, habituation, and sensitization to stimuli, pain, sleep, memory storage, and retrieval (Reus, 1989).

Anterior Pituitary Targets

Anterior pituitary targets are the *thyroid gland* (thyrotropin), and the *adrenal gland* (ACTH), which produces corticotropin-releasing hormone, controlling

ACTH and β–endorphin, significant stress hormones. ACTH in turn stimulates adrenal cortex production of cortisol and influences fat metabolism. *Gonads* [follicle-stimulating hormone, FSH; *luteinizing hormone* (LH); *growth hormone* (GH)] are controlled by two hypothalamic hormones, i.e., growth hormone releasing hormone (GRH) and somatostatin (growth hormone-inhibiting hormone). Growth hormone is stimulated by the same neural mechanisms that initiate deep sleep, and secretion is particularly high in children at puberty, when noctural rises in various sexual hormones are marked, and tend to decrease with age. This may account for the observation that children who have suffered impact, i.e., by inference, disconnection of the anterior pituitary, frequently have delayed or incomplete signs of puberty (Gill, 1985).

Posterior Pituitary Targets

Breast and lactation (prolactin and oxytocin of the posterior pituitary).

Neuroactive Hormones and Peptides

These are found in the HPA and elsewhere. Several hypothalamic nuclei (supraoptic and paraventricular nuclei, above the optic tract, in the wall of the third ventricle) secrete neurohormones that are transported via the *hypothalamo-hypophyseal* (supraopticohypophyseal) tract to the posterior pituitary gland. Then, hormones are released into the capillary blood, and transported by local blood supply (portal system) to the anterior pituitary, a true endocrine gland.

Releasing hormones (hypophyseotropic) are neurosecretory substances that act upon the anterior lobe of the pituitary, and are named according to the hormone they release. They are synthesized in various hypothalamic nuclei, whose axons terminate in the region of the *portal blood system* of the pituitary gland. Branches of the internal carotid arteries break up into sinuses, which transport releasing hormones into the anterior lobe of the pituitary gland (hypophysis). This also receives blood from the median eminence. (Diagrams of hypothalamic neural and vascular pathways, and nuclei, are found in Chapter 16, Carpenter and Sutin, 1983).

The following hormones are particularly significant for behavior or stress functions.

- *Thyrotropin releasing hormone* (TRH) controls thyroid-stimulating hormone, i.e., thyrotropin or TSH, and also growth hormone (see Chapter 4, Trauma, on enhanced bone metabolism).
- *Somatostatin* (inhibits growth hormone release), also known as growth hormone–releasing inhibiting hormone (GH-RIH).
- *Luteinizing hormone–releasing hormone* (LHRH), which stimulates luteinizing hormone (LH) and follicle–stimulating hormone (FSH, important in the sexual cycle and other sexual endocrine activities). This is also known as GnRH, or gonadotropin–releasing hormone. It is released by fibers in the region of the median eminence. Another effect of LHRH is on the secretion of prolactin by

the anterior pituitary. Hyperprolactinemia leads to hypogonadism, impairment of the menstrual cycle, and reduced libido, impotence, and infertility in men. It is associated with anxiety and depression.

• *Cortocotropin-releasing hormone* (CRH) is released into median eminence vessels (diencephalon), which carry it to the anterior pituitary, stimulating the release of ACTH or adrenocorticotropin (see Chapter 15 on Stress), which in turn stimulates the adrenal cortex to secrete cortisol. The CRH–ACTH–cortisol axis (Gill, 1985, p. 860) is discussed further in Chapter 15 on Stress).

Opiate–Like Effects

CRH also causes β–endorphins to be released, which project to the limbic lobe and brainstem. These affect learning and exert psychostimulant and neuroleptic-like effects. Cells of the periaqueductal gray matter bind these opiate substances (receptors). Opiate administration activates pain suppression mechanisms of the midbrain, medulla oblogata, and spinal cord (Livingston, 1985, p. 1141).

Pineal Gland

The pineal gland translates basic environmental information (light, heat, and magnetism) into signals and rhythms that modulate most neuroendocrine mechanisms. Alterations in the circadian synthesis and release of melatonin are associated with sleep disturbances, anxiety states, affective disorders, and psychosomatic diseases. Pineal-related immune reactions are disturbed if cancer and autoimmune diseases are present. Melanotonin stimulates antibody production. Low levels are associated with psychological and affective disorders, in which an increased incidence of infections, autoimmune problems, and cancers exists. It seems to buffer adverse immunologic effects of stress through circadian release of melatonin (Maestroni, Conti,& Pierpaoli, 1987). The pineal gland appears to be implicated in affective illness. It does not have a primary endocrine effect, rather it modulates the activities of hormones, enzymes, and neurotransmitters, and coordinates circadian biorhythms to environmental lighting conditions (Brown, Chik, and Ho, 1988; Brown, Steiner, & Grof, 1988).

Target Organs

The viscera, endocrines, and blood vessels are controlled through neural pathways, endocrine secretions of the anterior pituitary gland to other endocrine glands, neuroendocrine secretions of the hypothalamus posterior pituitary gland transported through the local circulation (portal system), secretions of the pineal gland, and diffuse control of viscera of the autonomic nervous system.

Visceral Functions

There is an exchange of energy between the organism and the environment, and maintenance of an internal environment that varies between homeostasis and mobilization for emergency. Specific functions include sexuality and reproduction, metabolism, respiration, temperature control, sleep, circulation, ingestion, secretion, excretion, reward, pleasure and aversive systems, motivation, etc. These functions are partially expressed in support of the somatic musculature (e.g., oxygen and nutrient supply).

Endocrine Considerations

See Chapter 15 on Stress and Psychodynamic Reactions and Chapter 19 on Children's Brain Damage. Endocrine and neuroendocrine secretion into the blood stream is detected by various areas of the brain, which in turn modulate the level of secretion by the neuroendocrine glands.

Representative Systems

Immune System

The immune system is conceptualized as a defense mechanism that monitors and mediates the balance between host and pathogens. Thus, experiences that are processed by the brain can regulate or modify defensive mechanisms such as susceptibility to disease (Ader & Cohen, 1984). The immune system must recognize and destroy both foreign environmental pathogens and self cells that are virally infected or neoplastically transformed (Gorman & Locke, 1989). Immunological cells must also inform neuroendocrine organs about their functional state, stimulating secretion of hormones, neurotransmitters, and neuropeptides, to interfere with immune cell function when required (Del Rey, Besedovsky, Sorkin, & Dinarello, 1988). This system is considered to be comparable in complexity to the nervous system itself.

Central control is through the hypothalamus, reticular formation, limbic system, and neocortex. The periaquaductal gray appears to be the locus for endogenous and exogenous opiates to induce immunosuppression and analgesia (Weber & Pert, 1989). Proximal control is primarily through noradrenergic sympathetic fibers on immune organs and nearby fields of lymphocytes and other cells. Immune reactions are subject to Pavlovian conditioning (Gorman & Locke, 1989). Target organs for the immune response (immune microenvironment) include thymus and other lymphoid tissue and bone marrow. It is sensitive to electrical, magnetic, and electromagnetic fields. Communication between neurons and lymphocytes is via chemical transmission, and involves a variety of biologically active substances, apart from neurotransmitters. Some neuronal signals may act via blood routes, in analogy to hormones (Jankovic, 1987). Lymphocyte products also act as messengers to the central nervous system. These are produced by bone marrow, which are the most ancient mosaic of cells providing immunity through identification and maintenance of "self" (Pierpaoli et al., 1987).

Impaired health can result from brain damage, due to impairment of the immune system, since there is an interaction between the HPA and the immune system (marrow and lymphoid tissue). Glucocorticoids (adrenal cortical secretion) reduce the deleterious effects of stress, but also reduce the immune response. Therefore, brain damage may impair the immune reaction because of reduced availability of intermediate circuits and neuroendocrine transmitters (Deschaux & Rouhabhia, 1987; Hadden, 1987). Lymphocytes secrete substances that increase corticosterone concentrations that are immunosuppressive. Thus, a massive overstimulation of the HPA can contribute to the establishment of infections (Del Rey et al., 1987). This becomes part of the stress response, i.e., oversecretion of glucocorticoids with potential inability of the body to maintain secretion within physiological limits.

Neuroendocrine Thymus–Lymphoid Interactions

Lymphocyte products "act as a messenger to the central nervous system" (Maestroni et al., 1987). There is a three-way interaction between nervous, endocrine, and immune systems, i.e., lymphocytes produce vasopressin and oxytocin, ordinarily produced in the posterior pituitary, and also ACTH and β-endorphin, produced in the anterior pituitary, creating a "neuroendocrine thymus–lymphoid axis"(!) (Geneen, Legros, Franchimont, Defresne, & Boniver, 1987). This modulates significant physiological and behavioral functions, probably including stress reactions.

Thymus and Other Lymphoid Organs

These components of the immune system are under the control of the ANS and other circulating products, and in turn act in consort with a variety of biological processes. These tissues produce T lymphocytes, which come under neurotransmitter influences (Hadden, 1987).

Sex

Sexual behavior and experience are very complex, and involve the brain and a variety of neural tracts. Significant pathways include the cerebral cortex, preoptic region of the hypothalamus, midbrain, pons, and spinal cord (see below for HPA dysfunctions).

In the male, potency problems evolving from psychological conflicts are well known, but their frequency in the older male is probably exaggerated, considering the variety of neural, vascular, endocrine deficits, and systemic illnesses that create potency problems (Krane, Siroky, & Goldstein, 1983). Sexual problems following trauma can evolve from damage to the brain, spinal cord, neuroendocrine glands, peripheral nerves, pain and restricted movement from somatic damage, etc.

In the male, erection is controlled primarily by the parasympathetic nervous system and ejaculation by the sympathetic nervous system. Ejaculation is a reflex involving sensation coming from the penis to sacral segments 2–4, and traveling in part to the upper lumbar spinal cord. The known pathways then leave the spinal cord in the upper lumbar region to the ejaculatory apparatus (Chusid, 1985, p. 169). According to Adams and Victor (1985, pp. 411–412): "All the neural apparatus for the control of sexual functions is organized through the lower spinal segments (sacral segments 3 and 4 and the nervi erigentes and pudendal nerves— "Pelvic nerve") and that the mechanism of erection may still be functional, even when completely removed from voluntary control, as in high spinal lesions."

Cerebral damage frequently is accompanied by sexual difficulties, e.g., reduced libido. The olfactory system, with its intimate connection with the limbic system, and the temporal lobe, are particularly implicated with sexual behavior (Torrens, 1983). Structures in the cortex, hypothalamus, and midbrain are also implicated (Siroky & Krane, 1983).

Disorders of the Hypothalamus

The following is restricted to potential sequellae of trauma. They can have other etiologies, and there are many conditions not listed (Adams & Victor, 1989, pp. 451–452): hyperthermia, adrenal, gonadal, and thyroid insufficiency, problems of appetite, and cardiac disorders consequent to subarachnoid hemmorrhage (see Chapter 4 on Trauma).

Hypothalamic–Pituitary–Adrenal Cortex Axis (HPA) Disorders

The incidence of deficits seems controversial, being assessed from rare (Epstein, Ward, & Becker, 1987) to "well-recognized" (Levin et al., 1982, p. 29). Severe head trauma is considered to be "an often-overlooked cause of anterior pituitary insufficiency" (Findling & Tyrrell, 1986). Symptoms depend on which hormones are affected (Pogach & Vaitukaitis, 1983). The thyroid and gonads are target organs (among others). See Chapter 13 on Cerebral Personality Disorders for behavioral effects. Depression, psychomotor retardation, and diminished sexual function have been attributed to damage to the HPA (Levin et al., 1982, p. 29).

Hypopituitarism

See also Endocrine Dysfunction in Chapter 19 on Children's Brain Damage. This is considered rare, but since it is usually not looked for, and its manifestations may take years to develop, it is no wonder that it is underdiagnosed.

Hypopituitarism is described as a subtle clinical event manifested by diminished or absent secretion of one of more pituitary hormones. Head trauma and child abuse are considered etiologic factors (Findling& Tyrrell, 1986). Pathological studies reveal hypothalamic hemorrhage or pituitary infarcts and hemorrhages. Lesions included interruption of the blood supply, transection of the stalk, and axonal damage. Hypopituitarism could be manifested by asthenia, depression, and altered sexual function, which could be misunderstood by a physician in a case of brain injury (Epstein et al., 1987). Traumatic damage to the hypothalamus, or the connections to the pituitary gland, can impair a variety of significant endocrinological functions (see Endocrine Function section in Chapter 19 on Children's Brain Damage). This can be "rarely" caused by head injury with fracture of the base of the skull. After many years, the symptoms include weakness, fatigue, sensitivity to cold, loss of libido (amenorrhea or impotence), and loss of weight, loss of drive, drowsiness, and impaired memory, with delirium, stupor, or coma (Lishman, 1987, p. 443). These conditions obviously can be confused with depression.

Hypothyroidism

Noradrenergic systems stimulate TSH and dopaminergic neurons inhibit it (Reus, 1989), making levels vulnerable to the integrity of nuclei and pathways. An epinephrine surge after TBI is related to reduced thyroid function (Marshall & Marshall, 1985). Some symptoms are consistent with those frequently found after traumatic brain damage, i.e., endogenous depression, and impaired memory, abstractions, comprehension and attention, peripheral nerve damage, headaches, confusion, peripheral neuropathy, and apathy. Chronic hypothyroidism can lead to a true organic psychosis (Reiser & Reiser, 1985; Reus, 1989).

Acute traumatic brain injury effects were studied by Woolf, Lee, Hamill, & McDonald (1988). Various thyroid hormone measurements fell significantly within 24 hours of injury, and the drop was proportional to the neurological dysfunction as measured by GCS. The changes were attributable to SNS discharge (circulating catecholamines), rather than a generalized stress response.

Hyperprolactinemia

The AP secretes prolactin (PRL), which increases lactation postpartum, but does not ordinarily regulate gonadal function. Its secretion is inhibited by the hypothalamus (Cocchi & Muller, 1988). Stress (Reus & Collu, 1988), head trauma or interference with the delivery of hypothalamic hormones to the pituitary stalk, and seizures (Rao et al., 1989) lead to enhanced release (Frantz, 1988). Hyperprolactinemia in turn leads to hypogonadism, reduced libido, impotence, infertility, anxiety, depression, stress intolerance, irritability, and some medical illnesses (Findling & Tyrrell, 1986; Reus, 1989).

Hypogonadism

Changes in gonadal function following TBI are attributable to hypothalamic damage (Woolf et al., 1988). See also Hyperprolactinemia, above.

Posterior Pituitary Disorders

Diabetes insipidus is accepted as a complication of closed head injury in children and adults, due to loss of vasopressin (Findling & Tyrrell, 1986). Interruption of the blood supply to the hypothalamus and pituitary leads to neurogenic diabetes insipidus (Ramsey, 1986).

Autonomic Nervous System Disorders

There are a variety of symptoms that may have different causes, including basilar skull fractures, traumatic lesions of the first and second thoracic spinal segments, and lesions of the lateral tegmentum of the pons and medulla (Adams & Victor, 1989, pp. 433–442). Some of the following symptoms can be generalized contralaterally or locally. These include enhanced and reduced sweating, hypotension, impotence, diarrhea, hyperthermia, disorders of urination (loss of awareness of fullness, bladder paralysis, loss of control), disorder of the colon and anus, and sexual problems (loss of libido, erection, and/or ejaculation).

Stress reactions: See Chapter 15 on Stress.

Spinal Injuries

These can result in impotence, ejaculation failure, failure of intromission, and absent ejaculation. The level of the injury will determine the nature of the reflex and symptom (Torrens, 1983).

Case of Sexual Problem after Spinal Injury

Radiculopathy was noted in the medical reports after an automobile accident. This implies that there was damage or irritation of sensory roots as they enter the spinal cord. The patient complained of pain and difficulties in ejaculating. The thoracic vertebral damage indicates the possibility that pathways from the brain to the sexual apparatus are damaged. Moreover, it is feasible that tracts from the brain were damaged at higher levels (as indicated in the L2 damage with radiculopathy). The same spinal tracts seem involved in ejaculation, with which the patient has difficulties. In addition to the above parasympathetic innervation, sympathetic innervation comes from the spinal cord via the hypogastric plexus. Thus, his sexual problems are consistent with difficulties attributable to pain, to restricted movement, and to known damage to the relevant areas of the spinal column.

9
Intellectual Functioning

Overview

This chapter will describe some dysfunctions of intellectual ability that occur after TBI, emphasizing deficits that impair adaptive functioning. Assessment considerations per se will be discussed in Chapter 21.

Definition of the System

Intelligence is a multifaceted, interactive process, involving different types of information processing and styles of problem solving. These processes are applied to

1. Learning procedures and facts of different levels of difficulty;
2. Solving problems at different levels of difficulty;
3. Understanding the relationship between facts and their context;
4. Comprehending the likely outcome of a given situation or action;
5. Forming concepts and generalizations;
6. Thinking abstractly (perceiving meanings beyond the obvious);
7. Creativity, i.e., generating and applying new ideas and alternatives;
8. Problem solving in structured and unstructured situations;
9. Special abilities, talents, and skills, which are relatively independent of general ability and other functions.

Neuropsychological Dysfunctioning

There are different patterns of intellectual loss: generalized loss of ability, ranging from barely detectable to dementia; loss of particular components (focal, e.g., spatial, verbal, calculations, artistic), within the context of generalized retention of mental ability; and pathognomonic responses found primarily in brain injury. The level of difficulty of problems that can be coped with is reduced, which may be apparent only under situations of increased or different demands. One should differentiate between reduced intellectual ability, as defined above, and inefficiency.

Reduced competence may be a consequence of inefficiency, which is a deficit of supportive functions (e.g., inability to concentrate), rather than mental ability itself. Significant impairment can be caused by relatively narrow deficits of cognitive ability, i.e., after what is called slight head injury, in the context of retained basic mental ability. Attention, ability to communicate, and all of the other systems affect the application of intelligence to daily living. Memory helps intelligence to express itself. During complex current operations it is advantageous to keep components of a task in short-term memory (McCarthy & Warrington, 1987). It is also useful to avoid difficulties mastered in the past (see Chapter 11, Efficiency and Control).

Primary Neural System

Although the cerebral cortex is traditionally described as the functional area for intellectual achievement, its interconnections are too profound to consider this more than a generalization. Gross loss of mental ability (dementia) is associated with cortical and/or subcortical mechanisms.

Intellectual ability probably is based on sequential processing, i.e., progressive elaboration of some stimulus or "idea" along a neural circuit, with simultaneous parallel functions providing input and modification simultaneously with activity in the primary circuit, e.g., memory, meaning, and monitoring. There is evidence for primary significance of nonverbal processing by the right hemisphere, and processing of verbal and sequential cognitive processes by the left hemisphere, although considerable overlapping occurs (Code, 1987; Joseph, 1988).

Components of Intelligence

General Intelligence

Wechsler (1981, pp. 7–8) stated that intelligence tests assess "an individual's potential for purposeful and useful behavior." General intelligence is a function of the personality as a whole, and is not always adaptive. There are influences from "personality traits, and other nonintellective components, such as anxiety, persistence, goal awareness, and other conative dispositions."

I define general intelligence as describing the range, difficulty, and complexity of *situations that can be understood, information and procedures learned,* and *alternative solutions to problems generated and selected.* Intelligence utilizes other functions, e.g., clear consciousness, mental control, attention and concentration, memory, health and stamina, good morale and sense of identity, and freedom from disorganization by dysphoric moods. Intelligence is differentially used in structured and unstructured situations.

Assessment is made by comparing IQ scales, factor patterns, and subtests, but formal measurements do not represent a complete picture of intellectual efficiency in the TBI victim any more than they do in the uninjured person. Much is to be learned from clinical observations of style, etc. (see Appendix 1).

Impairment usually reduces ability and speed of coping with problems, with greater difficulties in coping with complex or unstructured tasks.

Comparison of Verbal and Performance IQs taps the following functions (though in an overlapping fashion): previously learned information versus solving new problems, verbal versus nonverbal and holistic processing. Probably the verbal scale is more culturally loaded than the nonverbal scale, with relatively untimed versus timed tasks. I believe Picture Arrangement measures sequential processing (in Performance Scale).

The significance of a given score cannot be determined without reference to an estimated baseline performance (see Chapter 21 on Assessment). A given deficit may not be detectable when someone returns to a relatively undemanding environment. A person with an IQ of 135, functioning in an environment requiring an IQ of 80 might be able to solve all problems, even with a loss of 55 points of IQ. However, when more complex cognitive functioning is required, then the previously adapted individual will be ineffective.

Research for seven studies of head trauma victims who were administered the Wechsler Adult Intelligence Scale (WAIS) (Farr, Greene, & Fisher-White, 1986) found that the average Full Scale IQ was 90.5, Verbal Scale IQ was 94.8, and Performance Scale IQ, 86.4 (VIQ-PIQ = +8.4).

I will summarize my findings for TBI victims (BD), with comparison to a demographically similar group of Stress Victims (SD). All patients were ambulatory, and almost all were engaged in litigation. Characteristic BD trauma included vehicular accidents as passenger and pedestrian, falls in elevators, objects falling on the head (e.g., ceilings), and toxins. Stress victims suffered from incidents involving rape, false arrest, etc. Mean age: BD, 35; Stress 36. Mean level of education for both groups was slightly more than 12 years. Estimated pre-injury IQ for this demographic pattern (Matarazzo & Herman, 1984): VIQ: 97.4; PIQ: 98.6; FSIQ: 98.6. All results are from single measurements (see Table 9.1).

TABLE 9.1. WAIS−R Data by interval since injury: Brain damage and stress.

Group	Brain Damaged				Stress				P+
	I	II	III	Total	I	II	III	Total	
Number of Pts.	(75)	(39)	(47)	(161)	(13)	(9)	(13)	(35)	
SCALE									
Verbal	91.3	95.6	89.7	91.7	94.7	90.2	97.5	94.8	
Performance	86.4	87.3	84.6	85.9	90.6	93.0	92.5	92.4	.014
Full Scale	88.4	90.8	86.5	88.2	92.6	91.4	94.7	93.4	
FACTOR (See WAIS-R, below)									
Verbal	8.6	9.7	7.8*	8.6	9.6	9.2	8.8	9.2	
Perc-Orgn.	7.8	8.1	7.6	7.8	8.4	9.2	8.2	8.6	
Frdm/Dist.	8.0	8.6	7.6	8.0	8.8	8.3	9.1	8.7	

Interval: I. 1–8 months; II. 9–23 months; III. greater than 23 months (to 10 years).
*F = 4.13 (.018) 1-WAY ANOVA
+ (2-tailed t-test). Occasionally a bit of data was unavailable.

Verbal Scale-Performance Scale differentiated BD (5.7) from ST (2.4) at the .046 level. The patients were subdivided by the average length of interval since the accident or incident, i.e., 1–8 months, 9–23 months, and from 24 months to 10 years (Table 9.1).

For the BD Ss, the one way analysis of variance did not show any significant differences by interval for any WAIS-R Scales. The only significant difference between intervals was for the Verbal Factor. It will be observed that the average Verbal IQ for the group with the longest interval since the accident was actually less than the mean for the group tested after the shortest interval.

There was a significant difference between Performance Scale IQ of 6.5 points in favor of the Stress Group. This is consistent with previous findings (Farr et al., 1986, see above) indicating that Performance IQ deficit is characteristic.

Analogous results indicating non-improvement over time were also obtained for Rorschach variables based upon objective scoring categories. In ST group, there was a significant trend towards creating more poor Whole responses after a longer interval post incident, leading to the inference of deteriorated cognitive effectiveness.

The overall results were similar within a few points to the results of Farr et al., 1986, i.e., Full Scale IQ in the lower end of the Average range, with a 6 versus 8 point deviation in favor of Verbal IQ compared to Performance IQ.

The deviations between the estimated pre-injury IQ (see above), and current measurement were:

IQ	Brain damage
Full Scale	−9.1
Verbal	−6.2
Performance	−12.6

The findings indicate that after an injury (with the possible exception of some immediate recovery after trauma), over a period of 10 years, there is no improvement as measured by Full Scale IQ. Indeed, the only significant difference over time was a *reduction* in the Verbal Factor in the brain damaged group, with the lowest average in the patients measured during the longest interval after the injury. The Verbal–Performance score advantage is consistent with apparently all other reports of the effects of traumatic brain damage, i.e., the vulnerability to TBI of unfamiliar, less well learned holistic and nonverbal tasks when performed under timed conditions.

Information Processing

Incoming information, or ideas that are developed, are processed and then encoded in different ways on the way toward memory and problem solving.

Case 11. An 11-year-old girl is an example of the complexity of intellectual processing. She was comatose for 12 days after being thrown a considerable distance by an automobile. Her Full Scale IQ on the Wechsler Intelligence Scale for Children deteriorated in 4 years from 69 to 66. She performed fairly well on Math (Scaled Score = 7), and even Similarities (6). The required expression is relatively simple. However, when the level of verbal expression is more complex, e.g., Vocabulary, i.e., explanation of words, and Comprehension, e.g., a process, then she failed almost completely, i.e., 1 point Scaled Score each.

- *Encoded according to mode of input:* When sensory stimuli are received, they are progressively encoded in some characteristic way peripherally and centrally. Unless this type of information can be retrieved, for practical purposes it may be nonexistent. One may demonstrate indirectly that it may be present, but its utility is minimal. Ability to utilize information depends on recognition that it belongs to a class of objects. Mental processing then exchanges information between sensory input, working memory, and long-term memory. With impaired retrieval or processing (e.g., visual or verbal), new events are not stored and prior learning is not available. When use of particular kinds of information is impaired, the person cannot recognize classes of stimuli, or retrieve them from long-term storage.
- *Different patterns of special abilities:* Patterns of ability for the unimpaired person are a function of genetics and training. These are relatively narrow functions that are significant for mental processing, as applied to earning a living, education, independence, etc. They are relatively independent of general mental ability (there is always a positive, sometimes small correlation between special abilities and IQ). More narrow components of cognitive ability vary within somewhat narrow limits on both sides of the relative rank represented by general intelligence.

  Particular ability factors and skills (e.g., perceptual organization, verbal, calculations, etc.) are significant for certain kinds of educational training and special vocations. The engineer requires a high level of visuospatial problem-solving ability; the poet somewhat less so, with greater emphasis on sequential processing, without totally ignoring visual imagery and overall (holistic) organization. Nevertheless, modes of information processing sometimes alternate with each other, as the person copes with different phases of the solution to a problem, or alternate, or are utilized simultaneously. Special abilities may or may not be spared after TBI.
- *Different styles of problem solving:* This will be discussed in detail in Chapter 11 on Efficiency and Control.

Analysis and Synthesis

A new, complicated, or vague situation may be divided into meaningful parts, and then integrated into a new idea, or resynthesized for a better or different solution.

Abstraction and Concept Formation

The undamaged brain sees relationships between certain kinds of objects or ideas, forms categories, and understanding the implications of a situation beyond the immediate or obvious. Assignment to a category may yield a feeling of familiarity, so that prior experience (cognitive and emotional) is applied to a situation, and new events and stimuli are not experienced as totally different. Former experience is applied when events and things are seen as belonging to a certain category. Conceptual thinking also requires holistic processing, i.e., integrating information, concepts, or potential outcomes.

Coping with Structured and Unstructured Situations

Environments, including employment, make different cognitive demands, which may be differentially impaired.

• *Structured:* The situation and demands are familiar, and/or the requirements for success are relatively precise. An example is arithmetic, spelling, or a job with a detailed procedural manual.
• *Unstructured:* The situation is unfamiliar, and the requirements are not precise or subjective. Examples are the Rorschach, or entering a position in which little supervision is given.

Coding and Decoding Verbal Information

This is related to sequential processing, although verbal ability has some unique qualities: reception (auditory and/or visual channels), coding into words and concepts, offering meaning to the components, and finally expression in a grammatical sequence.

Sequential Processing

The individual perceives and adjusts ideas into cause-and-effect relationships, or arranges them in sequence to solve problems. Examples include placing words into a comprehensible and grammatically correct order for efficient thinking and communication, or receiving information in order: "How much is 3×3, and then subtract this from 15." A test example is Picture Arrangement (WAIS-R).

Simultaneous Processing

Certain types of information must dealt with all at once, although, as noted above, problem solving involves alternation between attention to more and less inclusive hierarchies of information. Examples of simultaneous processing include reading a map, chart, or diagram, forming complex concepts, or having a concept of a complete solution to a problem. Simultaneous processing can be a component of monitoring, i.e., alternating between an inner model of what the outcome should be, details of the solution as the problem is approached, overall view of the status of a solution (monitoring), and ultimately matching against the desired solution for suitability. Nonverbal, spatial, and simultaneous processing are somewhat overlapping concepts. In practical situations, internal speech and memory contribute to solution of nonverbal problems. This topic is further discussed in Chapter 21 on Efficiency and Control.

Representative Symptoms

Diminished Intellectual Productivity

The amount and quality of ideas are reduced. The person produces simple ideas because he cannot understand and process complex situations. Imagination is inferior, with lowered access to associations reflecting experience, creativity, or other socially valuable products (Ruff, Evans, & Marshall, 1986).

Dementia

This may be defined as a generalized reduction of intelligence in all or almost all measured areas of cognitive ability, sufficient to interfere with normal living, with no impairment in state of consciousness. Caution must be exercised to distinguish dementia from depression, a frequent symptom of TBI, which shares common characteristics with dementia: memory difficulties, apathy, anhedonia, social withdrawal, weight loss, anorexia, sleep disturbance, motor slowness, and hopelessness (Addonzio & Chamoian, 1986).

Dementia is associated with both cortical and subcortical lesions, and is caused by a variety of diseases and TBI. Chemical poisons causing dementia include alcohol; organophosphates; heavy metals such as arsenic, mercury, and lead; and trichloroethylene. Drug poisonings include haloperidol, bromides, phenytoin, lithium, barbiturates, atropine, and related compounds (Benson & Cummings, 1986).

Dementia with subcortical lesions is associated with movement disorders (chorea, rigidity, tremor, and bradykinesia). Cortical degeneration is evidenced by mental status alterations. The distinction between dementia with and without motor disorders was supported, with motor disorders associated with slowness of mental processing with the Stroop procedure, i.e., colors named and color names identified (Greiffenstein, Verma, Nichols, & Delacruz, 1989). Moreover, those with a motor disturbance seem to have a subcortical hypometabolism.

I identify dementia by a measured or estimated loss of ability represented by 15 points of IQ. Benson and Cummings (1986) suggest that this diagnosis be supported by a performance disorder in at least three of the following: speech or language, memory, cognition, visuospatial skills, or personality. Barth and Macciocchi (1986) point out the difficulty in examining demented patients because of their confusion and disorientation.

Apraxia

Apraxia is impairment of the ability to carry out purposeful movements, which were previously learned, in the presence of the basic motor skills, and sufficiently retained understanding of the nature of the task, not caused by weakness, sensory loss, or abnormal movements (Adams & Victor, 1989, pp. 46–48; Masdeu, 1985a; Reitan & Wolfson, 1985, p. 110). Apraxia may manifest deficits of planning, satisfactory plans but inability to carry them out, and/or lack of self-awareness.

Examples of apraxia include *dressing apraxia,* an inability to arrange clothing on one's body; *ideational apraxia,* an interruption in the logical succession of movements needed to carry out complex gestures, in the presence of an ability to perform individual movements; *constructional apraxia,* an inability to deal with spatial relationships; and *ideomotor or facial apraxia*, difficulty in pantomiming a task, e.g., combing hair, when they can use a real object correctly. Adams and Victor (1989) consider these symptoms to be descriptive, and attribute apraxias to disorders of association between the various parts of the cerebral cortex (often attributable to lesions of particular association pathways, see Chapter 2 on Neuroanatomy).

Loss of Conceptual Ability

The inability to see relationships and to generalize is one of the most characteristic cognitive deficits after brain damage. By loss of an abstract attitude is meant the inability to see beyond the obvious. If somebody is asked how "fly and tree are alike," the reply may be that they are "different," or that "they are high," or "they are not alike." Inability to see relationships hampers effectiveness since meaning is lost, and attention is paid to insignificant details.

Case 12. Example of Dementia

The patient was a 50-year-old immigrant with a poor knowledge of the English language. He was a high school graduate, married, had 3 years of military service, and was a blue-collar worker. Preexisting health and emotional problems were denied. His wife served as the interpreter.

Accident. He fell around 20 feet, and was unconscious for 6 hours. He was in the hospital for 12 hours, and left in a confused state, not knowing his address, only the county in which he lived.

Neuropsychological Summary of Medical Reports. Although the CT scan did not offer evidence for any mass, there was evidence of damage to the spinal nerves over a considerable distance as they leave the vertebral column (radiculopathy) and to the auditory tracts, indicated by brainstem evoked potentials of tracts between the hearing organs and auditory centers of the midbrain. Loss of left labyrinthine reactivity (nystagmus dysfunction) could be associated with brainstem damage.

The long fall made it likely that the angular and impact force of his fall stretched or tore neural synapses and/or tracts, impairing conduction, without necessarily creating the amount of bleeding that would appear on a CT scan. The follow-up hospital record indicates cognitive, sensory, somatic, and emotional deficits. Various somatic problems could be related to anxiety or to a disturbance of brainstem functions.

Current Condition. He has pain and does not want to think about the accident. He does not remember dreaming about it. He has not returned to work because of dizziness, pain in various parts of his body, fear of people, and anxiety about traveling alone. He sleeps during the day and is awake at night. His wife accompanies him when he travels. She describes him as being confused. He puts his shoes in the refrigerator, puts his keys in the door and goes away, and puts a bottle of rubbing alcohol near her bed, causing her to fear being accidentally poisoned. He cannot be trusted to go shopping.

Examination. During the examination he appeared pale, phlegmatic, restless, and spoke in a low voice. He was withdrawn and wanted to go home. He was depressed and wept when asked to do a relatively simple task such as copying the geometric Bender Gestalt figures. His right hand (preferred) grip strength (Smedley hand dynamometer) was 12 kg with a developmental age of 7, and left hand grip strength was 22.5 kg with a developmental age of 13. He saw the color violet as blue, blue and brown as black, and accurately identified red. He could not detect being touched on the left hand. When touched simultaneously on the cheek and hand (double simultaneous stimulation) he ignored the hand. When he heard a mechanical watch, the left ear sounded louder. He could not move each finger separately. Given the Block Design subtest of the WAIS-R Performance Scale, he missed the simplest assembly on the first trial. The prorated IQ (nonverbal reasoning and holistic informational processing) was 70. On the Comprehension subtest he failed all items. Asked "Why do we wash clothes?" he replied: "why wash clothes? Who? Wash?" Asked what he would do if he found an envelope on the street, he wept, and said: "From mother."

Taking into account all observations, it was concluded that he suffered from a general loss of intellectual ability, i.e., dementia, and was probably functioning in the retarded range of ability. Apparently he had suffered generalized nervous system damage, i.e., spinal cord (denervation of muscles in the range of C4–T1, primarily in the right, which would correspond to the loss of right hand grip strength), brainstem damage documented in nystagmus and hearing loss, right somesthetic area (loss of left hand sensitivity), right parietal area (inability to assemble blocks), etc. and possible left temporal verbal area (loss of verbal memory and comprehension).

10
Memory: Short- and Long-Term

Overview

Memory dysfunction is extremely complex, due to the variety of symptoms that occur, changes over time, and perhaps a dependency of symptoms upon location of lesion. In this chapter, adaptive problems created by memory deficits will be emphasized, i.e., frequently observed syndromes and symptoms, and some descriptive concepts that will be useful in understanding memory deficits of TBI victims.

It is estimated that persistent memory problems after head injury requiring hospitalization range from 43% at 23 months to 70% after 1 year for severe head injuries. These contribute substantially to poor outcome, including psychosocial functioning affecting the quality of life (Crossen & Wiens, 1988b). An extremely thorough research source including clinical findings, neuroanatomy, neurotransmitter functions, and disease syndromes is Oltron, Gamzu, & Corkin (1985).

Definition of the System

Memory is the process of storing and retrieving mental products and actions for use after different periods of retention, e.g., short, medium, and long term. It involves different kinds of encoding and retrieval for different stimuli and mental products (visual, verbal, dexterous skills). Memory gives meaning to experience and sensory information and enhances survival through remembering conditions of safety and danger. It contributes to efficient problem solving through rejection of previous unsatisfactory solutions, while saving partial products for temporary or long-term use if they are helpful.

Neuropsychological Dysfunctioning

Memory loss can be general, or related to special types of coded information (e.g., visual or verbal). Dysfunctioning includes inability to save short-term memory products and inability to retrieve information (of different kinds) from long-term memory storage. Lateralized lesions may create particular deficits of storage and retrieval. The significance of a given memory deficit depends on the demands on the individual for memory in practical adaptive functions. Sensory dysfunctions preventing reception or encoding can contribute to an apparent memory problem, although the deficit is conceptually different.

Memory and Trauma

Both isolated memory disorders and more general aphasias, created by even small lesions, interfere with mechanisms for learning and retrieving information. Since the temporal poles and orbitofrontal surface are most susceptible to trauma, and long fibers to shearing forces, the limbic and paralimbic areas and their interconnections may have a special vulnerabily in head trauma. Signoret, (1985, p. 182) has an excellent diagram of the limbic structures relevant to memory. If we assume that recovery and new learning are associated with sprouting of new connections between presynaptic and postsynaptic neurones, this is controlled by the ability of the target cell to invite sprouting and regulate the number and specificity of synaptic inputs. It does not accept synapses from every source (Schwartzkroin & Fuchs, 1989). The implication for optimal relearning and general restitution of function is presently obscure. See Chapter 15 on Stress for some physiological effects on memory and Chapter 4 on Trauma for neuronal regeneration and sprouting.

Primary Neural System

It is controversial whether different learning and memory functions are relatively localized, or whether areas and functions are inextricably related (Messing, 1987). Thompson (1988) asserts that the idea that memory is diffusely distributed in the brain is largely discounted. Rather, learning and memory involve particular systems and circuits, which are "hard wired," i.e., preexist, subject to modification (Thompson, 1988). Neuronal sprouting may occur during normal learning. Incoming axons fill available spaces, i.e., there is a change in the location and number of synaptic contacts (Schwartzkroin & Fuchs, 1989).

Structures implicated in memory include the temporal lobe [cortex (entorhinal and probably lateral), amygdala, hippocampus], frontal lobes, diencephalon (i.e., mediodorsal thalamus and mammillary bodies, see Nichelli, Bahmanian-Behbahani, Gentilini, & Vecchi 1988 for a detailed case example), bleeding into the ventricular system consequent to a caudate hemorrhage, with secondary irritation of the thalamus (Drake, Shuttleworth, & Kellum, 1988); and the region of the fourth ventricle with its noradrenergic secreting neurons (Corkin, Cohen, Sullivan, Clegg, & Rosen, 1985). Thompson (1988), in contrast to others, excludes the hippocampus and cerebral cortex as the locus for the memory trace, but the evidence presented is confined to conditioned learning in the rabbit. It is usually stated that hippocampus and amygdala are needed in memory consolidation.

One study of the global amnesic syndrome concluded that several nuclei and tracts of the thalamus and hypothalamus were involved. It is asserted (Signoret,

1985) that generalized memory loss (amnesia) occurs after bilateral involvement of limbic structures. Although memory is not located in any narrowly defined locus, comprehension and retrieval of verbal meaning are much hampered by deficits to the left temporal lobe, though not to the same extent in each person. Moreover: millothtalamic tract and internal medullary lamina were involved.

Limbic Structures and Memory

It is asserted (Signoret, 1985) that generalized memory loss (amnesia) occurs after bilateral involvement of limbic structures. Although memory is not located in any narrowly defined locus, comprehension and retrieval of verbal meaning are much hampered by deficits to the left temporal lobe, though not to the same extent in each person. The hippocampus and nearby infratemporal cortex are concerned with memory for recent events. Bilateral damage causes inability to learn new facts and skills, although intellectual level may remain relatively high. Less extensive damage can result in persistent inactivity, loss of initiative, and indifference (Carpenter & Sutin, 1983, p. 632). Skills are learned and retained without any sense of familiarity after removal bilaterally of the amygdala, hippocampus, or both (Pribram, 1980). Stress effects on hippocampal functioning are discussed in Chapter 15.

A generalization has been offered that limbic system lesions prevent the conversion of short-term into long-term memories, while lesions of the posterior thalamus create difficulties in acquiring short-term memories, but do not impair consolidation into long-term memory of what has been learned (Schwartzkroin & Fuchs, 1989). Nevertheless, the neuroanatomist Brodal (1981, p. 687) disputes the significance of amgdala and hippocampus in the consolidation of memories, and the neuropsychologist Thompson (1988) disputes the significance of hippocampus and cerebral cortex in the memory trace.

Different Kinds of Memory

This section is presented to orient the reader toward terms and concepts that are frequently used in research, which may also clarify any deficits experienced by their patients.

Loss of memory may be relatively great for particular content or categories (e.g., verbal or nonverbal, visual or auditory input), which can be related to the locus of brain damage. Visual memory tends to be impaired by right hemisphere damage, and verbal memory by left hemisphere damage (Fuchs & Phillips, 1989). (Although these are attributed to the temporal lobe, afferent pathways could be implicated, i.e., underlying visual radiation on its way to the occipital cortex, and auditory input to the superior temporal gyrus, i.e., auditory area.) Moreover, verbal processes aid problem solving in patients with visuospatial deficit. Also, left hemisphere lesioned patients can improve performance with visuospatial cues (Levin, Benton, & Grossman, 1982, p. 119). Different degrees of impairment may occur for different kinds of learning (Vilkki, 1987). (This point is seemingly disputed by Corkin et al., 1985, in cases of amnesia, see below.) Motor memory, i.e., complex acts that are built up by associations between sensory events and muscular output, has been attributed to a circuit from the sensory receptors (including vision, touch, and pain), via the inferior olivary nucleus (medulla) and inferior cerebellar peduncle, the dentate nucleus of the cerebellum, and motor output via the superior cerebellar peduncle to red nucleus, and then to motor nuclei (Thompson, 1988).

The following descriptive categories are frequently used in clinical and research literature (Baddeley, Harris, Sunderland, Watts, & Wilson, 1987; Nichelli et al., 1988).

Brief Sensory Memory Systems

These temporary stores of information include iconic (vision) and echoic (audition). Deficits could appear as perceptual difficulties, i.e., the impression that information is not received, although indeed it is not retained sufficiently long for processing.

Semantic or Declarative Memory

Storage of knowledge. Acquiring information about facts or episodes, some of which may have been learned in school, such as spelling, geography, names of objects, and verbs. Although there are numerous claims that facts are relatively spared in the presence of amnesia, long-term verbal memory (e.g., Information and Vocabulary) is often deficient relative to current processing (Similarities and Comprehension).

Procedural Memory

This refers to skills and procedures, e.g., perceptual, motor, and intellectual skills (complex cognitive learning), which tend to be preserved after brain damage (Squire & Zola-Morgan, 1985). The object of procedural memory can be to retrieve or utilize information stored in declarative memory.

Episodic or Autobiographical Memory

This is encased in the spatiotemporal context in which it is learned, e.g., memory of one's life's experiences. Personal experiences are often affected in TBI, e.g., amnesia.

Prospective Memory

Remembering to do something at a particular time.

Adaptive Functions of Memory

The significance of loss of memory refers to the demands made for particular kinds of learning in that person's life.

Retention of Personal History and Events

Mental activity is expected to have meaning within the person's history. Therefore, loss of a sense of familiarity interferes with one's relationship to individuals and events. Inability to remember the significance of various stimuli makes them meaningless, e.g., the sensory agnosias, inability to recognize faces, etc. One man described himself as "waking up to a brand new world every morning" (McMahon & Satz, 1981). So extreme a deficit prevents understanding of the full impact of this memory loss on his life, which he cannot express. Only collaterals inform him of the conditions of his life.

Learning New Procedures and Skills

These solve adaptive tasks in school, job, and daily life. Problem solving depends on integrated use of short-term memory and retrieval of information from long-term memory storage. The brain-damaged person does not learn from experience. There are deficits in cognition, foresight, memory, etc., which create repetitive unsatisfactory or self-destructive events (see Chapter 13, on Frontal Lobe Syndromes).

Retrieval of Skills and Information

Most daily activities are a function of long-term memory storage, including employment and household necessities, but many automatic or overlearned activities seem relatively invulnerable to memory loss. However, not remembering to turn a stove off, although simple, is life-threatening to the person and community. Not remembering which goods and customers are the specialty of a salesman is devastating to a sales manager. Not remembering changes in a patient's condition, or the characteristics of new procedures and drugs, would make a physician incompetent.

Loss of communications memory (e.g., word seeking) is related to aphasia (see Chapter 12 on aphasia). Apraxia, the loss of ability to perform familiar skilled movements, prosapagnosia, the inability to remember familiar faces (De Renzi, 1986), and other perceptual deficits have been considered in Chapter 7 on Sensorimotor Functions.

Some Functional Components of Memory

Memory Is Dependent on Concentration

Memory may be impaired as a consequence of an attentional disorder. It is necessary to attend to an event to remember it later, including selection of an event one is to pay attention to, ability to divide attention, and sustaining attention over a period of time. If a person is distracted, events will not register or be efficiently retrieved. Nissen (1986) states that memory requires alertness (a general process of readiness to react to information, capacity (conscious mental effort requiring intention or controlled processing), and selection (allocation of the limited capacity for attention to one stimulus or process rather than another).

One brain damaged patient pressed at an examination before trial (EBT) for information concerning an accident, could not recall facts due to confusion during the questioning by a defense attorney. He is oversensitive to noise and is unable to filter out signals.

Working Memory and Reference Memory

Some mental products are retained only long enough to complete a task. Working memory contains a limited amount of information, amounting to a picture of what is going on at the moment. It may be conceptualized as an executive system coordinating subsidiary systems, including verbal and phonological components, and a visuospatial sketch pad involved in imagery.

A deficit of working memory hampers the ability to solve problems and to retain directions.

• Complex or length problems: For example, on the oral arithmetic section of an intelligence test, as the problems become longer, the patient may ask the examiner to repeat the question, which has been forgotten before a solution is obtained.
• Retention of previous parts: working memory also permits the individual to remember which partial solutions have been tried and found insufficient so that they are not used again.

Different Periods of Retention Required

It is convenient to describe memory demands as

• *Short term* (a few seconds, perhaps up to a minute).
• *Intermediate or medium* (30 minutes and more, but this is a convention used due to practical demands of assessing longer retention than short term, e.g., with the Wechsler Memory Scale-Revised, 1987).
• *Long-term,* which for practical purposes means anything from 1 day to permanent retention. Information may be temporarily available, but if not placed in long-term memory storage it is as though there was no memory. Long-term memory is a conceptually infinite record of past experience (Hall, 1983).

Stimulus Modality

There is evidence that particular kinds of sensory input may be differentially impaired for new learning and retrieval, e.g., visual and auditory. The deficit may involve receiving, coding, placing in temporary or long-term storage, and retrieval. Interference with problem solving is discriminable from poor comprehension. Loss may vary with content, interval between learning and demand, and the locus of brain damage.

Some Syndromes and Symptoms

Posttraumatic Amnesia

This has been discussed in Chapter 6 on Consciousness. The remaining memory symptoms refer to the period after the patient becomes oriented, although, as has been observed above, orientation and consolidating memories may be independent. Therefore, the amnesic syndrome, discussed below, may overlap with posttraumatic amnesia (PTA), particularly if there has been a coma. Baddeley et al. (1987) determined that PTA greater than 1 day was associated with deficits measured 20 years later, including complex adaptive tasks such as vocabulary and arithmetic, various perceptualmotor tasks, and sorting tasks. PTA tended to be longer with penetrating than nonpenetrating head injuries (Korean Conflict Veterans). The duration of PTA correlated with measures of severity of injury, i.e., unconsciousness, medical complications, and seizures.

Retrograde Amnesia (RA)

This is loss of memory for events prior to accident (immediate and distant events and experiences). The writer's experience is in accord with Corkin et al. (1987), that RA is far less common than anterograde amnesia. It does not predict cognitive deficits studied 20 years later, while PTA does. As retrograde amnesia clears, it begins with recollection of memories from the most distant past (Levin et al., 1982, p. 81).

One extreme example was a youth who was asked whether he had any prior emotional or physical problems, and stated: "I forgot everything about me before the accident. I forgot who was my family."

Anterograde Amnesia

This is a loss of memory for events from the moment of injury onward. The person may slip in and out of consciousness, with some retention of memory in the "islands" of awareness. The length of anterograde amnesia includes reduced alertness and confusion. This can have forensic implications, since the victim is unaware of his actions after an accident, the presence of witnesses, or other details of an accident.

Amnesic Syndrome

This is an apparently permanent, or extremely long lasting loss of general memory. The greatest loss is in formation of new memories (anterograde amnesia), but there can be loss of stored memories (RA) as well. The patients are disoriented in time, confused, and continuously ask where they are (Strub & Black, 1988, pp. 287–288).

The nature of amnesia is controversial, i.e., whether it represents a unified system or a variety of deficits. It has been asserted that "amnesia does not represent a total breakdown in memory, but rather a disruption of specific memory functions" (Nichelli et al., 1988). In contrast, after neuropsychological study of global amnesia of different etiologies, including closed head injury, it was concluded by Corkin et al. (1985) that "Findings of quantitative but not qualitative differences. . .are consistent with the view that there is one form of amnesia resulting from invasion of a single neural system for fact learning."

Basic aspects of "bitemporal" amnesia are (McClelland, 1985):

- Damage to medial temporal lobe structures, which results in a correlated deficit of anterograde and retrograde amnesia;
- Not only a deficit in the acquisition of new knowledge, but more rapid loss of information once it has been acquired;
- Inability to access prior experience;
- Simultaneous recovery of the ability to acquire new experiences and remember lost ones.

Transient Global Amnesia (TGA)

This has been defined as a sudden and relatively reversible loss of the ability to record recently acquired information, from all spheres, into permanent memory. The onset is sudden, with confusion and repetitive questions, but without focal neurological features. During the attack it appears that there are no gross deficits of personality and behavior, language, cognition, visuospatial function, or neurological status (Hodges & Ward, 1989). It can be triggered by a mild blow to the head, possibly leading to a migrainous disturbance, followed by an amnesic attack grossly disproportionate to the degree of trauma. Short-term memory is preserved, but there is a sudden, temporary inability to store new memories for 2 to 24 hours, extensive retrograde amnesia (from a day to a month), queries about their condition, and disorientation for time. There is permanent amnesia for the attack, and permanent retrograde amnesia of ½ to 2 hours. Recovery is gradual, with subclinical memory impairment for some time. TGA must be differentiated from the dissociation found in hysteria (see below) (Drake et al., 1988; Haas & Ross, 1986; Hodges & Ward, 1989; Strub & Black, 1988, pp. 289–290).

Psychogenic Amnesia

This is reduced familiarity with, or experiencing the significance of, individuals and events, due to loss of associations. Emotional pain can prevent a person from remembering certain details about a trauma. Head injury, the conditions of the accident, and its after-effects could trigger this psychological defense. In hysteria, the victim acts normally, learns during the episode, but reports amnesia only when the episode is over.

Confabulation

This is an attempt to conceal gaps in memory by inventing details. It is associated with denial of memory loss.

Prosopagnosia

Not being able to recognize faces can be due to problems of perceptual processing or memory, or can occur when there is a particular kind of demand for performance (Ellis & Young, 1988, Chapter 4). It is associated with right posterior hemisphere damage, along with dressing apraxia, unilateral spatial agnosia or neglect, and poor nonverbal learning. As with other lateralized functions, some perceptual contribution is made by the left hemisphere to facial perception, i.e., recognition, associations, and semantic categorization, which seem independent of form organization (Landis, Regard, Bliestle, & Kleihues, 1988).

Clinical Examples

The following case illustrates significant anterograde and retrograde amnesia.

Case 13. A middle-aged man was struck by a wind-blown object. The neurological diagnosis of cerebral concussion evolved from the evidence for loss of consciousness, impact to head and neck, and subcortical damage (pupillary dysfunction), followed by a variety of cognitive and sensory deficiencies. The possible preexisting arteriosclerosis was insufficient to account for the symptoms experienced before the accident or currently.

The patient had military service, achieved a B.A. in art, and was currently employed in a job utilizing visual arts. He reports that he saw an object falling toward him. He was unconscious for minutes. It was 20 minutes before he felt like himself. He went to the hospital briefly. He believes that it was there that he lost his memory. He could not call anyone because he could not remember he was married. He is not sure how he got home, and he fell asleep in the bus. He recognized his wife, but not 2 of his children. "I recognized my wife more from her voice than her face. At church I didn't recognize the minister's wife whom I'd known for 15 years. I would introduce myself to people and they said: 'You know who I am.' I would go to stores and find myself 5 miles from the store in the opposite direction. When I finally realized and drove to the store, I didn't know what I wanted. I had problems getting back home. I didn't recognize the street where I lived for 20 years. It's getting better. Now I can walk again." He also had trouble keeping the days of the week in order. He would think Monday was Wednesday.

He was out of work for a while. His position requires visual perception, artistic ability, and manual dexterity. He states that he cannot take pressure, loses his temper, his hands are tremulous, and his productivity is half of what it used to be. Loss of efficiency will keep him from assuming a more lucrative and responsible position. Current symptoms include excessive urination and dizziness. At times he does not know where he is. He had seizures, resulting in confusion. Once he blacked out in a pool and had to be rescued. He has nightmares once a week, thinks about the accident every day, and forgot his native language.

Adaptability: "My wife has to take care of me. I can't function. I feel like a vegetable. She has to tell me when to take medication." He could double his income but cannot assume greater responsibility.

Identity: "I'm a different person. I'm more somber. I tried to commit suicide several times. I look at things from the bad side. I can't let myself laugh and enjoy life." He describes his feelings as weaker, and he hides them. Yet he has trouble controlling his temper. He flares up because he thinks his wife is checking on him. "I wish I had been killed instantly because I have suffered so much." He considers the future to be grim.

Case 14 illustrates inability to retrieve procedures for use in problem solving, and secondly, how the loss of associations, or intermediate steps, also hampers cognitive ability.

A man was in a 6 hour coma after he was on his bicycle and struck by a car. During the examination he repeatedly expressed frustration at the difficult items, which he claimed he could perform before the accident. "It's not there. There's a blankness in my mind and I can't figure nothing out. Sometimes its hard with the TV channels. I think of the program I want to watch but I can't think of the channel. I don't think of looking it up because I am used to knowing the channel."

Conclusion

The numerous cortical, subcortical, brainstem, and cerebellar areas to which functional importance has been attributed are reflected in the many kinds of memory processes in the unimpaired individual and deficits after traumatic brain injury. This situation reflects both the integrated nature of neuropsychological functioning and widespread neurological damage after TBI.

11
Efficiency and Control

Overview

Mental efficiency includes functions such as *problem-solving style, concentration, planning*, and *behavioral monitoring*. This chapter will illustrate component functions, and how their disorders contribute to impairment. Sometimes referred to as the "executive function" (Lezak, 1983; Stuss & Benson, 1986), the mental efficiency system involves many relatively narrow temperamental and cognitive functions, which are very vulnerable to damage to widely scattered areas of the brain. Deficits range from subtle, though impairing, to obviously disabling. Deficits of mental efficiency are related to problems of cerebral emotional disorder, including the frontal lobe syndrome. Patterns of emotional, motivational, and cognitive dysfunctioning are given in Chapter 13 on the Frontal Lobe Syndromes.

The role of the mental efficiency system in adaptation may be illustrated by the complaint of a patient: "I'm confused. I don't know if its all in my head or if it really happened. I can't understand why I can't dust myself off and start over again."

Cognitive control is relatively independent of level of intellectual ability, although it supports it. We have all met individuals, without outstanding education or high intelligence, who were admirable in the effectiveness with which they coped with personal or job problems. Similarly, memory is dependent on the integrity of other functions, e.g., attention, motivation, and programming (Bowen, 1989).

Definition of the System

Mental efficiency supports intellectual ability, relying on intact consciousness, attention, task selection, concentration, and motivation. Additional functions include efficient problem-solving skills, assessing one's status within the context of ongoing activities (monitoring), processing problems at a realistic pace, imagination in the form of planning and foresight to anticipate the consequences of an action, maintaining a satisfactory standard of performance, monitoring ongoing performance (recognizing, avoiding, and rejecting errors), flexibility to

178

adapt to change or unexpected circumstances, speed of informational processing, selection of activities for safety and well-being, style of cognitive operations (trial and error or preplanning), and initiating actions for necessity or pleasure.

Neuropsychological Dysfunctioning

Dysfunctioning of mental efficiency reduces problem-solving ability, even in the presence of seemingly unimpaired intellectual level (e.g., retained IQ). This can offer the false impression of reduced mental ability. It is characterized by inability to remain with a task, immature problem-solving approaches such as trial and error, inflexibility, perseveration of inappropriate activity, inability to monitor and improve ongoing activities, lack of concern about the results of actions, an apparent disconnection between intellectual awareness and what the person has actually performed or promised in the real world, and difficulty with performing adequately after a delay. Information is processed slowly, even if correctly. There are difficulties in suppressing an incorrect response among alternatives, and in responding correctly after a delay. Deficits of cognitive organization overlap motor programs, and have been categorized by Jason Brown (summarized by Bowen, (1989): (1) loss of initiative, with inertia, apathy, dyscontrol, and poor anticipation of consequences; (2) general defect in organization and self-monitoring; and (3) defects in final implementation.

Primary Neural Systems

Deficits of the executive functions appear to be maximal after frontal lobe damage (Stuss & Benson, 1986, p. 216). The frontal lobes, in particular the prefrontal area (rostral to the motor cortex), are believed to integrate the system of mental efficiency. Its rich interconnections with cortical, subcortical, diencephalic, brainstem, and spinal levels make it vulnerable to lesions elsewhere. It integrates sensory information after it has been processed in the occipital, temporal, and parietal lobes. Input is received from other integrative areas. Program ming of both cognitive and motor functions occurs here. These are further coordinated, and then transmitted to the motor area. Selective attention is dependent on the integrity of many higher cortical functions, so that a deficit almost anywhere can be impairing (Fowler, Richards, Berent, & Boll, 1987).

Special Contribution of the Frontal Lobes

Considerable details will be found in Bowen (1989) concerning anatomical and conceptual considerations concerning frontal lobe locus and cognitive or behavioral function. The frontal lobes seem to access possible concepts and programs, select among them, and then execute an integrated outcome. It receives information about ongoing activities (monitoring), which are considered to anticipate the consequences of plans and actions. Possible consequences of action are anticipated by the integrative capability of the prefrontal cortex. Ongoing responses are monitored for efficiency and match with a predetermined plan, and modified or discontinued in the unimpaired individual. Many mental functions can be carried out by the posterior systems, but are likely to be performed automatically and without the richness of the intact person (Stuss & Benson, 1986, pp. 248–249). Animal research suggests that the frontal lobes are essential to keep prior information in mind for a delay to make a correct response subsequently, and to retain information to perform an alternative (Fuchs & Phillips, 1989).

The dysfunctions of patients with frontal lobe lesions have been summarized by Fuchs and Phillips (1989): initiating behavior, switching from one strategy to another, using mistakes to alter performance, suppress incorrect responses, string together simple behaviors to produce a more complicated one, and deal with distractions.

Components of Mental Efficiency

It is useful to differentiate between the highest level of cognitive difficulty with which a person can cope without constraints of time, and the efficiency of problem solving with the ordinary demands of reality. The issue confronted here is which subsidiary functions contribute to effectiveness in solving a wide range of adaptive requirements.

Executive Function

How or whether a person engages in independent, purposeful and self-serving behavior involves executive function (see Lezak, 1983, p. 38). This is contrasted with cognitive functions, i.e., what a person does, or how well, e.g., specific functions, skills, and abilities.

Selective Attention

Targets of attention are processed at different stages of incoming stimuli, where centrally available information is brought to bear concerning the stimuli's relevance, or its own demand for consideration (Nuechterlein & Asarnow, 1989). Attention may be conceived of as having a limited capacity. We allocate our resources to a particular task according to its importance. At low levels of arousal, few available resources lead to failure of attention. At high levels of arousal, performance is impaired due to the necessity of discriminating between relevant and irrelevant stimuli.

The determinants of attention include

- *Categorization:* A concept is formed, to which attention is directed, from experience with certain kinds of objects, people, or ideas, expectation on the basis of prior experience, interest, danger, importance, and attractiveness.
- *Filtering:* These preselected targets are looked for and sustained in attention, and others are rejected.

- *Novelty.* New stimuli *activate* the brain; constant stimuli create *habituation*.
- *Danger.* Extreme stimuli, or representatives of particular classes, e.g., a wild beast, will grab our attention.

Goal-Setting, Planning, Initiative

The unimpaired individual can anticipate a future circumstance (for advantage or avoiding danger), which will be created if action is taken. Goal (I would like the house to look better), planning (I will need three cans of paint), and initiative (today is Saturday, so I will buy the paint and work until the job is finished).

Imagination

A mental image helps to estimate the *likely effectiveness* of a move before actually making a commitment. The alternative is trial and error, a problem-solving style characteristic of children or impaired individuals. A more mature problem-solving style, characteristic of unimpaired adults (regardless of mental level) is *preplanning a response.*

Concentration

Concentration is the ability to maintain attention and activity on a task for a useful period of time, while avoiding distractibility. This requires filtering out irrelevent stimuli, and maintaining incoming selected information or mental products in awareness for further processing.

Monitoring

Monitoring is observing ongoing activity to assess the situation, and detect errors, then making an appropriate move. Successful achievement of goals, and execution of plans generally, requires feedback (Pribram, 1980). The individual becomes aware of his environment, and then changes behavior to reduce any deviations from the mental representation of a goal. Concert pianist Van Cliburn put it well in a radio interview: "A performer must be 50% on the stage and 50% in the audience."

Flexibility

- *Changing our behavior as a situation changes:* This is required in employment, i.e., new assignments, markets, customers, supervisors, colleagues, etc., or in life, i.e., marriage, moving our domicile, changing schools.
- *Changing responses when an attempt is poor:* Recognizing errors or inefficiency to improve success or meet the standards of a particular goal.

Foresight and Judgment

Success and emotional well-being depend as much on avoiding trouble as efficient maneuvers (Parker, 1981).

Speed of Informational Processing

Effective processing is measured by the speed with which a task is completed, as well as the number of successes or their maximum difficulty. One's employer values productivity and performing cognitive and mechanical tasks at a speed that is useful.

Representative Symptoms

The following deficits are commonly observed after TBI. Representative procedures to assess efficiency and control are found in discussions of executive function (Lezak, 1983), frontal lobe function (Bilder & Goldberg, 1987), and Chapter 21 on Assessment.

Problems of Selecting an Appropriate Response

Reduced Flexibility or Perseveration

Inability to modify strategy or details of performance when circumstances change or an error is apparent. Perseveration is the tendency to offer the same response after it is no longer appropriate, fusing of a previous task with a new one, or inability to turn off a response after it has been initiated. One basis may be inability to generate new responses (Goldberg & Bilder, 1987; Bilder & Goldberg, 1987). It is a reliable indicator of brain damage (one of the few pathognomonic symptoms).

Inability to Divide Attention or Cope with Alternatives

• Selecting a correct alternative from several possibilities;
• Multiple stimuli or ideas cannot be considered simultaneously;
• Multiple ideas cannot be considered alternatively.

Impersistence

The inability to persevere in a task until it is completed.

Inability to Concentrate

The person is easily distracted and therefore unable to attend to a task continuously. The performance may be discontinued, or the mind wanders (Zomeren, Brouwer, & Deelman, 1984).

Improper Focus of Attention

Attention is given to an improper level of a hierarchy (either a higher level of organization or a detail, or an inappropriate detail among many).

Deficient Problem-Solving Style

Poor Standards of Performance

There is a reduced level of performance compared with preinjury status, with no effort to improve errors and inadequacies.

Recognizing Errors and Reality Testing

This is a component of monitoring. The brain-damaged person is less effective in recognizing errors in advance, before action is taken, or in recognizing an error after it has been expressed, and then nullifying it.

Regression

Many errors made by victims of brain damage are somewhat characteristic of performance of chidren, i.e., simplified, immature, or lacking details. This is differentiable from pathognomonic errors, which are more characteristic of brain damage alone.

Impaired Planning and Decision-Making

This involves poor selection of strategies, e.g., trial and error rather than pre-planning.

Poor Judgment

Defective Monitoring

As action or ideas are developed and expressed, the individual does not control ongoing action to ensure that results match the preplanned goal or inner model.

Feedback Is Ignored

Errors are not corrected and performance is avoidably poor.

Inability to Recognize Errors

Reduced cognitive ability, e.g., comprehension, and visuospatial ability, may be reflected in low level perceptual ability with deficits of monitoring.

The Person Does Not Learn from Experience

This is a common and disabling deficit in dysfunction of the efficiency and control system, and is frequently attributed to frontal lobe injury.

Autistic Reactions

Unrealistic perceptions, or overly personalized ideas, paranoid reactions, etc., can be release phenomena or secondary reactions to stress and impairment. The person may not recognize these deficits, and/or be unable to reject them as unrealistic.

Lack of Foresight and Judgment

Inability to predict consequences of one's actions, and to understand how others react to one's behavior, are commonly impaired after brain injury. This is discussed in detail in Chapter 13 on Frontal Lobe Syndromes.

Reduced Speed of Informational Processing and Problem Solving

Information is received and coded more slowly. The person is unable to keep up with others. Productivity, in the sense of amount of goods or ideas produced, is reduced.

- The author recently examined four individuals who had completed professional school, but needed documentation for the Board of Examiners that they had "dyslexia," to qualify for more time to complete the licensing examination. They had the ability to complete professional training, but from childhood required extra time to complete examinations. Histories included trauma, high fever, etc.
- Slow thinking is characteristic of brain damage. I was told of this example by the wife of a patient who was suffering from dementia after a head injury, and was confronted with rapid-fire questions by a psychologist who was retained by the defendant's attorney. He ignored the request to slow down, and the patient's increasing distress and suspiciousness. Result: The stress precipitated a grand mal seizure!

Clinical Examples

1. Case 15 suggests a *deficit of monitoring*, i.e., a woman was very ineffective when she had to match her performance against a mental image of the correct response. During the examination, she made frequent errors in following instructions, as well as deficits in copying models by drawing them. Her Wechsler Adult Intelligence Scale-Revised Perceptual Organizational Factor scores (closely related subtests) were particularly low.

2. Case 16 represents a *deficit of planning and initiative*. A professional man, who was in an automobile accident in which he struck his head against the windshield, described his inability to organize himself. On a given day he cannot decide what he must do. He can waste the whole day in a decision. His morale

is low because he cannot count on himself. He does not generate any plans for himself, but acknowledges that he does well in a structured situation, i.e., when others set up a plan for him. Therefore, he wants to reprogram himself (in the sense of a computer doing what a program determines). If somebody tells him what to do he performs it well. After expressing pride in teaching himself how computers work, he stated: "If you slip a disc in me, and press 'enter,' I will know what to do. I am missing the drive, the program, the diskette, the commands, everything it needs. I have the hardware, i.e., feet, eyes, hands."

3. Case 17 represents a *deficit of decision making*. A woman had a slight accident, not requiring her to go to the hospital, while driving her car. She thinks about the accident every time her back hurts, i.e., several times per day, but has not had any dreams about it. Asked what was the worst effect of the accident, she replied that she is frightened by driving, will not use a cab, and has severe anxiety about activities unrelated to the accident, and depression. Asked about the effect of the accident on her life and goals, she stated that it was necessary to cancel a variety of plans. She could not make a business presentation. She was asked if she saw herself as different, or not her real self. "I was at a business meeting. I was not there. The words had no meaning. I couldn't make a decision when asked. I was someplace else. I wasn't functioning. I couldn't think. I was important and I couldn't be part of it. In another professional matter I could not come to a decision." Are there any changes in your feelings since the accident? "I feel terrible. I can't drive home to be with my daughter. I also broke a plan with a friend." How do you feel about the future? "I hope I'll be all right, emotionally more than the pain. I hope I'll get over my fear of driving. I feel out of control of my life. I'm doing stupid things."

12
Communications Problems—Aphasia

Overview

Communications, verbal expression, and comprehension in particular may be our most significant adaptive skill. We use it to exchange information with the world, to signal ourselves during problem solving, and to encode memories. Loss of communication ability is a common after-effect of brain damage, i.e., difficulties in understanding others and expressing oneself verbally. Aphasia often improves over time, being most common immediately posttrauma with severe brain damage (Levin, 1981; Sarno, 1981b). Loss of ability to communicate may vary with the mode of expression, e.g., writing or vocalizing.

Some Linguistic Definitions

The reader will find these definitions and concepts useful in further study of the aphasic literature.

Phonemes: The minimal sound units that constitute meaning.
Phonology: The science of speech sounds, including *phonetics* (production and reception of sounds, emphasizing written symbols) and *phonemics* (the study of the phonemes of a language).
Grapheme: The sum of letters and their combinations representing a single phoneme.
Morpheme: A linguistic unit that cannot be broken down into smaller units, e.g., short words, modifiers (ly), and letters creating a plural (s).
Lexicon: The morphemes of a language.
Syntax: The structural relationship among words in sentences.
Semantics: The relationship between *signs* (pointing to the presence of something that is not immediately evident) and *symbols* (e.g., a material object, in this instance perhaps a printed word, representing an idea).
Grammar: The rules of a language.
Pragmatics: Patterns of language use.

Prosody: Prosody refers to rhythm and intonation and other nonverbal qualities, which convey emotional and attitudinal information about the speaker.

One may contrast *language* (a system of units and rules for applying them, structured in components such as phonology and syntax), and *communication* (which includes nonverbal components such as prosody and pragmatics) (American Heritage Illustrated Dictionary; Berndt & Caramazza; 1981; Blumstein, 1981). Nonverbal, expressive-communicative forms of behavior include symbolic, paralinguistic, and affective events (Golper, 1985).

Symbolic events: Hand gestures, body movements, facial expressions, pantomimes, sign language, etc., substituting for words.

Paralinguistic events: A nonverbal communication including nonlexical spoken utterances (e.g., "um"), speech rate, pitch and stress, hand, body, and eye movements, and gestures in tempo with speech or expressive movements (Golper, 1985).

Affective events: Expression of feelings through facial expressions, vocal tone, speech rate, pitch, stress, various hand and body movements, as well as verbal statements consistent with affect.

Definition of the System

The system involves understanding information and instructions, and expressing one's thoughts and feelings so as to respond to others or express one's own needs and ideas. Included are (1) reception, (2) processing, (3) comprehension, (4) expression, (5) ability to structure and comprehend language according to basic grammatical rules, (6) learned skills such as reading, writing, and spelling, and (7) motor capacity, i.e., clear speech. Although primarily involving language skills and comprehension, communications also utilize nonverbal emotional qualities such as facial expression, prosody (tone of voice), and comprehension of the context within which an event occurs. This is discussed in detail in Chapter 13 on Cerebral Personality Disorders.

Basic Neural System

Communications utilize varied sensory circuits for input, central processing, and motor output, regardless of the content of the information or response, whether language or nonlanguage (Reitan & Wolfson, 1985, p. 12). Although the left temporal lobe is traditionally described as the prime generator of verbal ability, right hemisphere involvement in processing aspects of language is well established. To some extent it substitutes for the brain-damaged left hemisphere, particularly in very young brain-damaged children. Moreover, the right cerebral hemisphere plays a significant role in aspects of communication requiring visual perception (recognizing patterns such as words, faces, etc.). Almost the total area of the cortex, when lesioned, can contribute to language disorders, if one considers the various diagrams offered by Benson (1985). Strub and Black (1981, p. 262) emphasize (with examples) individual differences in language localization and dominance. Damage to the frontal lobes bilaterally contributes to dysarthria, i.e., loss of control over the speech musculature, and to the left frontal lobe permits normal muscle control but there are deficits in programming of speech sounds (1985). Subcortical lesions (left sided thalamic and basal ganglia lesions) also create serious aphasic problems, i.e., deficits of voice control, timing, speech initiation and modulation, Tourette's syndrome, etc. (Van Lancker, 1985). The left peri-Rolandic area usually controls speech production (damage leads to articulation problems). The right peri-Rolandic area seems to substitute for the transmission of articulatory impulses to the speech muscles after damage to this region on the left (Murdoch, Chenery, & Kennedy, 1989). The motor speech area is expressed through cranial nerves VII, X, XI, and XII, which control the muscles of articulation. Many cortical, brainstem, and cerebellar areas can also be involved (upper motor neuron) (see in particular, Cranial Nerves, Chapter 2).

Two Phases of Language Have Neuroanatomical Correlates

Propositional speech: Transmitting ideas utilizes the supplementary motor area (SMA) and right Broca's area (see Chapter 2 on Neuroanatomy). The latter area is also involved with prosody, or the emotional content of speech (Bowen, 1989).

Nonpropositional speech: Relatively automatic verbal usage, e.g., counting, frequently used phrases. Nonpropositional speech can access the motor cortex in the presence of lesions of the SMA and Broca's area.

Neuropsychological Dysfunctioning

Symptoms vary considerably with the extent, location, age at injury, and elapsed time since the injury. Deficits may be receptive (decoding incoming information), expressive (comprehending and organizing and communicating ideas), or motor. Impairment can be related to lesions in particular sensory systems (e.g., auditory or visual), to association tracts between them and other areas offering meaning and organization into programs, or to motor expression at the cerebral level. Overt aphasia is a characteristic syndrome after major brain damage. However, except for anomia, in outpatient professional practice it is rare. Rather one sees "subclinical" deficits of communications that are easy to miss (see below). This is discussed in greater detail in Chapter 16 on Expressive Deficits.

Reading and writing are among the language abilities most vulnerable to TBI, and are difficult to study because of the complex range of abilities on which they depend (Van Lancker, 1985). A pragmatic rating scale has been offered, which reflects useful components of communication. It appears to be useful in assessing inpatients, recent victims of brain damage, and the lower end of the outpatient

TBI continuum (Ehrlich & Barry, 1989): intelligibility, eye gaze, sentence formation (grammar and complexity), coherence of narrative, topic (maintaining direction), initiation of communication.

Complexity of Language Skills

Parallel Distributed Processing

There are various components of language processing, i.e., semantic, linguistic, phonetic, etc. When one module is removed, the deficits result from the residual function of that network, with no implication made concerning the association of an aspect of processing with a given neural structure (Lytton & Brust, 1989).

Relationship to Memory

Deficits in language skills illustrate the interrelatedness of cognitive functions. Communications problems can be due to loss of memory, which in turn can be attributable to inadequacy of higher level comprehension functions (McCarthy & Warrington, 1987).

Reading

Reading is an example of the concept that different kinds of processing simultaneously contribute to comprehension and memory. Learning to read involves phonological processing and visual processing. Visual processing requires a subsequent process of transformation into a sequence and then phoneme (sound decoding, Code, 1987, p. 54). Reading can involve two systems (Lytton & Brust, 1989).

Direct, i.e., a visual route from the word form to the semantic system. Words are interpreted as whole symbols (e.g., Chinese ideograms), and comprehension precedes verbalization.

Phonological, i.e., letters are converted to sounds to construct words, and pronunciation precedes comprehension.

Anomia

Anomia (word finding difficulty) also illustrates the complexity of higher processes (Kirshner et al., 1987). Identification of objects requires integrated input from various systems. Different locations of anatomical damage contributed different reasons for anomic errors. Perceptual (visual) errors were associated with right-hemisphere strokes. Patients' verbal and/or communications problems did not lead to many visually related errors compared to semantic ones. With impaired visual input, the stimulus is inadequately conveyed to verbal processing areas, leading to reduced accuracy of identification or to misidentification.

Subclinical Deficits

Aphasia is usually followed by significant improvement. Therefore, overt aphasic difficulties are more characteristic of the most severely injured patients, or acute patients with lesser impairment, than most outpatient TBI victims some time after the injury.

The professional involved with the brain-damaged person in the community should be alert to subtle signs of communication disorder after TBI. Subclinical aphasia has been described by Levin (1981). Communications seem normal with superficial examination, yet subclinical verbal deficits often exist. Careful observation, perhaps with the challenge to respond to difficult verbal problems or tasks, reveals significant deficits. Careful listening may be needed to detect inability to express ideas with full complexity. A person may use single words to substitute for appropriate richness of expression, and yet get a full score on some tests of verbal ability (Wilson, 1986).

Traditional aphasia batteries may lack sensitivity to the particular problems of the victim of closed head injury, which differs from the language population of other aphasic patients (Penn & Cleary, 1989). Many aphasic syndromes are infrequent in traumatic brain injured patients after a period of recovery. There is evidence that head injured adult language symptomology differs from that of aphasics with vascular etiology. There is a more generalized language deficit associated with global cognitive impairment. This contributes to reduced effectiveness in communications in therapeutic and social situations, and is a poor prognostic indicator for return to work (Ehrlich & Barry, 1989).

General comprehension deficits should be differentiated from aphasia (more narrow deficits in the use of language or communications). The extent of the loss of ability to comprehend and to express complex ideas will vary with the extent and location of the injury.

Compensation

There can be many reasons why a person will deliberately cover up, including embarrassment at word seeking, loss of mental ability, etc. (see Chapter 16, Expressive Deficits). Therefore, unless the listener challenges the brain-damaged individual with relatively complex verbal ideas and problems, a deficit may not be detected. Embarrassment causes evasiveness in content and manner of speech, ultimately leading to social withdrawal. This is considered by some to be the most common after-effect of brain damage.

With careful testing, the following problems of communication can be detected even when the patient seemingly has recovered:

1. Reduced ability to comprehend and express ideas, information, and other communications;
2. Inability to repeat what one hears;

3. Inability to associate visual stimulation with verbal meaning;
4. Unclear speech (see dysarthria, below).

Subclinical verbal deficits are masked by seemingly adequate conversation, since it requires relatively little intelligence to maintain a simple conversation, e.g., current events in the person's life, how one feels, or daily activities. The examiner, interviewer, or teacher can be deceived by the statement that all is well and that normal activities are participated in.

A Taxonomy of Compensatory Strategies
(Penn & Cleary, 1989)

Simplification: The message is condensed, simplified, unmeaningful words inviting further comment by the other speaker.
Elaboration: Expansion and circumlocution to ensure effective transmission.
Repetition: To help processing and hold the listener's attention.
Fluency: Place holders (nonmeaningful utterances) and pauses.
Sociolinguistic: Sensitivity to the needs of the other speaker, e.g., taking one's turn, self-corrections.
Non-verbal: Words, gestures, intonations that support, substitute, or add to a message.
Interlocutor: This refers to actions by the nonpatient that facilitates conversational flow, e.g., assistance, changes of speed, cueing.

Symptoms and Syndromes Associated with TBI

Difficulty in understanding and expressing language, resulting from a newly acquired disorder of the central nervous system, can be associated with a deficit of comprehension, of physiological mechanisms to control and express speech, or of understanding or expressing the structure of language (syntax). The author is in full accord with Benson (1985) when he describes the aphasia literature as "chaos" with proliferation of classification schemes. Therefore, this presentation is to orient the reader, without subscribing to any particular taxonomy. Benson (1985, p. 33) offers a chart with types of aphasia listed with their characteristics on these dimensions: spontaneous speech, paraphasia, comprehension, repetition, and naming. Some conditions described in the aphasia literature are eliminated here as not generally occurring after TBI.

The following description of aphasic symptoms and syndromes includes concepts found in clinical reports and research literature (Benson, 1985; Damasio, 1981; Goodglass & Kaplan, 1983; Strub & Black, 1981; Stuss and Benson, 1986, Chapter 11). A close association between lesion and symptom is not attempted, except where it illustrates a previously discussed principle of neurological or neuropsychological functioning. *The description begins with relatively limited symptoms.*

Word Naming Deficit (Anomia)

Anomia is considered to be a variety of fluent aphasia, and often appears subclinically. There is reduced ability to retrieve the name of objects, people, and places when confronted with them (e.g., a picture), and also in finding appropriate words in ordinary conversation. The patient is verbose, offering circumlocutions (substitute words and phrases) for what cannot be retrieved from memory.

Dysarthria

Dysarthria is a disorder of the cerebral motor mechanism of speech articulation (not loss of understanding, or damage to the nerves or structure of the muscles, larynx, etc.). As a motor problem, dysarthria should be differentiated from inability to organize the motor components of the verbal expression. Comprehension deficits (dementia) should be differentiated from aphasic deficits more narrowly attributable to the use of language or communications. Dysarthria can be caused by defective speech production and planning. It is also attributable to the mechanics of speech, i.e., as opposed to its syntax and complexity.

Paraphasia

Paraphasia is "the central sign of aphasia, consisting of a substitution of an incorrect and unintended word or sound for a correct one" (Damasio, 1981). It is not identical with a dysarthritic inability to pronounce words. Expression of language occurs through unintended syllables, words, or phrases.

Agrammatism

Agrammatism is a loss of ability to speak grammatically due to brain disease. There is telegraphic verbal output. Nouns and verbs may be used, but indicators of tense, person, and number, and other parts of speech are lost. Comprehension is impaired.

Agraphia

Agraphia involves deficits in producing written language due to problems of syntax, spelling, and word choice, i.e., not motor problems per se.

Alexia

Reading ability is hampered by a brain lesion. Alexia may be due to a deficit of visual perception, or in associating visual symbols with an auditorily presented word. The patient may write a letter, but be unable to read what he has written.

Aphemia

This is a deficit of purely vocal output, i.e., motor aspects of speech, without language peculiarities (paraphasia). The patient is able to use written language to express ideas. Initial muteness is followed by hypophonia and then return of grammatically correct speech. Comprehension and writing may be normal. It is considered a speech problem, rather than an impairment of language. Some evidence is presented that this motor expressive problem is caused by damage to the subcortical connections of the peri-Rolandic region of each hemisphere (the operculum), or to impairment of speech motor planning due to damage to the basal ganglia (Murdoch et al., 1989).

Mutism and Hypophonia

This involves total loss, or reduced voice volume, of widespread possible neurological origin, which must be differentiated from disease of the larynx or its innervation. From the description of Stuss and Benson (1986), it seems poorly differentiated from aphemia when Broca's area is involved. The various types of aphasia usually refer to more complex functions and generalized impairment.

More Generalized Aphasic Syndrome

Among the parameters that have been offered for classification, and are useful in the conceptualization of aphasia, are the following:

Expressive versus Receptive

Communications processing, retrieval, and expression can be dichotomized into actual communication and phonological competence, versus sensory decoding, analysis, and comprehension.

Motor (Anterior) and Sensory (Posterior)

Anterior and posterior lesions are dichotomized. Presumably anterior lesions impair motor programming and expression (upper motor neuron deficit within the motor cortex and elsewhere in the frontal lobes), and posterior lesions impair receptive ability and initial transmission to association and comprehension areas.

Fluent Aphasia ("Wernicke's Aphasia")

Speech may be in connected sequences, easily expressed, well articulated, but accompanied by poor comprehension, and paraphasic. It is associated with posterior brain lesions.

Nonfluent Aphasia ("Broca's Aphasia")

Language is sparse, interrupted, awkwardly expressed, interrupted, and produced with great effort. Comprehension is relatively intact. Patients appear to understand speech with little difficulty, but subtle comprehension deficits can be detected. Although Broca's aphasia is usually classified as an "expressive" deficit, there is evidence of deficits of comprehension and many aspects of sentence structure that contribute to comprehension (Berndt & Caramazza, 1981). There are deficits of written and spoken language, writing (agraphia), and repetition. Since it is associated with left posterior frontal cortex lesions (not far from the motor cortex), perhaps extending into the insula, white matter, and basal ganglia, it is associated with right sided motor weakness, including hemiplegia or hemiparesis of the upper extremity. The lesion is typically, though not exclusively, in the inferior frontal gyrus. Prognosis is considered good, because of retained comprehension, although deficits of fluency and grammatical proficiency remain. Residual depression, frustration, and irritability may be the consequence of awareness of the deficit and frontal lobe damage.

Receptive ("Wernicke's") Aphasia

Verbal output is fluent, with semantic substitutions (paraphasia). There is a disturbance of comprehension, reading, writing (use of real letters to make nonsense words), and ability to repeat what is heard. Varieties include "word deafness" (reading is intact in the presence of loss of auditory comprehension), and "word blindness" (reading comprehension is worse than auditory reception). The auditory area may be disconnected from Wernicke's area with which comprehension processing is associated. Typically there is no motor deficit, since the lesion is posterior (superior temporal gyrus). Nevertheless, Wernicke's symptoms can be observed with anterior lesions.

Conduction Aphasia

Fluent paraphasic output, with substitutions of one sound for another (phoneme), relatively normal comprehension and reading, but severe disability in repetition. Since it is associated with damage to the arcuate fasciculus connecting the auditory receiving area with the motor area, it is considered to reflect a distinct anatomic separation between higher level conversational speech, and more rudimentary verbal skills of repetition.

Global

All aspects of language are severely impaired, with the possible exception of articulating a few words or utterances. There is nonfluent output, a severe comprehension deficit, and little or no ability to repeat, read, or write. Most patients are hemiplegic.

Subcortical or Thalamic Aphasia

The symptoms include mutism, with little spontaneous speech, hemiplegia, hypophonia, and deficits of comprehension, naming, reading, and writing. Repetition is usually spared, with a tendency for echolalia (repeating what is said). In some cases, thalamic lesions impair attention, making the patients distractible, leading to incoherent and garbled speech when not forced to pay attention. Hemorrhage is a common cause, and as such the TBI victim is vulnerable. Lesions can be very diverse, but it is claimed that there is a correlation between the site and the syndrome of language or speech disorder (see Alexander, Naeser, & Palumbo, 1987, for a thorough review).

Transcortical Motor Aphasia

Speech expression is similar to nonfluent aphasia, but there is better ability to repeat spoken language, missing in Broca's aphasia. There are deficits of articulation and writing, but reading comprehension is retained.

Transcortical Sensory Aphasia

Comprehension is severely limited, with fluent output, and echoing of what has been said by the examiner, with additional nonrelated words.

Word Deafness

Word deafness is the inability to comprehend incoming information, in general, or through particular sensory channels, e.g., sensory agnosias. It may be associated with more complex deficits involving speech and reading.

Aprosody, or Right Hemisphere Speech and Language Involvement

Aprosody is the inability to express or understand nonverbal aspects of communication (Ross, 1985): prosody, melody, rhythm, emotional expression of faces, gesturing, etc.

Jargon Aphasia

Jargon aphasia is a variety of speech disturbance in which neologisms occur. Some are similar to the target word (paraphasias), and some to another word used in a nearby context. Still others are phonologically dissimilar to the target but similar to other neologisms. These strategies, and stereotypes, serve the function of concealing inability to retrieve words, but do not aid in communicating one's desires (Panzeri, Semenza, & Butterworth, 1987).

Dyslexia

Dyslexia refers to difficulty in reading. It may be *developmental* (defined here as of unknown origin) or *acquired*. Acquired dyslexia is further subdivided (Lytton & Brust, 1989):

Deep dyslexia: Difficulties with phonological processing, e.g., nonsense sylla-
    bles, substitutions of related words, with some retention of comprehension.
Surface dyslexia: They can read orthographically regular words, but those with
    phonological peculiarities (e.g., "tough") will be broken up.

Clinical Examples of Communications Problems

Case 18: An Accident in an Elevator that Fell

A woman worked as a community mediator to bring people to a workable agreement. She states that her "coordination" is not correct (she meant communication), i.e., she used the wrong word (paraphasia). Sometimes she recognized that
she cannot find the right word (anomia). "I don't want to talk. Words come out,
I don't want to say the wrong thing. I will say one thing and mean another. My
conversation does not flow. I could not remember what I was doing to do it." Anomia, i.e., inability to retrieve nouns from long-term memory was confirmed by
the WAIS-R. Her average age-scaled score for prior learning (Information and
Vocabulary) was 6.5, in contrast with current verbal processing (Comprehension
and Similarities) of 9.5. On the Boston Naming Test, her score of 36 was about
equal to a 2nd grade student, or a developmental age of 7½.

Case 19: A Woman Whose Car Was Struck from the Rear While Stopped

A woman in her 40's was a college graduate, married with children, and performs
office work. Her Full Scale IQ of 124 was 11 points higher than the estimated
premorbid IQ, and Verbal IQ exceeded Performance IQ. Despite this apparently
retained verbal ability she complained of not being able to communicate. On
the Symptom Checklist she asserted she had difficulty with verbal organization,
difficulty enunciating some words, and does not understand other people. There
was also loss of social interest, with embarrassment because of loss of verbal
skills.

She asserts that she is unable to work because of these deficits: verbal ability
and communication loss. She loses words and loses her train of thought. "I don't
have organizational skills I had. When I speak to somebody I lose my train of
thought. I have to rehearse and even that doesn't always help." Although she
seemed able to express herself adequately, a subclinical verbal deficit was
revealed by her inability to relate her job history sequentially.

Conclusion

Recognizing and assessing communications deficits are difficult and primary tasks of the professional concerned with the brain-damaged victim. The details of neural and linguistic deficit are complex, and in many instances poorly correlated. For many purposes, the most significant task is assessing the significance of communications problems for pragmatic and adaptive functions.

13
Cerebral Personality Disorders and Frontal Lobe Syndromes

Overview

Emotional distress and dysfunctioning are so common after brain damage that the author considers it unlikely that TBI can occur without damage to the emotional apparatus directly, and/or some form of posttraumatic stress.

Studies after intervals of up to 15 years show that one-half to two-thirds of very severely head injured patients show personality disturbances (Grant and Alves, 1987). Relatives who live with the patient see their psychopathology as intensifying over time (Levin, 1985). It has been asserted that emotional stress is associated with litigation, and disappears afterward (Alves & Grant, 1987), but this point is doubtful.

In any event, the state of being impaired creates distress, which in turn will affect adaptive functioning. Unfortunately, emotional distress is often not documented after TBI, and this chapter is designed to help the reader understand the dimensions of this problem. To review the neurological functioning associated with cerebral emotional disorders could be like attempting to review all of neuroscience, but an overall guide will be attempted!

This chapter will emphasize disorders directly caused by trauma to the brain, including the frontal lobe syndrome(s). The vulnerability of the frontal lobes and their fiber connections has been discussed in Chapter 4 on Trauma. The next chapter (deficits of adaptability) will concern itself with sexuality (in part because it is a a social problem, contributing to deficits of self-esteem). Naturally, TBI also affects motivation and performance. Chapter 15 on Anxiety, Stress, and Psychodynamic Reactions will offer a further overview on dynamic emotional disorders frequently occurring after TBI. The difficulties found in determining accurately the emotional life of TBI victims (and other deficits) due to their inability to express their problems are discussed in Chapter 16 on Expressive Deficits.

Some Conditions Affecting Emotional Expression

Level of arousal: Reticular activating system, portions of the thalamus, and medial frontal cortex.

Vegetative functions: These are mediated by the hypothalamus and frontal cortex.

Retrieval of previous experience: Limbic system, particularly the hippocampus.

Comprehension: Left hemisphere is most intimately involved. TBI victims with severely reduced intelligence frequently also seem somewhat unreactive to the consequences of their dysfunctioning.

Right hemisphere processing of emotional communication: Verbal information and nonverbal information are received and processed differently.

General context: Ability to retrieve information for meaning and familiarity is involved.

Moods are affected by neurotransmitter transport: Catecholamines (norepinephrine, epinephrine, dopamine), serotonin, endogenous opiates, etc. There is a "complex interplay" with steroid hormonal systems, e.g., the HPA axis (Arato, Banki, Nemeroff, and Bisette, 1986). Their regulatory role in opiate and adrenergic receptor functions, taken into consideration with what is known about changed levels during stress and injury, would affect emotional functioning (see Chapter 2 on Neuroanatomy and Chapter 15 on Stress).

A balance between facilitation and inhibition: For example, the dorsolateral frontal system versus orbitofrontal limbic system (Lee et al., 1988).

Emotional Dysfunctioning After TBI Is Very Complex

Premorbid level of adjustment: This affects the ability to cope, and, most likely, creates a ceiling to adaptive functioning after rehabilitation.

Dysfunctioning consequent to brain damage: A variety of modes of expression, dysfunctioning, and loss of control are discussed below.

Posttraumatic stress: The flood of neurotransmitters accompanying injury and fear have long-lasting effects on brain circuits and thus behavior.

Reactions to being impaired, injured, scarred, and loss of status: Morale is affected, with difficulties in rehabilitation, social relations, attempting to solve adaptive problems, etc.

Age of injury: When brain damage occurs in a child, there is reduced ability to develop controls and monitor socially dangerous behavior (to others and by inference to self).

Neurological Contributions to Emotions

Definition of the System

The brain generates emotions, motivation and drive for action, a sense of one's self, and adaptive functions such as self-protection, anger, sex, and love. The unimpaired person experiences and expresses a range of feelings, within normal limits, toward an appropriate target, that evolve from personal history and the current situation. Personal emotions are communicated clearly, and those of others are understood. The balance between feelings (internally experienced), motivation (intention to take action), and expression (motor action and nonverbal communication) contributes to one's welfare.

Neuropsychological Dysfunctioning (Organic Personality Syndrome)

Emotional life in the brain-damaged accident victim reflects complex dysfunctioning and distress:

1. Positive disorders directly caused by brain damage, i.e., release phenomena (irritability and poor control over anger), seizure disorders, and associated cognitive and emotional dysfunctioning;
2. Hyporeactivity (dulled expression; reduced motivation);
3. Conditions mimicking psychogenic conditions such as immaturity, psychopathy, depression, and anxiety;
4. Emotional disturbance at being impaired;
5. Various posttraumatic stress reactions.

Basic Neural System

The association between emotional functioning and brain structure is complex and incompletely established. However, so many stuctures are involved, that brain damage is almost certainly accompanied by emotional dysfunctioning (refer to Chapter 2 on Neuroanatomy). Emotional expression is intimately involved with the regulatory apparatus of the autonomic nervous system: the frontal lobe cortex, the limbic lobe system and amygdaloid nuclei, and the hypothalamus. Additional structures involved in mood and emotional expression include the cortex, caudate nucleus, thalamus, limbic lobe system (e.g., the amygdala), brainstem, and autonomic nervous system. The role of neurotransmitters, and the tracts that carry them, is very complex, as illustrated by the interrelationship between depression and anger, which is well known clinically (Mann & Stanley, 1986).

Limbic structures and the Papez circuit are involved with loss of control after TBI (irritation and aggression), passivity, and depression (Depue & Spoont, 1986).

• Stimulation of the amygdala can cause a fear or anger response. Different structures within it play a facilitatory or inhibitory role. A dopamine pathway into the amygdala facilitates irritability. This is the mesolimbic dopamine system (ventromedial mesencephalon, see Kalivas & Nemeroff, 1988), which is significant for rewards processes, psychostimulant drugs, drug addiction, neuroleptic responses, stress, etc.
• Stimulation of the hypothalamus can lead to aggressive behavior.
• Ablation of the rostral cingulate gyrus (part of the same Papez circuit) produces tameness and reduced aggressiveness in some species (Adams & Victor, 1989, p. 428), perhaps by interrupting a circuit contributing to aggressiveness.

• *Septal nuclei:* This plays an inhibitory role in aggression and serves a pleasure–reward function. Lesions contribute to hyperreactivity and hyperemotionality, including response to frustration, and are expressed as aggression.

Laterality differences have been proposed. It has been generalized that the right cerebral hemisphere processes negative emotions and the left cerebral hemisphere processes more positive feelings (Heilman, Watson, & Bowers, 1983). However, there is no clear-cut neurological model. Ross (1985; Ross, Anderson, & Morgan-Fisher, 1989) has hypothesized that the right hemisphere is dominant in modulating the affective components of language in ways comparable to the left hemisphere's control over propositional aspects of language. Ross' table comparing various aspects of aphasia (fluency, repetition, comprehension, reading comprehension) with aprosodia (spontaneous prosody and gesturing, prosodic repetition, prosodic comprehension, and comprehension of emotional gesturing) for many types of aphasia is repeated in Ruckdeschel-Hibbard, Gordon, and Diller (1986).

Dysphoric reactions and uncontrollable crying occur with greater frequency after left than right hemisphere and more anterior than posterior injuries (Robinson & Benson, 1981; Starkstein, Robinson, & Price, 1987). It is asserted that the remaining functional right hemisphere processes negative feelings and nonverbal emotional expression. Laterality differences were not supported in recent experimental studies of patients with focal brain lesions (Weddell, Trevarthen, & Miller, 1988) or primarily vascular accidents (Moehle & Fitzhugh-Bell, 1988).

Subcortical mechanisms are significant in emotional expression, e.g., the amygdala in aggression and self-mutilation (Lee et al., 1988). Neuroendocrine effects are significant, e.g., damage to the HPA can lead to hyperprolactinemia and consequent depression and anxiety (Findling & Tyrrell, 1986). See also seizures and anger dyscontrol syndrome below.

Depression

Endogenous depression is a direct consequence of head injury (Peck, Ettigi, Narasimhachari, & Mishra, 1986) that may be associated with left cerebral damage, other lesions, or reduced arousal due to depletion of neurotransmitters. Dull affect is sometimes caused by damage to the dorsolateral aspect of the frontal lobes, and has also been attributed to right cerebral hemisphere damage (Heilman et al., 1983). Lack of noradrenaline, secreted by the locus ceruleus for example, could contribute to a depressive condition. Anterior lesions may be more disruptive of catecholamine pathways than posterior lesions, producing more depression (Robinson & Benson, 1981).

Hypoglycemia

Violence may be triggered by hypoglycemia, and accompanied by memory disturbances (Roy, Virkkunen, Guthrie, & Linnoila, 1986). It is noteworthy that one cause of hypoglycemia is categorized as deficiency of contrainsulin hormones, all of which have been discussed in the section on the HPA or other areas affected by trauma (glucagon, cortisol, growth hormone, epinephrine, thyroid hormones, Merck Manual, 1987, p. 1085). The presence of violence in the context of hypoglycemia makes one consider the possible presence of epilepsy or a structural disease (Elliott, 1986). Yet, social control (e.g. the 5-hour glucose tolerance test) does not characteristically lead to violence.

Reduced Serotonin

Reduced serotonin may be related to violent behavior toward others, including arson, or toward oneself (suicide). It seems implicated with reduced impulse control, including explosive behavior when drinking alcohol, a known vulnerability after TBI (Banki, Arato, & Kilts, 1986; Roy et al., 1986).

Left Hemisphere Lesions

A study (Starkstein et al., 1987) of patients with a variety of cerebrovascular disorders led to these conclusions: severe depressions are more frequent with left anterior hemisphere lesions and left subcortical lesions relatively close to the anterior pole are equally associated with depression, particularly when frontal dorsal structures (caudate nucleus) are involved. The caudate nucleus is in a feedback pathway between cortical centers. It also reciprocally innervates the dorsomedial nucleus of the thalamus, known to affect mood. It is a way-station for catecholaminergic neurons (energizing) from the brainstem via the median forebrain bundle, which then pass to the frontal cortex.

Lesions of the Lentiform Nucleus

Lesions of the caudate and putamen cause a depressive-like condition, which also closely resembles a frontal-like syndrome, i.e., inertia, akinesia, and slowness (Laplane et al., 1989).

Reduced Motivation

Reduced motivation has been attributed to damage to the cingulate gyrus (Livingston, 1984, p. 1152) and to the basal ganglia, as a frontal lobe-like syndrome. The mechanism proposed for hypometabolism of the frontal lobe cortex illustrates the complex effects after trauma. Damage to the globus pallidus caused deafferentiation, i.e., input into the prefrontal cortex (Laplane et al., 1989).

Cognitive Contributions to Emotional Dysfunctioning

Ruckdeschel-Hibbard et al., (1986) contrast the "catastropic reaction" (resentment of deficit) with the "indifference reaction" (including unawareness of deficit). These may be more descriptive of behavior than emotional state.

Although associated with left and right cerebral damage, respectively, emotional expression or its deficit is affected by the presence of anterior, posterior, and subcortical lesions.

Inappropriate Responses

Brain damage may be accompanied by inability to recognize emotional feelings in others, and difficulty in comprehending and expressing emotional aspects of language. Therefore, inappropriate behavior might be continued after another person would recognize negative feedback. Behavior that is considered to be inappropriate is likely to be categorized as part of a disturbed emotional reaction. Cognitive deficits impairing appropriateness include inability to recognize emotional feelings in others, inability to comprehend and express emotional aspects of language, and decreased sensitivity to others' responses.

Reduced Verbal Ability

The aphasic individual, despite language deficits, sometimes can grasp the meaning or intent of a speaker. Paralinguistic and emotional features of language are analyzed by the intact right hemisphere. Reaction to a fraction of emotionally significant information can create inappropriate behavior. The expression of feelings becomes primarily nonverbal and nonpropositional, with reliance upon intonation and facial expression.

Defective Monitoring of Behavior

Self-defeating actions may exist, in the absence of conspicuous intellectual deficiencies, due to inability to monitor behavior. The patient cannot determine whether actions are in accord with long-term goals. Social and vocational problems stem from loss of foresight and inability to recognize errors, and have a variety of consequences. These have been called the frontal lobe syndrome (though, as will be detailed below, there are other types of dysfunctions as well). A mistake may not be recognized, or the patient cannot size up a social situation appropriately, or in general, to correct errors once they are made. Poor judgment leads to reduced standards of performance in employment and personal behavior. Even after recognizing errors, a brain-damaged individual may be slow to learn from experience and inappropriate behavior is continued indefinitely.

Reduced Emotional Understanding and Communication

The person may not understand or express nonverbal and emotional components of speech and communication, e.g., prosody, facial expressions, emotional tone of the voice, particularly recognition of the semantic content of the communication. Right cerebral hemisphere lesions are considered to be more significant than left cerebral lesions. When this process is studied with auditory input, there is a left ear advantage for nonverbal sounds and emotional content, reflecting the fact that most auditory tract impulses decussate to the contralateral side (Bisiach, Ballar, Perani, Papagno, & Berti, 1986; Etkoff, et al., 1986; Golper, 1985).

Paranoia

This disorder is consequent to an inability to recognize faces and emotional expression (mechanics of emotional expression, intonation, prosody, etc.), after damage to the right hemisphere. There may be paranoid ideation about imposters, difficulties in expressing one's feelings convincingly, misinterpretation of others' reactions, and deviant thought and verbal expression.

Some Affective Symptoms of Brain Damage

The following personality factors were detected in victims of severe head injury, studied by the Coma Data Bank through the Katz Adjustment Scale:

I. Social Obstreperousness (e.g., belligerence and negativism);
II. Acute Psychoticism (e.g., anxiety, bizarreness);
III. Withdrawn Depression (withdrawal and helplessness); also Suspiciousness, nervousness, confusion, and stability (Grant & Alves, 1987).

Another taxonomy (Eames, 1988) classified brain damage symptoms as follows:

I. Active (aggressive, impulsive, disinhibited, antisocial);
II. Passive (insightless, driveless, lacking in motivation, slow and anhedonic);
III. Syndromal (manipulative, hysterical, ritualistic, cyclothymic, fantasizing or confabulating, paranoid).

Summary of Brain Damage Syndromes

Disinhibited and poorly targeted anger: Anger and in its extreme the dyscontrol syndrome (see below) are common.
Autistic anxiety: The conditions and after-effects of brain damage will create anxiety except in some grossly impaired individuals.
Reduced motivation with inability to cope: Lack of drive and loss of competence are common.
Pseudopsychodynamic expression: Obsessive-compulsive disorder may be preceded by increased arousal, which would lead the septohippocampal system to become oversensitive and label neutral stimuli as aversive (Drummond, 1988). Significant psychiatric symptoms may be an expression of neural dysfunctioning or a means of behavioral control against behaviorally disorganizing neural stimulation recognized as maladaptive.

The following symptoms and patterns are common after TBI.

Anxiety

It was with some astonishment, while reviewing material for this chapter, that I realized that by consensus, anxiety is not presented as a prominent symptom of traumatic brain damage! Of epilepsy, yes, but of brain damage, no! Therefore, to draw attention to this quite common after-effect, it is listed first, with the note that an entire chapter will be devoted to it. Since generalized fearfulness is a common after-effect, any brain damage reducing the ability to express or experience anxiety would also prevent the victim from calling attention to other forms of impairment.

In a review of "organic mental syndromes" (Horvath, Siever, Mohns & Davis, 1989) (primarily disease related but including traumatic injury), anxiety is summarized as follows: an irrational anxiety in panic or persistent form manifested by motor tension, autonomic hyperactivity, apprehensive expectation, and hypervigilance; and/or avoidance of objects of situations associated with anxiety. The relationship to a posttraumatic stress like syndrome is clear (see Chapter 15 on Anxiety and Stress).

Identity Changes

Depersonalization: Loss or change of one's identity, i.e., one feels that the sense of self is unfamiliar.
Disorientation: Loss of a sense of familiarity with one's person or surroundings.

Changes in Level of Emotional Expression

Feelings may be experienced more or less deeply: See Kandel and Schwartz, (1985, p. 609).
Loss of impulse and emotional control: Feelings can be experienced as being out of control, e.g., crying, anger, and irritability.
Emotional lability: Loss of control over the emotions leads to mood swings.

Multiple Symptoms

After brain damage, there can be a myriad of affective abnormalities, in particular lability and depression (Joseph, 1988): indifference, hysteria, gross social-emotional disinhibition, florid manic excitement, childishness, euphoria, impulsivity, and abnormal sexual behavior.

A correlation, though small, was established between "postconcussion symptoms" (PTA, headaches, anxiety) and elevated scores on the Minnesota Multiphasic Personality Inventory (MMPI). Experiencing multiple symptoms may reflect difficulties in coping, and serve as a signal for therapeutic intervention

(Novack, Daniel, & Long, 1984). As observed, however, in Chapter 4 on Trauma, headaches need not indicate an emotional disorder, since they can result from trauma that simultaneously caused soft tissue injury and brain damage.

Seizure-Related Emotional Expression

Anxiety, depression (with increased suicidal risk), decreased libido and impotence associated with temporal lobe seizures, a different report of increased libido, and controversial claims of increased aggression (Heilman et al., 1985) have all been noticed. Endocrine changes are reported, probably related to stimulation of the hypothalamic–pituitary axis: gonadal hormones varying from normal to increased; decreased and elevated prolactin.

There are personality changes that have been associated with temporal lobe epilepsy, i.e., deepened emotions, concern for details, and sometimes paranoid qualities. Seizure-related emotional reactions could be a conditioned reaction, i.e., the induction of response through limbic stimulation could be the unconditioned response, which becomes associated with an accidental occurrence of some environmental event (Heilman et al., 1985). Unrelated environmental events then would trigger emotional reactions associated with the seizure experience.

Between seizures, electrochemical activity may not be normal, i.e., persistent focal electrical discharges, creating sensitization to further discharge (kindling). There may be a progression of any underlying neurological disorder, and further damage resulting from anoxia and trauma during seizures, and toxic effects of medication.

In cases of temporal lobe epilepsy, in addition to hyposexuality, disrobing and sexual-like activity during seizures may occur. Elevated prolactin postseizure may be related to impotence (Pritchard, 1983). Damage to the HPA can result in sexual problems, as well as a psychogenic reduced self-esteem as a secondary consequence of impairment. Sexual problems may lead to social withdrawal.

Depressive-Like Conditions

Depression is an umbrella title for many different conditions that are not clearly differentiated from each other (see Chapter 8 on Neurophysiological Functions for discussion of damage to the hypothalamo–pituitary axis. Further discussion is in Chapter 15 on Stress). The manner and intensity of display of dysphoria may be unrelated to the context, of unpredictable intensity, or mood (Damasio & Van Hoesen, 1985, p. 105). Depression may result from hormonal, structural, or neurohumoral causes (see laterality; hypoglycemia and reduced serotonin, above). Its close clinical connection with hostility is well known, and physiological changes that encourage hostility also are associated with suicide (many references in Mann & Stanley, 1986). The interaction of depression and stress is illustrated by the elevation of CRF (controlling ACTH) during depression (Arato et al., 1986).

Traumatic depression is expressed as hyporeactivity and apathy, rather than unhappiness (a realistic source and emotionally appropriate expression).

Reduced affective expression, e.g., a form of endogenous depression, should be distinguished from apathy (Weintraub & Mesulum, 1985), and from the specific expressive deficit caused by brain damage (Etkoff, 1986).

Emotional Flattening, Endogenous Depression

Emotional flattening, i.e., lack of nonverbal expressiveness, should be differentiated from indifference (see indifference reaction below). Emotional flattening is quite common in TBI. One may observe a bland, and sometimes pleasant demeanor, and evidence of serious suffering in the personal statement or Rorschach (stress-related or depressive content). The depressed person may seem to be calm and indifferent, and not communicate intense emotional pain and hopelessness. One must be aware of the lack of emotion in the voice, or the low level of energy, offering a false impression of mental retardation or indifference.

Lack of emotional communication contributes to the observer's inability to recognize the presence of brain damage and its ill effects (see Chapter 16 on Expressive Deficits). Behaviorally, the results of depression can be inconspicuous, i.e., such negative symptoms as apathy, lethargy, little spontaneity, unconcern, reduced sexual interest, little overt emotion, and inability to plan ahead.

Emotional indifference can result from stimuli coming from a single sensory modality, e.g., vision. Some right hemisphere victims may state that they are now "okay" or "much better"—even with physical disabilities, or emotional behavior reminiscent of a child or zombie (McMahan & Satz, 1981).

Apathy, Loss of Motivation and Planning

Reduced expression of these functions occurs: activity is expressed; initiative or drive to pursue valued goals; ability to be independent, purposive, and self-serving (Lezak, 1983, p. 38); ability to initiate all motor activity, motivation to work (Thickman & Ranseden, 1986); sexual interest, overt emotion, ability to plan ahead (Stuff & Benson, 1983).

Indifference Reaction

Lack of complaints may be unrecognized as a sign of brain damage per se. The indifference reaction includes such symptoms as anosagnosia (indifference to or unawareness of a neurological deficit), indifference toward failure or events concerning the family, minimization of hemiplegia through attributing it, or other symptoms, to some other cause. It is associated with right brain damage (Ruckdeschel-Hibbard et al., 1986).

Blunting of Social Skills and Inappropriate Sexual Behavior

See Heilman et al. (1983) and Wood (1984). Social problems arise from decreased social sensitivity to others' responses to them, and loss of ability to express one's own feelings. There may be public genital exposure, fondling, masturbation, delusions and confabulation, inappropriate joking, and sexual references (Blackerby, 1987).

Release Phenomena

Pathological laughing, euphoria, crying, rage, fear, temper, and irritability can occur. Gross loss of emotional control is associated with damage to subcortical lesions in nuclei and tracts (Brazis et al., 1985, pp. 323–324; Heilman et al., 1983). Uncontrolled and inappropriate expressions of pleasant feelings, with restlessness, are sometimes observed. Euphoria and uncontrollable outbursts of laughing are more common after right hemisphere damage. Episodic outbursts of rage and fear can be stimulated by threat, restraint, or frustration. Between outbursts the behavior is normal, and the patient may apologize for it. This is attributed to lesions of the hypothalamus (ventromedial), orbitofrontal cortex, or temporal lobe (Brazis et al., 1985, p. 262).

Loss of Control over Anger

Anger is expressed in TBI as irritability, fear of loss of control, and overt dyscontrol. Brain-damaged victims may react in paradoxical ways to threat, i.e., with rage when there is frustration or trivial issues, or blandly when threatened or given pain (Brazis et al., 1985, pp. 323–324). There is evidence concerning neurological dysfunctioning as a contribution to violent crime. After head trauma, the individual may go through an aggressive and combative stage that may last for weeks, followed by headaches, lightheadedness, loss of energy, irritability, etc. Children may exhibit hyperkinesis (Elliott, 1976).

Rage outbursts are particularly associated with

1. *Damage to the amygdala,* which is involved "in a definable neural system which organizes effective and directed attack behavior" (Mark & Ervin, 1970, p. 85; also Livingston, 1985, p. 1282);
2. *Impairment of cortical control* (Mark & Ervin, 1970, p. 59);
3. *Stimulation of the hypothalamus and the area around the fornix* in the diencephalon. Hypothalamic elicited aggression can be inhibited by stimulation of the ipsilateral frontal cortex (Trimble, p. 115), illustrating cortical inhibition over limbic affective mechanisms.

Dyscontrol Syndrome

The dyscontrol syndrome has been related to wife and child battery, motiveless homicide, unprovoked assault on a friend or strangers, sexual assault, dangerously aggressive driving, and senseless destruction of property. It can be expressed as verbal violence, leading to disrupted marriages, careers, and parental relationships. Of 70 cases in private neurological practice, 12 were attributed to head injury after age 15. Explosive rage takes over, which can be controlled with difficulty, or be expressed when provoked. Physical violence can have a primitive quality, such as biting, gauging, spitting, and use of a knife or hammer (Elliott, 1976).

The victim is frequently aware of this deficit, but cannot exercise self-control. It is considered to be due to brain damage upsetting the balance between the limbic system and the neocortex (see information on amygdala, above) (Mark & Ervin, 1970, pp, 59, 127). Hypersensitivity to external stimuli, accompanied by sympathetic hyperarousal and inability to habituate, seems related to the explosive expression of anger. Such patients frequently complain of hypersensitivity to loud noises, rhythms of audition or vision, and bright lights. Bilateral amygdalectomy, which reduced episodes of aggression and rage, seemed to be followed by diminished autonomic responsiveness (Lee et al., 1988).

One young man described his emotional life in terms of his difficulty in controlling his feelings: "I'm afraid to hurt somebody . . . I don't want to think of what might happen . . . Temper, too many tempers. Sometimes nobody does anything and I am mad. It's been better; don't be in my sight because I could tell you a few things. I used to be a quiet guy."

Propensity to Violence and Neuropsychological Impairment

A review of the literature and personal investigation of adolescent and adult criminals (particularly violent-aggressive and psychopathic) implicated bilateral dysfunction of the frontal and temporal lobes with a dominant hemisphere emphasis in about 72% of the cases. Persistent juvenile, nonviolent offenders had a greater involvement of the nondominant hemisphere (Yeudall, 1980). Lewis, Pincus, Feldman, Jackson, & Bard (1986) studied 15 death row inmates, chosen for examination because of the imminence of their executions, not because there was prior reason in individual cases to suspect neuropsychopathology. All had had severe head injury, five had major neurological impairment, and others displayed blackouts and "soft" signs of neurological dysfunction. In addition six had preexisting schizophrenoform psychoses, and two were manic-depressive. Elliott (1976) observes that the dyscontrol syndrome is not revealed by the conventional neurological examination if the cue of "soft signs" is ignored. Explosive rages, he notes, are more common with diseases of the limbic system than the neocortex.

Regression to Diagnosable Emotional Disorders

Grant and Alves (1987) reviewed the literature on incidence of diagnosable emotional disorders after head injury. There is some increase in the incidence of psychosis, though not necessarily schizophrenia (since this possibility is not considered by the *Diagnostic and Statistical Manual*, 3rd ed.). The situation is not much improved in the revision, since neither trauma, head injury, nor brain appears in the index! Under Axis III (Physical Disorders) neurological disorder or "soft neurological signs" are mentioned, but nothing related to brain trauma.

Obsessive Compulsive Neurosis

There are reports of obsessive-compulsive neurosis following head injury (Drummond, 1988; McKeon, McGuffin & Robinson, 1984), though, as noted above, this could be a physiological alerting reaction to actually neutral stimuli, causing needless searching or checking. Tics, mental stereotopies, and obsessive-compulsive behaviors (rechecking, peculiarities of counting, turning light switches on and off) were observed after lenticular nucleus (basal ganglia) lesions (LaPlane, 1989, see case #6).

Schizophrenia

Head injury seems to lower the threshold for psychosis: The likelihood of schizophrenia increases (Wilcox & Nasrallah, 1987). These patients had a disproportionate rate of head injury compared to patients with bipolar emotional swings, depressives, and surgical patients.

"Catastrophic Reaction"

A "catastrophic reaction" occurs when patients become aware of deficits in their mental ability. It is in contrast to emotional blunting, i.e., loss of control with tears, swearing, fear, and anger. It is a reaction to impairment, i.e., the inability to perform cognitive tasks, named by Goldstein (Bruno, 1984). Rorschach criteria are offered by Piotrowski (1937). The patient is depressed and pained that tasks are now beyond his or her capacity (Heilman et al., 1985; Lezak, 1983, p. 61).

Perplexity, anxiety, and despair when a patient cannot perform an assigned task is associated more with left than with right hemisphere lesions. It contrasts with the indifference reaction. Symptoms include restlessness, hyperemotionality, and vegetative signs of anxiety, crying, aggressive behavior, swearing, displacement of anxiety or aggressiveness, compensatory boasting, refusal to continue, depression, discouragement, and anticipation of inability to succeed (Bruno, 1984; Ruckdeschel-Hibbard et al., 1986).

The catastrophic reaction is generally attributed to damage to the left cerebral hemisphere. The particular reason is controversial, i.e., whether the more functional right hemisphere processes the residual "negative" emotions, or merely expresses feelings in a nonpropositional, nonverbal manner. With loss of verbal comprehension, emotional distress would be characterized by a nonlinguistic awareness that something is not right.

Frontal Lobe Syndromes

The frontal and temporal lobes are particularly susceptible to closed head injuries in which the inertia of the blow is received by these areas impacting with the skull. Since the prefrontal cortex and tips of the temporal lobes are intimately connected with the limbic system, basal ganglia, thalamus, etc., a wide variety of symptoms can ensue, and different syndromes (see below) can coexist (Adamovich et al., 1985, pp. 20–23; Trimble, 1988, p. 164). It has been observed that it is difficult to find a neuropsychological definition of the frontal lobe syndrome accepted by all authors (Laplane et al., 1989), but this is comprehensible in view of the fact that there are several "frontal lobe syndromes," see below).

Frontal lobe damage is likely to be undetected by classical neurological and psychodiagnostic tests. It is possible to attribute frontal lobe symptoms to functional causes or psychopathy. Interviewing friends and relatives (Strub & Black, 1988, p. 286) is important in the diagnosis, and change in behavior is especially significant. Multiple deficits occur, i.e., affect, loss of efficiency, cognitive deficits, etc. Cognitive deficits are subtle, but impairing. They are manifested in reduced efficiency, i.e., loss of flexibility to meet a changing environment, and deficits in placing ideas in temporal sequence.

Motor dysfunction may accompany damage to the lateral areas, i.e., those abutting the motor cortex. More posterior lesions are linked with difficulties with the organization of movement, while anterior ones result in difficulties of motor planning, and dissociation between behavior and language (Trimble, 1988, p. 167).

Personality Changes

The frontal lobe-damaged victim is characterized by personality changes and deficits in cognitive control and efficiency. Voluntary behavior is not under control. These patients are intolerant of stress, and have difficulty in dealing with novel situations. An overview suggests decreased drive, self-monitoring, and lack of control, all conditioned by the premorbid personality (Stuss & Benson, 1986, p. 129).

There is no consistent reaction. Polar opposites in personality patterns may occur: reduction of emotion (pseudodepressed, see above), or an apparent antisocial reaction (pseudopsychopathic). Both types of behavior may coexist, creating confusion about the presence of brain damage. Large frontal lesions commonly cause a mixture of both personality types, with the paradoxical description of frontal lobe personality as "apathetic, irritable, and euphoric."

One boy when bicycling down a hill hit a tree and lapsed into brief unconsciousness. He was described by himself and his family as different thereafter. His physician stated that he would overcome any difficulties, so even into adult life he was unable to connect the personality change with the accident.

Expressive Deficits Can Create Confusion as to Whether TBI Exists

Indifference to the consequences of one's actions, or emotional blunting does not lead to a request for treatment and gives the impression of indifference. The alert is offered by Strub and Black (1988, p. 286) that "apathy" (disinhibition and short temper) without sadness, tears, self-depreciation, and vegetative signs should strongly arouse the examiner's suspicion of organic and particularly frontal lobe disease." Thickman and Ranseden (1986) point out that *since frontal lobe damage is often unrelated to specific cognitive impairment, detectable by standard tests, relatively preserved cognitive skills mask the profound disturbances that these patients exhibit in significant aspects of their lives.*

Indifference to the Consequences of One's Actions

Brain-damaged individuals may not understand the consequences of their decisions and behavior and may be unable to monitor, or to learn from their own experience (Haas & Ross, 1986). Inappropriate feelings, e.g., laughing, seeming indifference, and inability to understand the emotional reactions of others, and also emotional dulling, can exacerbate social problems by outraging others. Poor judgment is concealed from a consulting professional or examiner unless a collateral complains or informs. In this context, individuals described as psychopathic and antisocial (lacks emotion, callous, remorseless, failing to learn from experience, cannot anticipate consequences) manifest autonomic hyperactivity (skin conductance, anticipatory heartrate, biochemical indicants of fear) (Mednick, 1980).

Needlessly Immature Behavior

Unknowingly immature behavior often accompanies frontal lobe damage. Behavior is impulsive, childish, and repetitive, inappropriate, poorly controlled, exaggerated, puerile, or jocular. Symptoms include sexual disinhibition, increased activity, self-indulgent attitude, and little concern for others. Poorly planned behavior is not in accord with the individual's expressed goals or usual personality. It can be socially unacceptable or self-defeating, with the person unaware of, or not remembering, serious criticisms and rejection.

In the adult, this can be recognized as a severe personality change. In the child, up to around age 13, it may be considered to be mere immaturity. However, lack of development of normal functioning, due to frontal lobe injury, can lead to delinquency, antisocial acts, or psychiatric disorders.

Self-Destructive Behavior Is Persistent

Frequent and persistent inappropriate behavior continues despite considerable social feedback. This is attributable to a deficit in self-monitoring (ongoing, future, and past behavior), and to difficulty in remembering emotional information (Levin, 1985). Even with verbal acknowledgement of problems, he may be unable to correct it, impairing his own life and that of his family.

The Question of Crime

Whether the deficits of the frontal lobe victim increase the likelihood of crime (violence or property) is not fully established. The relationship between general physiological factors and violent behavior has been discussed above. There is inconclusive evidence for frontal lobe dysfunction to be involved in crime (Kandel & Freed, 1989). Stuss and Benson (1986, p. 134) point out the similaritiy between sociopathy and delinquency, and some frontal lobe functioning, i.e., lack of cognitive control leading to uninhibited hedonistic action. A systematic approach to neuropsychological examinations where frontal lobe impairment is offered as a defense, utilizing known symptoms, history taking, and selected neuropsychological procedures, is offered by Hall and McNinch (1988). Autonomic hypoactivity has an asocial behavioral pattern associated with it (see below).

Syndromes of Frontal Lobe Damage

Disinhibited

The *orbitofrontal* cortex receives input from the basolateral component of the limbic system, and through it from parietal lobe and olfactory pathways. It is concerned with the sensory-receptive and interpretive cortex. This results in the so-called "positive" symptoms found in frontal lobe damage. This has been described as "pseudopsychopathic." Behavior is restless, explosive, distractible, hyperactive, and inappropriate. Mood is labile and jocular. "Witzelsucht" may occur, i.e., inappropriate facetiousness and a tendency to pun. Judgment is poor. Paranoia may ensue. These patients are more impaired than others by drugs or alcohol, i.e., they overreact to the disinhibiting effects of these substances (Golden, 1986).

Apathetic

Dorsolateral prefrontal area: The medial limbic system is concerned with the reticular core. This has been described as "pseudodepressed." Angular acceleration injuries are associated with coma, followed by posttraumatic confusion, and a pattern of "negative" symptoms. The results are inconspicuous, i.e., apathy, lethargy, little spontaneity, inattention, slowness, and long latency of response, unconcern, reduced sexual interest, little overt emotion, and inability to plan ahead. There may be little or no conspicuous sensorimotor or intellectual deficit. Prefrontal lobotomy severs fiber tracts between the frontal lobe and the dorsomedial nucleus of the thalamus. What was observed was difficulties in anticipating the future, lack of concern for pain and obsessions, and perseveration.

Akinetic

Medial frontal area: This involves a paucity of spontaneous movement, gesture, and verbal output. Somatic signs include lower extremity weakness and loss of sensation, and incontinence (Trimble, 1988, p. 164).

Additional Cerebral Personality Syndromes

Thalamic Syndrome

The thalamus contributes an emotional tone to sensory experience. When it is damaged, the threshold for touch, pain, and temperature is raised on the other side of the body, but sensations are exaggerated and disagreeable. A pinprick may be experienced as burning, and ordinarily pleasing music becomes disagreeable. Spontaneous pain and emotional instability (laughing and crying) may ensue (Barr & Kiernan, 1988, p. 193).

Kluver–Bucy Syndrome

Removal of both temporal lobes, with damage to the hippocampus and amygdaloid bodies, is characterized by voracious appetite, increased, and sometimes perverse, sexual activities, and docility (Barr & Kiernan, 1988, pp. 272–273). Lesions to the nearby temporal association areas can lead to loss of learned patterns of behavior. Clinical features are considered to be the opposite of those found with temporal lobe epilepsy (decreased sexuality and heightened emotionality) (Kandel & Schwartz, 1985, p. 624) (refer also to the hypothalamus, in Chapter 2, Neuroanatomy).

Secondary Mania

This is defined as the occurrence of a manic affective disorder resulting from a medical condition with no previous personal or familial history. Manic symptomology can be documented shortly after trauma, at a later state of life than would normally be expected. This is attributed to damage to the limbic portions of the frontal and temporal lobes, in particular the subcortical regions of the brain, not necessarily a release of the right hemisphere (Schneider & Kaplan, 1989).

Some Clinical Examples

Case 20: Loss of Control over Anger

An auto accident victim was asked about his temper: "It gets me into a shouting match. I grab my daughter, hold her, but haven't punched her. I have a hard time putting things into perspective. Little things bother you." Are there any changes in your feelings since the accident? "I deal with things, not feelings. I'm impatient. I don't have control anymore. I can't control my anxiety. I forget what I'm going to do after carrying out one errand. I can't deal with people, noise and movement. I can't hold back my feelings." Do you see yourself as different, or not your real self? His reply indicated that overtly, his feelings are weaker, and he tries to hide them. However, he has difficulty controlling his feelings. "I'm a different person. I'm more somber." He hit bottom at 3 months and he is on the upgrade now. "I tried to commit suicide three times. I look at things from the bad side. I can't let myself laugh and enjoy life. I flare up because I feel my wife is checking on me, even if she's only doing conversation." He acknowledges that he doesn't show his feelings. "I wish I had been killed instantly because I have suffered so much." He regards his future as grim.

Case 21: Depression Leading to Suicide

A middle-aged man was knocked down by a bus, with a brief period of unconsciousness. He was well-educated, with a normal family life. His only preinjury emotional distress was a drug-related psychotic reaction to a prescribed medication for arthritis. He had built a hobby into a business that requires both business judgment and a variety of fine manual skills. He states that he had a brief loss of consciousness, in contradiction to medical records. He was alert when medical personnel arrived so he was recorded as no LOC. His body was considerably jarred, and he was disabled for several months, and still unable to recover his previous skills. He described himself as sufficiently depressed to consult a psychiatrist, anxious, with bad dreams, and poorly motivated. A subsequent psychotic attack suggests that he could not cope with his impairment. This degree of reaction is sometimes seen. His loss of ability to enjoy himself and sense of changed identity are frequent reactions to disabling head injury. He was examined by another physician, who felt that he was being insufficiently medicated for his depression, and shortly thereafter he committed suicide by shooting himself.

Case 22: A Fall Backwards Contributing to Reduced Emotional Responsiveness and Dementia

Five years before the current (second examination) a man with 11 years of education and no contributing medical history had a work-related accident in which he was turning a heavy box upside down when the handle ripped off, he hit the side of his head, and then hit the back of his head on falling (which side is unclear from the patient's report and many medical examinations). However, there was evidence for left cerebral hemisphere and left midbrain lesions, with reports of memory deficits, emotional blandness (intepreted as "conversion hysteria with hysteria and schizoid features," depression, a variety of motor and cognitive dysfunctions, etc.).

Before the accident he supervised 11–12 people, and was being trained for a manager's position. He drove home, which he does not remember. He cannot describe the details of his life after the accident. (It was necessary to have his wife's assistance during the interview.) Subsequently he developed blackouts, seizures with a metallic taste in his mouth, and loss of control over his bladder, dizziness, and right-sided weakness. He describes himself as irritable, depressed, anxious, damaged, and feeling like a different person. He states that his future is damaged and his life has lost meaning. His wife describes him as quiet and secluded, and he states that he does not remember what is going on, i.e., does not recall what happens from one day to the next.

His current Wechsler Adult Intelligence Scale-Revised Full Scaled IQ was 62 (Verbal, 62; Performance, 67). This is a drop, conservatively estimated, of 27 points from the preinjury estimate of 89 based on age and education. This is the third WAIS-R (one was administered by a different examiner) and there is no sign of a practice effect. He could not read the simple word names on the Stroop Word and Color Test. His report of bumping into things was confirmed by evidence for an inability to detect right sided visual targets on the Mesulum Verbal and Non-verbal Concellation Test (Mesulam, 1985). The examiner could not administer a Rorschach, but a previous examiner reported an impoverished record, and a "blood" response, which points to gross regression, poorly controlled anxiety, and a sense of being damaged.

Conclusion

Emotional reactions are the best example of the integrated functioning of the nervous system. A plethora of disturbances have been attributed to wide-ranging lesions, and all the evidence and suitable models are not yet in. It is time to lay to rest the canard that emotional distress after traumatic head injury is attributable in most cases to malingering, neurosis, preexisting conditions, or secondary gains. These exist, and it is the duty of the examiner and therapist to recognize and expose them, but for most victims of TBI, emotional dysfunctions, posttraumatic stress, sensitivity to impairment, and loss of self-esteem add to other forms of impairment.

14
Adaptability, Independence, and Daily Functioning

Overview

One of the most shocking experiences to victims of TBI is the loss of capacity to take care of themselves. In a moment, individuals may be changed from normally functioning people, adequate in reality and self-esteem, to dependent individuals incapable even of properly defending themselves or of obtaining assistance. Since employment has been prevented the victim of trauma may rely on government resources or compensation through litigation. Income is cut off and medical bills can be considerable.

Cost of Head Injury

One study indicated the following costs for a head injury, with the family responding 6.7 years later on the average (McMordie & Barker 1989). The victims were seriously injured, i.e., the mean LOC was 62 days. Doctor and hospital bills, $92,811; drugs and other medical expenses, $11,278; legal, $31,278, structural modifications in the home, $3,324; specialized therapy, e.g., speech and physical therapy, $14,817; other (some unspecified data), $162,757. Many respondents indicated that some victims who needed service were not receiving any. The above costs do not include loss of earnings, nor the necessity for family members to go to work, borrow money, and lose possessions (declare bankruptcy, sell house).

Of the respondents 26% received a legal settlement (the range was from $1,300 to $3,600,000 with a mean of $346,238) and 43% received some yearly benefits, with a mean of $7,398. Treatment can cost more than $100,000. Non-residential programs may cost $3,000/month, while residential programs may cost $10,000/month. The cost of specialized therapy (speech therapy, cognitive rehabilitation, etc.) may be from $65 to $150/hour.

Governmental agencies at all levels are frequently unsympathetic to the disabled person, who, by definition, is unable to cope with reality, including the very agencies who as official resources for the disabled, or employers with some residual responsibilities for injuries incurred on the job, might be expected to

217

handle these matters efficiently. I know of one case in which, after 5 years, a disabled governmental employee has not had a resolution of a claim for disability with the Workers Compensation Board incurred when a crazy hospitalized patient injured him in the course of his job. A teacher was knocked down a flight of stairs and rendered blind, and her Board of Education is claiming it never happened. I have examined many applicants for Social Security Disability, referred by attorneys fortunately, who could not have stage-managed their own claims without an interested family member making proper arrangements. Of course, if somebody is too disabled to file suit after another's negligence has caused an accident, then a potential defendant has escaped the costs of careless or reckless behavior.

Neuropsychological Dysfunctioning

The disabled person cannot take care of himself in a practical way, loses independence, and cannot fulfill responsibilities to employer, family, and community. Efficiency is reduced by loss of cognitive, motor, sensory, and executive dysfunctions, and previously learned skills, and the impairing effects of gross emotional distress, e.g., depression, anger, anxiety, and pain. Reduced judgment increases the likelihood of further accidents that may result in brain injury or other hazard. Each trauma also reduces reserves so that subsequent injuries have greater effects than single ones. Responsibilities cannot be handled, and mobility is reduced.

Adaptive Deficits

Dysfunctions after TBI have far-reaching consequences on the quality of the patients life, i.e., inability to handle practical matters. In addition to neuropsychological deficits of cognition and efficiency, impaired mobility, pain, and anxiety reduce the ability to perform many activities. Common problems with generalized effects include poor memory, inability to use time well and scheduling, planning and decisions, and loss of skills, e.g., writing, reading, calculations, spelling, typing, vocational processes, driving, and sports.

Rehabilitation is hampered by cognitive deficits that prevent relearning and performing former functions, i.e., slow learning, loss of foresight, or poor relationship between comprehension and behavior (Golden, 1986). Inability to understand the consequences of one's actions results in self-destructive antagonism of community members. Emotional disorders create antagonism or social distance.

Increased Vulnerability to Further Accidents

Reduced mental ability, flexibility in coping with circumstances, and somatic capability contribute to further head and other injuries. After a first head injury the incidence of repetitive injury is three times, and after a second head injury, eight times that of the general population (Miller, 1986).

Poor Health

Brain damage causes impairment of the immune system and hypothalamopituitary axis, hyperarousal of autonomic and somatic functions, etc. This hampers resistance to disease, and decreases comfort and the ability to concentrate. Somatic symptoms, change of weight, inability to sleep, etc., are common. My clinical experience suggests that fatigue, for example, creates a vulnerability in any area of the person's life, including the potential for severe psychiatric illness.

One man stated: "I feel less viable. I used to be very athletic. I gained 25 lbs. I have terrible colds."

Inability to Enjoy Use of Leisure Time

Quality of life is impaired by emotional distress, loss of dexterity and range of motion, embarrassment about scarring, anxiety that restricts travel, etc. One cannot enjoy leisure time, e.g., hobbies, sports, reading, movies, social relationships games, reading. Brain injured people often cannot utilize public places, e.g., library, church, clubs, movies, theatres. Problems with leisure time put particular stress on family relationships.

Disturbance of Family Life

The patient is described by the spouse as not the person they married. Mental rather than physical deficits offer the most stress, although problems such as incontinence are significant (Bond, 1983b). Although physical symptoms may improve, the family experiences the patient's emotional disturbance as unimproved. Particularly troubling are irritability, temper, tiredness, aspontaneity, tension, anxiety, and restlessness. The TBI victim may require so much attention that this limits the freedom of other family members. Examples would include unsafe behavior when unsupervised, visits to professionals, etc. On the other hand, the impaired person may not wish to travel and participate in family or social events in or outside the home, because of self-consciousness. This causes the family to become less cohesive.

Loss of earnings may occur precisely when there are higher medical bills. This further disturbs leisure time pleasure. Wives are described as becoming depressed, lonely, isolated, and assuming their husbands' roles. Spouses of brain-damaged victims are disturbed by an inability to perform, a reduction in their mates ability to be affectionate, childishness, dependency, aggression, irritability, etc. The patient may be experienced as being like a child. Professional persons may not take the trouble to explain the permanency of the condition, particularly to a less well-educated family (Brooks, 1984). The course of family reactions to its changed status may go through denial and hope, then depression, despair, and finally emotional equilibrium brought about by acceptance of the reality of the problems.

Sexual Life Is Disturbed

Sexual activity can be affected by lesions at any level of the CNS, or in the divisions of the ANS serving the lower half of the body. The level of sexual drive can be unchanged, reduced like other aspects of motivation, or disinhibited. There is a marked trend, however, for sexual drive to be reduced, including reduced self-confidence and sex appeal, depression, and decreased erectile ability, drive, and frequency (Kreutzer & Zasler, 1989). Previous personality characteristics may become accentuated. On the other hand, disinhibited sexual behavior may not yield to increased control (Bond, 1984).

The injury may be experienced as the loss of the partner, yet since the person is alive he or she cannot be mourned properly. Increased isolation, loneliness, and responsibility result in depression. Depression is enhanced by the physical, mental, and personality changes manifested by the spouse (Bond, 1983b).

Emotional Disorders

The rate of mental illness is increased since resources to avoid and cope with stress are impaired. Anxiety and depressive reactions are extremely common, including posttraumatic stress disorder, and cerebral personality syndromes. Regression to formerly abandoned drug habits takes place. Depression results from unhappiness concerning social adjustment and reduced quality of life, e.g., loss of friends, feelings of impairment, and loss of attractiveness (see Chapter 15 on Stress and Psychodynamic Reactions).

Impaired Independence

McKeny (1983) describes the special problems of the acutely and severely injured TBI victim differentiating between skill levels, e.g., basic (feeding, dressing, personal hygiene, mobility, toileting) and advanced (financial management, driving, social skills).

After TBI there is an interaction of impairment and emotional distress (reduced attractiveness and disturbed self-esteem). Reduced mental ability may prevent the victim from devising strategies that make life pleasant and constructive. Daily coping is unpleasant and unrewarding.

Ways of coping can be subdivided into strategies, with individuals varying in their use of different components (Moore, Stambrook & Peters, 1989):

Direct action: confrontation; planful problem solving;
Palliative: accepting responsibility; distancing; self-controlling, escape avoidance; positive reappraisal;
Both direct action and palliative: seeking social support.

Low use of coping strategies may be a form of denial in closed head injuries. Although this is usually considered to be maladaptive, including loss of insight, it is associated with decreased distress, and serves to increase self-esteem and hope.

Impaired mobility and other sensorimotor problems lead to further deficits, since traveling and personal safety become problems. The patient cannot use public transportation, drive, or avoid getting lost.

Impaired Personal Responsibilities

The TBI victim may be unable to take care of household and children due to reduced comprehension, headaches, and immobility. They have problems with cooking, cleaning, repairs, and taking care of dependent family members.

Driving and Use of Power Tools

A variety of deficits may make it unwise or impossible for the TBI victim to continue to use or learn to use machines that are dangerous to himself or others. Epileptic seizures in particular should be considered. Although seizure victims are not involved to a great extent in collisions with another vehicle (0.03–0.1%), they are involved in a somewhat great number of personal vehicular accidents (Andermann, Remillard, Zifkin, Trottier, & Drouin, 1988).

McKeny (1984) asserts that a traumatic head injury renders most victims incapable of operating a motor vehicle, temporarily or permanently. Assessment should include motor problems, seizures, visual abiliy including scanning and peripheral vision, judgment of depth and distance, colors, and speed of response, overall judgment, and medications that slow responses or impair consciousness.

Problems with Time

Loss of time sense leads to problems of planning and scheduling, or difficulties with ongoing activities.

Loss of Skills

Deficits of calculations, writing, reading, spelling, typing, vocational processes, driving, sports, etc. prevent employment and also hamper domestic responsibilities (taking care of clothing, hygiene, shopping, budgeting, banking).

Reduced Work Efficiency

Even relatively minor accidents often have severe and permanent effects, due to reduced concentration and mental level, and emotional problems. Whether TBI causes employment problems is partially determined by the demands a job makes on particular functions. When a person succeeds with employment postinjury, it is due to retention of social skills, nonintellectual abilities, and use of previously learned skills. Work deficiencies can be hard to detect by the employer and colleagues may cover up.

The employee may not realize the seriousness of an accident. The writer has examined many patients who were unaware of deficits represented by an estimated loss of 30 points of IQ. Some of them were professionals or executives, who complained of headaches, memory problems, or poor coordination, inability to concentrate, etc.

The supervisor may see the impaired employee as a misfit, a complainer, someone with emotional problems, or a malcontent. Termination or reduction can occur without any proper examination or assessment concerning disability.

Characteristic Deficits Impairing Employability

Many functions vulnerable to TBI are precisely the areas in which impairment occurs after brain injury!

Reduced Efficiency (Executive-Type Functions)

This includes deficits in planning ahead, judgment, foresight, and monitoring ongoing actions.

Special Functions

Special skills, e.g., calculations, processing verbal, nonverbal, and holistic problems, functioning in either structured or unstructured situations; creative thinking, dealing with complexity, appropriate level problem-solving style, and short-term and long-term memory are affected.

Inflexibility and Inability to Cope with Change

Victims of TBI may have impaired ability to learn new ideas and to adapt to change.

Loss of Social Ability

Incapacity to relate to others at all levels, due to depression, irritability, temper problems, anxiety, social withdrawal, inappropriate jokes, anger, loss of interest, etc., is manifested.

Loss of Ability to Assume New Responsibilities

These deficits cause inability to be promoted to new or more responsible duties. They are augmented by difficulties with intraorganizational changes, or changes in social and environmental matters that affect an organization's success and efficiency.

Definition of Impairment

Capacity to return to work depends on many conditions, including motivation, anxiety, residual functions, presence of pain, scarring, muscular, and orthopedic injuries, availability of social support, transportation, etc.

Adults

Impairment may be defined as a reduced capacity to function in the areas of employment, social, and family life, to be independent, and to enjoy life, as the result of some event or illness.

"Disabled" means "not able," i.e., unable to work or function, primarily inability to work, and secondarily to take care of one's personal responsibilities such as health care, shopping, preparing food, taking care of bills, and ambulation without assistance. This is an extreme condition, which can be brought about by relatively narrow impairment in particular functions (vision), or general factors (dementia or health). It is also affected by emotional problems (e.g., embarrassment due to scarring, anxiety, loss of motivation, irritability, and temper).

Children

Impairment may be defined as an inability to perform school and domestic responsibilities, as well as personality problems in getting along with peers, family, teachers, etc. It may be expressed immediately as cognitive or personality problems, but delayed development or unattained maturity of functions is common. It is expressed variously:

1. Development may proceed initially at a normal rate, with reduced effectiveness appearing later.
2. There may be a reduced rate of development from the time of injury.
3. Immediate deficits, with an inability to catch up to the preinjury level and rate of development may appear.
4. The lead poisoning data (see Chapter 17 on Neurotoxins) suggest that there may be an initial loss followed by a plateau without further loss (as represented by percentile rank on general tests of intelligence).

Levels of Impairment

The professional who wishes to evaluate a brain-damaged impairment from the viewpoint of the employer might consider this informal scale:

1. *Minimal:* Can return to original job essentially without limitation.
2. *Reduced reserves:* A person may be unimpaired after a single minor injury, and resume his or her life. However, when an unexpected problem or organizational or environmental change occurs, the person is simply less intelligent or flexible.
3. *Reduced competence:* Unable to perform original duties but can perform a less demanding or essentially different job.
4. *Unemployable:* General lowering of ability to the point of unemployability.
5. *Mental retardation:* An IQ of 69 or below may be assumed to be a result of some kind of brain damage.

Disability as a Legal Entity

The Federal Government defines disability as follows: "The inability to engage in *any* substantial gainful activity by reason of any medically determinable physical or mental impairment that can be expected to result in death or has lasted or can be expected to last for a continuous period of not less than 12 months (Social Security Administration, 1986, p. 8).

Cerebral trauma as a cause for disability is considered under two categories (Social Security Administration, 1986, pp. 56–75).

Neurological impairments (epilepsy, major and minor motor seizures; and central nervous system vascular accident): Impairment is determined by persistence despite the fact that the individual follows prescribed anticonvulsive treatment.

Mental Impairments: Organic mental disorder is defined as psychological or behavioral abnormalities associated with a dysfunction of the brain. The required level of severity is met when the requirements in both categories A and B are satisfied:

A1. Disorientation to time and place;
A2. Memory Impairment (short-term or long-term);
A3. Perceptual or thinking disturbances (hallucinations, delusions);
A4. Change in personality;
A5. Disturbance in mood;
A6. Emotional lability (explosive temper outbursts, sudden crying) and impairment in impulse control;
A7. Loss of measured intellectual ability of at least 15 IQ points from premorbid levels, or overall impairment index clearly within the severely impaired range on neuropsychological testing (Luria–Nebraska, Halstead–Reitan batteries).

Resulting in at least two of the following:

B1. Marked restriction of activities of daily living;
B2. Marked difficulties in maintaining social functioning;
B3. Deficiencies of concentration, persistence, and pace;
B4. Repeated episodes of deterioration or decompensation in work or work-like settings.

In practice, the determination is frequently totally unrealistic. Since the impaired person can perform some work, disability may be denied. The availability of the unskilled work is often not taken into consideration. Frequently the person is too disabled to even apply or carry through the needed procedures.

Kodimer (1988) provides a very useful statement concerning the definition of disability, the procedures of the Social Security Administration, and the numerous problems of having a disabled person adjudicated as such. Puente (1987) lists the six stages of Social Security Disability Procedures from initial application to Federal Court.

Since the brain-damaged and psychotic person has serious problems in expressing impairment, the requirement that they first apply for disability, and then engage in a cumbersome litigation process if denied, is unjust. Many disabled individuals are incapable of processing applications and appeals. The patient's therapist may have to fill out the forms or to stage-manage contacts with attorneys, governmental officials, and insurance companies.

Clinical Examples of Reduced Adaptability After "Mild" TBI

Case 23: Passivity

A man, age 44, reported tenderness in the left temporal area after a high speed automobile accident. His wife stated that "The thing that most bothers me is that he doesn't want to do anything. He wants everybody to be unhappy because he is unhappy." She is trying to improve his habits, i.e., sleeping and waking. He is resisting. They moved into a new house 1½ years ago, and he has not helped to set up. He was formerly very handy in repairing household appliances and furniture. Now, nothing interests him. He is willing to sit on a broken chair. He uses excuses not to do things at home. He starts something but does not finish it. He never asks the children what is new or what they have learned. He does not take part in parent–teacher meetings. He takes no responsibility. He is helpless. He does not want to do anything. He is rejecting of family members.

He describes his condition as follows: "I feel 100% different. I don't know what I am doing. I forget what I have in my pocket. I'm scared of everything. At night I can't sleep. When I close my eyes I remember the accident and think that somebody wanted to kill me." He cries privately and feels guilty because his condition has not improved.

This appears to be the frontal lobe syndrome, i.e., loss of motivation, inability to finish tasks, and deterioration of personal habits. He experiences a change of identity, intrusive thoughts, guilt, and paranoid ideas.

Case 24: Reduced Competence

A woman, a high school graduate, who did responsible office work, was struck by a falling object. She was briefly unconscious. This is her daughter's description: "Her eyes kept rolling from the time she was picked up, for 45 minutes on the way to the hospital. She was not completely conscious until the next day. The first dramatic change was in the hospital a day or two after the accident. She used her maiden name to sign some hospital forms, although she was married for 37 years. She couldn't remember her birthdate. She couldn't count backwards from 100. She couldn't count forwards."

Now, she gets easily excited and cannot tolerate loud noises. She gets angry and is very picky. She is frustrated because she cannot do what she used to, e.g., gardening due to inability to hold tools. She is not as quick. She denies people have told her things. Everything bothers her. She is overly nervous concerning her grandchildren. She was the backbone of the whole family. She is nervous, e.g., traffic bothers her. She hates to go in stores. She goes out infrequently. She doesn't pick up on intellectual problems such as analogies. She does not understand crossword puzzles. She cannot write so she cannot fill out checks. She cannot type or do housework. She cannot use a can opener. She has an anxiety attack when she is physically unable to operate a vacuum cleaner or duster. She gives up more easily.

Examples of Employment Problems

Case 25: Deficits of Higher Level Functioning

A man with a technical position was out of work for a month after a minor head injury. When he returned he felt weak and concealed his condition. He inadvertently filled out an expense account in duplicate. Dizziness prevented him from driving, which was needed to visit subordinates. He also had light flashes. He was less effective in planning, organizing, and research. He felt lazy but was turning reading over to others. "I have done no research in the laws, i.e., planning strategy and innovations."

Case 26: Inability to Make Decisions

A woman in her mid-30s, a highly paid executive, was responsible for supervision of a large staff of office workers, cost reduction, public relations, etc. While walking in the street she was struck by a falling object on the head and shoulder, was stunned, but not unconscious. After a number of hours in the hospital she was released. "I didn't realize the seriousness. I couldn't sleep for nights and nights, had awful nightmares and woke up with a cold sweat." She feels that her personality has changed: "I am more reserved, less outgoing or witty, and more tired. I go home instead of going to a health club or dinner with friends. I have less outside professional interests."

Concerning work, she said "I can't sit too long. I get all kinked up, more than previously. It takes me longer to make decisions and to get things accomplished. My attention span is hampered. It is difficult to work with a violent headache. I close the door and sit quietly. Sometimes I have to function with a headache. If I don't sleep, its hard to work the next time, because I drop things, e.g., computer books. I just forget things; I get halfway there and I don't remember what I was doing; 10 minutes later I remember. Mathematical problems take longer."

Neuropsychological examination revealed an estimated loss of IQ loss of 32 points from 129 in the superior range to a slightly below average Full Scale IQ of 97. On the Wide Range Achievement Test-Revised, she had deficits in Reading, Spelling, and Arithmetic, which, along with other cognitive problems, impair her effectiveness. It appears that she has lost considerable ability to keep up with new situations.

Case 27: Communications Problem

A licensed professional woman in her mid-30s has to make convincing presentations before groups. In an auto accident she struck her head on a hard object, damaging her teeth, nose, and jaw. She cannot see on the right side due to double vision. She also has a visual–perceptual disorder of which she is unaware. Although she has retained an IQ in the superior range, her reality testing (estimated by Rorschach extended form accuracy percent), memory, judgment, and conceptual thinking have suffered. She continues to work, although she is anxious, depressed, and fearful of many forms of transportation. Her efficiency has been greatly reduced.

Case 28: Loss of Psychomotor Skills

The 40-year-old pilot of a plane that crashed wanted to resume his profession. He appeared to the examiner to be well related, pleasant, and cooperative. His problem-solving style was independent and precise. Yet, he was unaware of a deficit, represented in part by an estimated 10 point IQ loss. Considering his occupation, it is significant that he had a one-sided loss of strength, slower psychomotor speed and processing of information, loss of ability to suppress irrelevant information, and reduced intellectual efficiency in unstructured situations. Since a year and a half had elapsed since his accident, not much further improvement could be expected. It was apparent that it would be imprudent for him to resume his career as a pilot.

15
Anxiety, Stress, and Psychodynamic Reactions

Overview

Brain damage is a distinctive form of stress since the very organ of coping has been damaged, i.e., an impaired ability to maintain vocational, domestic, or academic responsibilities with loss of quality. It is also accompanied by frightening experiences at the time of injury, or the period of recovery. Ultimately, the victim may have the experience of being unable to cope with usual demands and being unable to earn a living, and also have problems with ambulation, scarring, rejection, sexual problems, and so on.

One of the most characteristic features of stress reactions, in general, and TBI, in particular, is that a single event may be impairing. TBI instigates a profound stress reaction, with contribution from both physiological and psychological factors, perhaps associated with multiple bodily trauma. These account for long-lasting cognitive and emotional dysfunctioning through changes in neuronal circuits, which create continuous anxiety and conditioned avoidance reactions.

Definition of the System

The unimpaired person conducts his or her life relatively calmly, with good emotional control. There is a sense of self-esteem, capacity to enjoy life, and ability to make plans for the future. Problems are faced without excessive fatigue, anxiety, depression, illness, emotional or bodily reactions, or a belief that one cannot cope with problems.

Neuropsychological Dysfunctioning and Definition of Stress

A stress reaction may be defined as a persistent maladaptation to a brief or long-lasting event, that was actually or potentially damaging and was experienced as overwhelming. Persistence is related both to characteristic neurotransmitter and hormonal effects, and the experience of feeling threatened and impaired. Emotional reactions to having an accident are usual, as well as to the period of recovery, being impaired, and having one's life interfered with. Significant features of posttraumatic stress reactions include various forms of anxiety, intrusive thoughts, and being preoccupied by the trauma; denial, alone or alternating with anxiety; loss of self-esteem; feeling like a victim; feeling less attractive due to impairment, loss of status, and scarring; a view of the world as dangerous and bleak; dysphoric moods (depression and anger); hyperarousal or hypoarousal of various somatic functions; sexual problems; inability to enjoy life; inadequacy; social withdrawal; and regression. New trauma is reacted to maladaptively.

One should differentiate among the original stress reaction, the emotional changes directly caused by brain damage, and the reaction to being impaired. Frequently, symptoms after stress are more extensive than those indicated for posttraumatic stress disorder (PTSD) by the *Diagnostic and Statistical Manual, 3d Ed. Rev.* (1988) (DSM-3R). Guidelines for obtaining information from stressed individuals are suggested in Chapter 23 on Therapy and the Appendix ("Intake Procedures").

The Significance of Stress

Danger

Stress may be real or imagined, physical or psychological (Herrenkohl, 1986). The identifiers of stress are the experience of powerlessness, within the context of immediate or ultimate bodily damage, and the feeling that the danger experienced is inescapable (van der Kolk, 1988). An overwhelming experience of terror can lead to its organization and preservation in memory, through primitive cognitive mechanisms. These include prelinguistic representation that is expressed through anxiety attacks and panic. The symptoms are influenced by the level of personality development and the degree of physiological disorganization (van der Kolk, 1988).

The Overwhelming Event

TBI is likely to be experienced as overwhelming because of the particular events, or the circumstances of recovery. Being inside a vehicle when it crashes, being knocked down by a car or bus, falls of great distances, having a ceiling fall on one's head, being assaulted, etc., are extremely frightening.

Sometimes, the person has no forewarning, e.g., a falling ceiling, or there is posttraumatic amnesia, and the person wakes up with pain and blood in a damaged vehicle, or in a hospital bed in a state of confusion, with multiple soft tissue and bony injuries, tubes coming from bodily orifices, or a "halo" brace screwed into the skull to protect a broken neck, awakening from a coma with bandages, tubes, lack of awareness, pain, and confusion, followed by a long dependency, a period of isolation from normal activities and social support, and the experience of being impaired and less attractive. Confusion, anxiety, and problems of identity are common.

Emotional Stress Is a Process

The frightening experience, followed by somatic injury, constitutes an extended stressful period. A gradual process of maladaptation, with symptoms varying with time and personality changes, may occur before a final breakdown (Alexander & Ax, 1951). The period of impairment with failure and rejection can be of sufficiently intense and long-lasting duration to constitute significant stress by itself. The pattern is influenced by the patient's level of recovery from injury and support from the environment. Mood characteristics, e.g., anxiety and depression, can be cyclical. Neither the initial response nor the ultimate symptom pattern can be immediately predicted.

Stress Dimensions After TBI

Accompanying Somatic Injury

Traumatic brain damage can be accompanied by severe somatic injury. Healing of the brain and internal organs, limbs, skin, and body may be slow and only partial, with the period of stress extended due to pain, embarrassment, isolation, etc.

Length of Exposure to the Stressor

Stressors vary between a single, momentary event, such as an accident, and lengthy exposure to conditions that are extended (combat, internment in concentration camps).

Passivity or Activity During the Period of Danger

Whether one has had an opportunity to prepare, or to respond with appropriate and effective behaviors (Reus & Collu, 1988), can influence the content of frightening memories, feelings of being overwhelmed, or putting up a struggle, etc. In most cases of TBI, the situation is either beyond the person's control, or totally unexpected, or both.

The Meaning of the Experience

The significance of an accident plays a role in stress and recovery (see Chapter 1 on concerning meaning). Reus and Collu (1988) assert that the psychological perception of the stress is more significant than its physical characteristics in determining increase of glucocorticoids (adrenal hormonal response to stress, in particular making glucose available, the primary brain energy source). Religious attitudes and interference with plans are significant contributors to the meaning of the experience.

Susceptibility and Claims of Prestress Influences

One should take into account stress resistance (see Chapter 3) as a modifier of postaccident reactions. I disagree with the frequent assertions that the emotional reaction to stress is related to a preexisting personality condition. Asked to justify this impression, one would state that the events, and impairment, have a more powerful influence on mood than earlier psychodynamic considerations. Indeed, there is little evidence that the posttraumatic reactions of TBI victims in particular relate to prior personality considerations. There appear to be individual differences in response to psychological and physiological stressors (e.g., response of the HPA axis) that may be constitional, but these did not seem related to psychometric variables (Bossert, Berger, Krieg, Schreiber, Junker, & von Zerssen, 1988). Styles of coping with distress certainly do shape reactions, but the meaning of the experience to the victim seems far more shaped by the nature of the accident, and its consequences, than preexisting personality dynamics. Nevertheless, others have disagreed with this conclusion.

- A pre-existing cerebral injury can predispose to neurosis (PTSD) (Trimble, 1988b, p. 191);
- "Psychological attitudes pertaining to injuries of the head" (Schilder, 1964, p. 326);
- Ineffectiveness of the victim's mother as a mediator or soothing influence on arousal in the child. Under stress, this would lead to physiological disorganization with extremes of under- or overarousal, which would influence the intensity of the stress reaction, and interfere with the capacity to assimilate and accommodate new information;
- Prior trauma predisposes individuals to develop PTSD (van der Kolk, 1988, citing T. Field);
- High anxiety as a steady personality trait, with a contribution from the meaning of the event (Kreitler & Kreitler, 1988);
- Predisposition toward emotional stress due to few resources to cope with difficult or novel situations;
- The accident's special significance, how it is integrated into the personality structure, and unconscious motivations and fantasies (Schilder, 1950).

My experience in performing a comprehensive neuropsychological examination, and subsequent counseling sessions, indicates that accident victims rarely if ever offer any evidence that a preexisting neurosis shaped the symptoms. Associations of the accident to particular prior experiences seem extremely rare. In most cases of brain injury, the overwhelming event, accompanied by fright, injuries, and reduced adaptability, is usually of far greater significance to the outcome than the meaning of the event to the victim. Prior employment status seems not to be a predictor of external stressful events (Rimel et al., 1981). However, one may regress to pre-existing emotional dysfunctioning, e.g., depression, psychosis, anxiety attacks, and the like.

Neurophysiological Characteristics of Stress

Survival

A high level of bodily reactions supports overt action and emotions. Stress responses meet the body's demands to survive, e.g., meeting the brain's and body's metabolic requirements, and contribute to analgesia. Eventually normal or pathological functions terminate the stress response. Injury also creates neuropathological processes that have serious, pervasive neuropsychological effects (see Chapter 4 on Trauma). For details concerning neural pathways participating in the stress response, the reader is referred to Palkovitz (1987).

The Stress Reaction and the Hypothalamic–Pituitary–Sympathetic Nervous System Axis

The response to stress is integrated by the nervous system, in particular the CRH–cortisol axis, i.e., the hypothalmic–pituitary–adrenal–sympathetic nervous system. This axis is part of a general neuroendocrine response to noxious environmental stimuli, e.g., pain and trauma. CRH stimulation is regulated by different afferent nervous impulses, arising in various regions of the nervous system, with a sequence of steps leading to activation of the sympathetic nervous system, stimulation of ACTH (leading to cortisol secretion by the adrenal gland cortex), and β-endorphin secretion (Gill, 1985, p. 860).

Incoming stimuli inducing CRH secretion occur in three major groups of pathways (Palkovitz, 1987; refer also to Chapter 2 on Neuroanatomy): (1) pain signaling systems include the spinothalamic, spinoreticular, spinocervicothalamic, medial lemniscus, and spinal trigeminal tracts; (2) special sensory stimuli (e.g., vision and audition); and (3) emotional stimuli through limbic projections, e.g., hippocampus, septum, and amygdala, whose stimulation elicits a rise in corticosterone levels. Elimination of input to the hypothalamus abolishes this rise, i.e., it integrates the stress response. The hippocampus also plays a role in stress feedback (see hippocampus, below).

The cerebrospinal fluid also takes a role in integrating brain and peripheral endocrine functions insofar as hormones or hormone-releasing factors from the hypothalamus are secreted into the extracellular space or into the CSF (Carpenter, 1985, pp. 18–19).

There are various glandular products released into the bloodstream including hormones, adrenal cortex products (glucocorticoids, primarily cortisol, and mineralocorticoids, secreted by the adrenal cortex), and catecholamines [epinephrine (adrenalin) and norepinephrine (noradrenalin)], secreted by the adrenal medulla (core) and nerve endings. High levels of cortisol seem to act as a barbiturate and depress brain nerve cell function (Barnes, 1986). Continued stress is accompanied by catecholamine turnover and eventual depletion, and secretion of opioids (endorphins) with eventual depletion. The consequences include anxiety, irritability, explosive outbursts, insomnia, hyper-alertness and emotional lability (Kolb, Burris, & Griffiths, 1984; van der Kolk, 1984; van der Kolk & Ducey, 1984; Carr, 1984; Kolb; 1987; van der Kolk, Boyd, Krystal, & Greenberg, 1984).

Neurotransmitter Effects

During stress there is an outpouring of biologically active substances. Head injury and/or multiple trauma are accompanied by "a tremendous catecholamine surge," which instigates electrocardiographic changes, depression of thyroid function, and hypoxia (Marshall & Marshall, 1985). In addition, there is an out-pouring of other neurotransmitters, neurohormones, neuropeptides, and hor-mones involving the hypothalamic–pituitary–adrenocortical axis, and sympathetic nervous system, limbic cortex, and lobe, etc. Corticosterone levels, i.e., a major response to stress, are influenced by the levels of another stress-related substance, the level of the neurotransmitter norepinephrine, which modu-lates in the hypothalamus input from the hippocampus and reticular formation. Yes, the brain does function as an integrated organ!

The hypothalamic stress response of the adrenal cortex is balanced by the anterior pituitary (ACTH) and pineal gland (melatonin). See Chapter 4 on Trauma for additional neurotransmitter effects related to dysfunctions of the CSF.

The reader interested in the latest research concerning neurotransmitter effects consequent to stress may explore varied effects of stress on dopamine utilization in frontal cortex regions with mesocorticolimbic connections (midbrain, e.g., sub-stantia nigra, to caudate nucleus, putamen, and frontal cortex). This is a very com-plex area, and for further information see the symposium edited by Kalivas and Nemeroff (1988, e.g., Preface, and articles by Fallon et al., 1988, and Holson et al. 1988).

Memory Effects

Neurotransmitter Contribution to Long-Term Memory

During stress and moderate emotion, the sympathetic branch of the ANS stimu-lates a rapid heart beat, dry mouth, increased cardiac output, etc., which are associated with ongoing events. There is also ongoing secretion of cortisol, epinephrine, and norepinephrine, all of which have known memory-enhancing functions (Thompson, 1988). The combination of enhanced neurotransmitter presence, afferent feedback from the body, and sensory reception of the trauma synergistically imprints the experience. Moreover, other events that stimulate enhanced bodily reactions could be associated with the greater trauma, creating generalization. In contrast, it is well known that athletic individuals, e.g., jog-gers, are stress resistant because they do not consider increased feedback from the body associated with high levels of stress-type endocrine substances as being unnaturally dangerous.

The Stress Role of the Hippocampus

The hippocampus (which plays a role in memory), contributes to feedback to the adrenal cortex to modulate the stress response, together with the pituitary, amygdala, septum, and reticular formation. It is sensitive to glucocorticoids (for which it has the greatest concentration of receptor sites) and vasopressin. Circulating glucocorticoids (e.g., cortisol) are released, and influence fat and protein metabolism and muscle tone, inhibit inflammatory responses, influence CNS functioning, etc. They exert feedback effects via the hippocampus (Sapolsky et al., 1984). Therefore, hippocampal damage, or depletion of receptors after chronic stress, leads to an increase of adrenal cortical secretion via corticotropin hypersecretion.

Chronic stress contributes to oversecretion by the adrenal cortex, followed ultimately by depletion. There is evidence that loss of adrenal secretion leads to loss of hippocampal granule cells (dentate gyrus), which could account for deficits of learning (Sloviter, Valiquette, Abrams, Ronk, Sollas, Paul & Neubort, 1989).

Neurophysiological Effects on Behavior

The condition exists in various forms—acute, delayed, and chronic—but the long-term psychopathological effect is claimed to be essentially the same for all PTSD sufferers (Kolb, 1988). Nevertheless, some of the subjective symptoms vary according to the circumstances of the stress. The reactions of the U.S. soldier in WW II (Raines & Broomhead, 1945) was not the same as the Vietnam War (Glover, 1988; Salley & Teiling, 1984; Spiegel, 1988), and both differ from the accident victim.

Enhanced Arousal

Arousal is a state of heightened activity "shared by the physiological components of a number of naturally occurring states, including anger, excitement, sexuality, fear and even sadness" (Neiss, 1988). It is measured through autonomic activity, ACTH, and corticosteroid levels (Levine, 1986). Somatic stress reactions are reminiscent of anxiety (urination, heart rate, sweating, etc.). Arousal provides the enhanced attention, emotion, and excitement that is described as being "psyched up." Extremes of arousal affect the ability to perform effectively.

The effect of arousal on performance varies with task difficulties, the nature of the stress, the nature of the subjects, the level of arousal, the ongoing psychological state, and the nature of the task involved, e.g., attention or memory (Gale & Edwards, 1986). Arousal, effort, and range of comfort tolerated by the individual are controlled by brain receptor sites sensitive to peptides, which ultimately control the adrenal cortex. Feedback from the body regarding hormonal levels affects the level of pituitary hormones secreted (Pribram, 1980).

Anxious patients have slower rates of habituation and higher baseline levels of physiological reactions (Gale & Edwards, 1986; Levine, 1986; Schwartz, 1986; Zahn, 1986). The prestress level of arousal (physiological functions) does not return to the baseline. The baseline levels of headaches, chronic back pain, and temperomandibular joint disorders (common after traumatic head injury) are not detectably higher than control subjects. However, stress-related increases in bodily reactions causing pain are slow to return to baseline levels (Flor & Turk, 1989).

During conditions of arousal, physiological, emotional, and cognitive processes, which ordinarily function within particular limits, are under less control due to the after-effects of stress (and brain damage). This interferes with calm assessment of a situation and adaptive reactions to reality.

Reduced Functioning

This relates to neurotransmitter and endocrine depletion, and in the case of trauma, to damage to the limbic and autonomic nervous systems, and tracts within the spinal column. This contributes to deficits of sexuality, motivation and impairment of endocrinological functioning, and impairment of the immune response.

Long-Lasting Emotional Reactions

Persistent anxiety, anger, and depression are consequent to biological reactions (Dunn, 1987; Keefe, Wilkins, Cook, Crisson, & Muhlbaier, 1986; Taylor, 1984; Trief, Elliott, Stein, & Frederickson, 1987; van der Kolk et al., 1984; Weiss & Glazer, 1975; Weiss, Glazer, Pohorecky, Brick, and Miller, 1975).

Opiate-Like Reactions

- *Stress–induced analgesia* is equivalent to an injection of morphine, i.e., an endogenous opioid response (van der Kolk, 1988), whose depletion ultimately can create opiate withdrawal symptoms.
- *Symptoms of opiate withdrawal.* Depletion of endogenous opioids after long-term demand for their secretion occurs in posttraumatic stress disorder. The consequence is central noradrenergic hyperactivity, i.e., reaction to a loss of opiate presence.
- *Fugue states.* These may occur during partial seizures. The temporal lobe limbic system is considered to be particularly sensitive to peripheral sensory changes leading to clinical and neurochemical symptoms of stress (Kolb, 1988).

Physiological Dysfunctions

Endocrine Disorder

Vegetative functions are often impaired after brain damage and somatic injuries occurring through accident or illness, consequent to trauma to neural tracts between the hypothalamus and the anterior pituitary gland, causing endocrine disorders, e.g., insufficiency of the gonads and thyroid. Irritative lesions can cause hyperactivity with symptoms similar to those of psychogenic anxiety. Stress is a multifactorial phenomenon acting on the whole hypothalmic–pituitary–gonadal axis (Reus & Collu, 1988) (see also Chapter 19 for developmental problems of children).

Mood Changes

Cortocotropin-releasing hormone (CRH) manufactured in the hypothalamus and many brain regions, is implicated in affective conditions common after brain damage, i.e., depression with reduced libido and panic attacks (Gold, Avgerinos, Kling, Loriaux, Calabrese, Chrousos & Kalogeras, 1987). CRH secretion is stimulated via pain and other sensory pathways, and emotional stimuli via limbic lobe pathways (Palkovitz, 1987).

Neuronal Depletion and Dysfunctioning

Stress reactions are intense, physiologically, cognitively, and emotionally. Overload leads to a variety of effects, including neuronal death. The latter is considered to be a definite possibility in intense and chronic PTSD (Kolb, 1988). Hypoarousal may be related to catecholamine depletion (diminished motivation, affect, and occupational functioning) and hyperarousal to subsequent hypersensitivity (startle, outbursts, nightmares, and intrusive recollections).

Immune Dysfunctions

The neuroendocrine axis mediates between the CNS and immune systems. After stress, disturbances both in the body's immune system and in interpersonal relationships occur, leading to further vulnerability in the body's ability to handle illness and difficult social situations. (Beutler, Engle, Oro-Beutler, Daldrup, & Meredith, 1986). Glucocorticoids modulate stress responses and suppress immune function (see Chapter 8 on Neurophysiological Functions). In particular, depression, which is accompanied by high cortisol levels, and loneliness (both characteristic of TBI) are known to reduce various immune responses (Meltzer & Lowy, 1986).

Some Cognitive Aspects of Stress

Primitive Thinking

Intrusive memories have the characteristics of early memories, i.e., without symbolic and liguistic representations or an autobiographical context (van der Kolk, 1988).

Dissociation

Defenses fail when the victim is reminded of the event by internal or external stimuli (this discussion is continued below under Personality Reactions). The consequences may be episodic rage attacks (Salley & Teiling, 1984) or fugue states (Spiegel, 1988). In brain-damaged victims, the possibility of partial seizures must be explored (see below).

Long-Term Persistence and Avoidance

A two-factor learning theory (Kolb, 1988) suggests the following.

1. The role of conditioning: Situations reminiscent of the original trauma result in a startle response, i.e., hypersensitivity of the sympathetic nervous system.
2. Avoidance: Through principles of instrumental learning, the individual learns to avoid cues that arouse anxiety (see avoidance, below). It is acknowledged that learning theory is insufficient to account for all of the physiological disturbances.

Reduced Intellectual Effectiveness

Reduced concentration due to anxiety and avoidance of a variety of activities impairs new learning and problem solving.

Complex Memory Effects

Intrusive Memories

After a "biologically important event . . . all recently active circuits may be 'printed'" (Livingston, 1985, p. 1270) by neurotransmitters and allied substances. This creates sensitization to dangerous stimuli, or generalizations that are reminiscent of them, repeating the trauma and creating new synaptic connections fixating it.

Short-Term Memory Losses

Patients with PTSD manifest deficits of short-term, though not long-term memory (Everly & Horton, 1988). Whether this is due to interference by ongoing neurological hyper- or hypoarousal, or merely more routine concentration problems, remains to be determined. (Note: Mental products not stored on short-term memory cannot be imprinted into long-term memory storage.)

Stress-Related Amnesia

Retrograde amnesia may have either a neurophysiological or psychogenic contribution. The hippocampus, which participate in locating experiences in space and time, can be suppressed after severe stress with its high corticosteroid levels (see also Golden, Moses, Coffman, Miller, & Strider, 1983, p. 39; Beutler et al., 1986; Flood et al., 1987; Epstein et al., 1987; Marshall & Marshall, 1985; Mishkin & Appenzeller, 1987; Sapolsky et al., 1984; Gill, 1985, p. 892).

Stress-Related Transient Global Amnesia (TGA)

Although TGA has been discussed as a consequence of TBI, it apparently occurs after severe stress, and might be mistaken for hysterical amnesia (HA) (Merriam, 1988). One differentiating factor is that TGA is characterized by anterograde amnesia, i.e., the inability to retain information currently obtained, whereas in HA there is a memory loss for significant identifying information, in the context of functionally intact recent and remote memory. It is hypothesized that a severely disturbing or emotionally arousing event results in the liberation of natural benzodiazepines, which disturb hippocampal functioning. The latter structure's contribution to fixing events in memory has been discussed above in Chapter 10, on Memory.

Dreaming

Contrary to some reports, it is claimed that the amount of dreaming after head injury increases, provided some time is allowed for readjustment. There is a marked increase in dreams of threatening content, though a comatose head injury victim has no registration of the traumatic event (LOC and disturbances in memory). The loss of self-esteem and self-confidence creates a permanent state of stress, which could be reflected in the patients' threatening, frightening, and anxiety-provoking dream content. On the other hand, dreams with sexual content decrease, perhaps related to functional problems being of a higher priority (Benyakar, Tadir, Groswasser, & Stern, 1988). In addition, the reader is reminded of the range of neurological structures, potentially damaged during TBI, that participates in sexuality (fact and fancy). It is reasonable to assume that dreaming is in part an expression both of neurological functioning and of feedback of intention and action. Consequently, the sexual deficits experienced at many levels by TBI victims might easily be reflected in reduced sexual dreaming.

Categories of Personality Reactions to Stress

Gross Anxiety

The stress victim is preoccupied with the trauma, either through constant reminders, flashbacks while awake, bad dreams, nightmares, impairment that prevents usual activities, social embarrassment from scars and unemployment, etc., psychodynamically generated "working through" anxiety.

Hypervigilance

Hypervigilance is a true defense against recurrence, which develops due to continued intrusiveness and associations to the trauma.

Intrusive Ideas and Nightmares

The victim is hyperalert, feels scrutinized or paranoid, has flashbacks, is easily reminded of the accident or of his or her condition, is preoccupied with the trauma, and consciously reenacts it. There are symbolic associations to the trauma and dread of reoccurrence and reenactment of the trauma. There may be sleeplessness, bad dreams, or nightmares.

Nightmare

A man who dismounted from a truck was struck three times by an automobile from the rear, on the third occasion hitting the windshield of a car, and then finally thrusting himself under a nearby car after hitting a windshield: In his nightmare: "After I hit the ground I'm all alone and there is nobody there. I'm all alone. What happened?"

Flashback

Flashback involves a reexperience of the trauma. Here are some examples.

- *A fall of 480 feet on an industrial platform:* "I relive the accident. I hear the screams and the roar of the air. Everything reminds me of it. I see skyscrapers and guys working on it and I think of the accident. I see it all the time. I can't get rid of it."
- *His car was struck from the rear while stopped* The night of the accident: "I would want to go to sleep and as I started to go to sleep I would reexperience the accident in vivid detail, 7–8 times until I sat up. I tried to avoid falling asleep. Finally I fell asleep sitting up."
- *A Marine Vietnam veteran with flashbacks mistaken for hallucinations.* The patient underwent long periods of mortar bombardment, and apparently incurred a head injury by striking an object in a rapid entry into a foxhole under attack: "I have flashbacks with violent thinking and feelings, without memory as to why. Once I saw a guy acres away, he was standing with a girl trying to pry a box open . . . I saw a profile of someone in black pajamas in a palm tree. I saw two Japanese business men, one had on black glasses and the other wore a grey suit . . . holding hostages . . . chained to a tree, and a guy in a car was thinking about picking them up. These scenarios went on for an hour or two. These visions were real, they were there . . . I opened a door into the scenario. I heared a voice and I thought they might be shooting a scene . . . I was frightened sometimes, and at other times just felt myself a spectator."

Rorschach Examples of Intrusive Thinking

The Rorschach, with extensive inquiry, is routinely administered to TBI victims, because of its utility in eliciting the cognitive level of functioning, and personalized reaction to the stressful experience and post-injury life. Personalized experience of aggression by the projected figure seems not to have been previously described. Examples of Rorschach stress-related content are included in Appendix 3, Neuropsychological use of the Rorschach Inkblot Test.

Hyporeactivity

Avoidance reactions: Activity is reduced due to fear of specific locales or activities that remind them of the accident.

Reduced affect: Emotional life is overcontrolled, suppressed, or constricted, depression is experienced, trauma is denied, motivation is reduced, and emotional numbing is experienced, to avoid reexperiencing the trauma and its effects. Life is not meaningful and what other people care about does not make sense (Laufer, Brett, & Gallops, 1984).

Learned helplessness: Prolongation of the stress experience leads to "learned helplessness," characterized by constricted affect, decreased motivation, and decline in occupational functioning, attributed to depletion of norepinephrine systems. Since endogenous depression is common after traumatic brain injury, it is noteworthy that increased HPA activity is the most consistently reported abnormality associated with major depressive disorder. It is inferred that HPA hyperactivity is followed by depletion (Asnis & Lemus, 1987; Laufer et al., 1984; Kolb, 1987; Dor-Shav, 1978).

Change of Identity and Morale

The TBI victim has experienced a change of identity. Frequently, the sense of self is far less articulated than before. As Dr. Ravella Levin described this phenomenon (in a personal communication): "I am a stranger to myself. This person with aphasia, memory problems, seizures, etc., really isn't Me!"

Vulnerable

The stimulus barrier most of us develop that gives us the illusion of invulnerability can be shattered in a moment. The sense of vulnerability increases defensive behavior to avoid recurrence of injury (Janoff-Bulman, 1985).

Unattractive, Damaged

The self is experienced as damaged, mutilated, unattractive, conspicuous, and an object of contempt.

Acute Sense of Shame

Scarring, impairment, loss of income, etc., reduce self-esteem, motivate social isolation, and attempts to conceal damage. Nobody should know of one's condition. After a "mild" head injury a woman was asked if she felt like a different person: She said she felt less attractive, i.e., damaged. She wanted somebody else to take care of her. Others told her that she was no longer interested in her appearance. She felt that her life has lost meaning since she could not work, had no means of income, and felt handicapped.

Incompetent with Poor Morale

The brain-damaged person often feels incompetent to deal with such a difficult environment, i.e., his sense of self is incompetent and victimized, and his future is bleak.

Helplessness

The victim feels that the injury occurred as a result of overwhelming force. There can be a cry for help, i.e., a need for assistance, nurture, shelter, and dependency. Although other stress victims may feel that they could have done more to protect themselves at the time of injury (Spiegel, 1988), accident victims are frequently taken by total surprise.

Discouraged

There is little self-confidence that one can improve things with one's own efforts, and the feeling that one must give up valued goals. Repeated failure, rejection, and inability to obtain help from the system may lead to "learned helplessness," or reduced initiative.

Depersonalization

Depersonalization is considered by Grigsby (1986) as a defensive response to a potentially life-threatening danger after even minor closed head injury. ("Almost like a separation from my body. Something is knocked out of kilter.")

Weltanschauung

To the accident victim, the world is dangerous, and ungiving, and one's future is bleak. It is experienced as dangerous, with forces too violent and overwhelming to be coped with. The victim feels trapped in an unhappy life. There is a search for the meaning of one's experience, i.e., "Why me?" or "Why has my life been changed so rapidly and destructively, with no fore-warning for no good reason?"

Reactive

There are various psychological modes of experiencing the trauma and impairment, defenses against distress, and restitutive efforts.

Guilt

Guilt may be experienced because of an inability to fulfill important obligations, the belief that one has brought problems on oneself, and the inability to meet responsibilities. The guilt of survivors, when others have been injured or worse have died, is familiar.

Depression

Depression with anxiety is not considered a direct response to brain injury, but rather a reaction to the stress of impairment and injury. It is experienced as an inability to enjoy life, and a sense of feeling damaged and of hopelessness. Loss of cognitive and adaptive functions makes significant goals unattainable (Atteberry-Bennett, Barth, Loyd, & Lawrence, 1986). There is a concern with death, and perhaps a wish to die. When pain is substituted for depression, there may be no suicidal ideation, loss of appetite, or guilt feelings (Hendler, 1981a, p. 85).

Anger

See also amygdala functions and organic brain syndrome (Chapter 8). Anger is a reaction to trauma, impairment, and the perpetrator of the accident, against whom one cannot strike back because of the constraints of law, the inaccessibility of the perpetrator, the need to be discrete during litigation, and the general indifference of society to perpetrators and victims of many avoidable injuries.

Inability to Enjoy Life

Associated pain can prevent bodily mobility, the ability to enjoy or to participate in former activities, due to reluctance to travel, problems of mobility, health, and neuropsychological deficits, withdrawal, pain, loss of relationships, impairment, and embarrassment (Oddy, 1984).

Regression to Former Levels of Adaptation

Regression refers to returning to a prior level of adaption, using means of coping that were given up as circumstances changed or the individual matured, or behaving in a less mature or more primitive fashion, after some stress, injury, or brain damage.

Dissociation

This may be a warding off of the traumatic experience during the event, as well as subsequent defense against memories. The sufferer may even reenact the event. The potential for intellectual dysfunctioning is particularly great when mind-altering drugs are being used.

Case 29: A woman who struck her head when a small plane crashed at sea, and was threatened by sharks, had an out-of-body experience: She saw a blinding light like the sun, saw Christ, her children, her whole life, felt forgiven, was told by Him she had to go back, and He would call her, but not now. Suddenly she was back in her body, lost consciousness, and woke up in the hospital.

Denial

This is a common means of coping with a damaged life-style. Although psychotherapists can understand how this will hamper some aspects of rehabilitation, when one considers the long-lasting effects of stress, as well as the deep loss of ability occurring in many accidents, this is not a totally maladaptive response in all cases (see also Chapter 14 on Adaptability, concerning the role of denial in recovery).

Psychogenic Amnesia

No doubt this occurs, but anterograde and retrograde amnesia is a more likely explanation of memory loss after brain damage.

Restitutive Phenomena

Restitutive phenomena include wish-fulfilling fantasies, concealing damage or impairment from others, a wish to return to a happier world, pleasant and constructive plans and fantasies, denial of trauma, injury, and dysfunctioning, awareness of the need to compensate for deficits, and constructive efforts at rehabilitation.

Secondary Gain

Obtaining advantage from an illness, e.g., attention or dependency is a secondary gain. This interacts with the possibility of malingering, passive reaction to problems, overprotectiveness, and guilt feelings on the part of one's family, all of which could contribute to a less than active approach to overcoming impairment.

Complex Interaction of Injury and Personality

This includes an emotional displacement in people unable to recognize (Taylor, 1984) or express feelings. It is affected by the physiological level of arousal at the time of injury, is associated with prior experiences (Beutler et al., 1986). There may or may not be demonstrable pathological findings related to depression when guilt is experienced because of failure to get better (Trief et al., 1987).

Pain

Psychic Component of Pain

Pain is more than a signal of tissue damage (see headaches, Chapter 4 on Trauma). It is a complex experience, including emotionally aroused muscular tension, cognitive, affective, and behavioral components (Flor & Turk, 1989), with an interaction between pain, depression, anxiety, bodily symptoms, and anger. Its components are somatogenic, anxiety, depression, social stress, secondary gains, and modifying cultural factors (Black, 1982). If pain recedes after electroconvulsive therapy, or antidepressant medication, depression is considered to be the primary problem (Adams & Victor, 1989, p. 114). It may be a final common pathway by which personality conflicts and deficits, in the context of stress, find expression (Acklin & Bernat, 1987).

Since chronic pain is a manifestation of depression and anxiety, the patient does not reveal the basic affect (Hendler, 1981b); depression affects the way pain patients express their feelings to doctors (Keefe et al., 1986).

Chronic pain is part of a syndrome including depression, guilt, self-criticism, a sense of failure to meet the expectations of others, and social alienation. The distinction between "functional" and "organic" pain is not supported (Trief et al., 1987). It is influenced by prior experience as well as contemporatry reactions to being impaired and a victim.

Pain contributes to a wide variety of subsequent illnesses and maladaptions (Hartig, 1984): inability to sleep, loss of appetite, decreased libido, bodily concerns, drug dependency, constipation, irritability, isolation, loss of interests, work, and family relations, and feelings of helplessness and hopelessness. These lead to suicidal thoughts (see Depression Leading to Suicide, Chapter 13).

Influences on Pain

1. If emotional arousal at the time of the accident was low, and there was some time to prepare for the accident, pain may primarily give information that the person has been injured. However, if emotional arousal is high, and there have been prior experiences with pain or danger from a similar source, then pain is experienced as "excruciating" or "unbearable."

2. Feeling angry, and the nature of the pain, further shape the postaccident emotional state. Thus, pain may be more or less intense than an outside observer would consider to be "appropriate." Hendler (1981b) described "exaggerated posttraumatic headaches" that are often attributed to psychological causes in a patient whose symptoms are triggered by an accident. Their premorbid adjustment is described as tense, anxious, or "high-strung," and they may not give an accurate history. Their symptoms include decreased efficiency, and problems of concentration, memory, depression, etc. If they are suffering from an organic brain syndrome they may use pain to attract attention.

3. Pain is affected by its emotional context, i.e., a variety of situational and personality factors. Experiencing and expressing chronic pain and depression may be influenced by prior experience. It may reflect disturbance of, or failure to, process current intense emotional experience. The victim does not react in what would appear to be an appropriate manner.

4. Many depressed individuals suffer inwardly. They do not communicate their feelings and thus might appear not to be seriously suffering. Inability to express feelings normally contributes to the use of pain as a signal for help. The experience of pain, bodily reactions, and depression can be due to an inability to express intense anger and/or fear directly. When depression is experienced it is more likely that pain will be experienced more intensely (Keefe et al., 1986).

5. Alexythymics (people who cannot express their feelings, or distinguish between bodily sensations and different emotional states) communicate distress by means of physical complaints. An inability to express pain and other dysphoric moods, e.g., fear and anger, would lead to doubt as to the victim's sincerity. Pain is enhanced by impairment. It can substitute for other emotional distress, making assessment of emotional injuries difficult.

6. Opiate-like effects are noteworthy. Chronic pain, in apparent excess of injury, could be due to a drug-like withdrawal reaction (see opiate-like reactions, above). The stress reaction can include both immediate alleviation of pain and enhanced experience of pain. Prior arousal, not trauma, may be the major determinant of the need for analgesics (Goldstein & Halbreich, 1987). Pain level after surgery is inversely related to presurgery β-endorphin levels.

Social Distress

Active Withdrawal

The sense of shame due to impairment contributes to the preference to be alone. There is loss of social interest in both family and friends, evolving from reduced self-esteem, status, and economic problems; impairment and reduced mobility, which reduces participation in work and play; scarring, which causes embarrassment; and anxiety and pain, making transportation difficult. Disfigurement is common after traumatic injury: bones can be permanently set in disfiguring positions. In one case I saw an obviously broken clavicle. One 2–year–old child had a disfigured elbow. Participation in work, community, or social life with friends and family are reduced or eliminated.

The Experience of Isolation or Alienation

Social contacts are reduced because others find the patient less attractive, causing feelings of isolation and alienation. Deficits or dysphoric moods make it difficult to reestablish one's life, which impedes making new friends and seeking employment. The outcome of withdrawal may be earlier mortality (House, Landis, & Umberson, 1988).

Somatic Reactions

Hyperarousal, Release, and Somatic Forms of Anxiety

These include startle, diarrhea, frequent urinating, sweating, tremor, rapid heart beat, headache, panic, and nausea.

Sleep Disturbances

There is an inability to sleep, with bad dreams and nightmares.

Pain

See above.

Somatic Conversion

Somatic reactions mimic illness (Schilder, 1964; Herskowitz & Rosman, 1982, pp. 139–140).

Parental Vulnerability

There is evidence that prenatal stress feminizes the sexual behavior of males, and reduces fertility and fecundity in females (Herrenkohl, 1986). Children of stressed mothers may be irritable and hyperactive and have gastrointestinal disturbance.

Health Risks

Although stressful life events are associated with health risks, a recent review characteristically did not provide information concerning brain injury and its role in disease (Miller, 1988). However, abnormally high corticosteroid concentrations injure the immune system, leaving the person vulnerable to oncogenic viruses and other pathological processes that are ordinarily held in check (Livingston, 1985, p. 1261).

Sexual Problems

Libido changes occur, including reduction and enhancement, perhaps accompanied by impulsivity and insensitivity, or reduction. The person may be passive and nonreactive. Both varients are baffling and frightening for a sexual partner (Neistadt, 1988). A survey of the National Head Injury Foundation suggests that brain injury has its greatest impact in the area of sexuality (1987; *Headlines*, 1988). I have also seen this statement made for social relations). The effects of damage to the brain are loss of control over endocrine functions, with reduced levels of drive and self-control, loss of social skills, cognitive functioning, self-image, and self-esteem, poor judgment, egocentricity, inability to delay gratification, impairment of social factors leading to isolation, depression, role changes, and altered bodily image and self-concept, and loss of preinjury social skills and general knowledge. These are compounded by apathy and loss of sexual interest, stemming from damage to frontal areas that regulate motivation and initiation of behavior.

The effects of reduced sexuality depend on the age and emotional development of the person. Immaturity and instability compound difficulties in satisfying a partner's needs for affection and emotional intimacy.

Cognitive Defects

Even emotional trauma, without any documentable history of head injury or brain damage, may impair intellectual abilities to the point that performance is very difficult to distinguish from brain injury. See Chapter 9, Intellectual Functions, and Gill, Calav, Greenberg, Kugelmass, & Lerer (1990).

Reduced Intellectual Level

Some confirmatory evidence is found in Chapter 18 on Recovery, in which stress alone was associated with a reduction from estimated prestress IQ. There are two types of poststress cognitive deficits:

1. *Effects on concentration* (distracted by stress-related intrusive thoughts), guilt, poor morale, etc.
2. *Damage to neuronal circuits* caused by stress-stimulated neurohumoral effects.

Adaptive Consequences of Stress

Grave maladaptive difficulties accompany symptoms of stress resulting from an incident of TBI.

Diagnosable Psychiatric Disorders

Resources to avoid and cope with stress are damaged. In children, for example, over 50% of head injury victims develop significant emotional problems: schizophrenia, paranoid psychosis, affective psychosis, and suicide. There may be a predisposition for schizophrenia when it occurs immediately upon injury (Lishman, 1987, p. 164). I have observed regression to schizophrenia that had been in remission.

Decline in Occupational Level

Victims of TBI often give up goals due to loss of competence and motivation, cosmetic injuries, etc. Inability to maintain responsibilities on the job causes reduced efficiency, loss of status, and potential unemployment.

Inability to Maintain Domestic Responsibilities

Accident-related problems that impair ability to take care of one's home and family are extremely distressing.

Regression to Former Levels of Adaptation

Regression can involve use of tobacco, alcohol, and drugs that had been rejected, dependency, and unemployment.

Clinical Examples of Posttraumatic Stress Response

Case 30: Adult Automobile Victim

"I was crossing the street. I saw myself go up in the air. In a matter of a second I said, 'Oh my God.' That was it." He was unconscious for about 5 minutes, awoke, and somebody was asking him if he knew his name. He was in the hospital about 4 hours and needed assistance to leave. "They had to cut off my clothes because I couldn't move my left side. The left side of my face was scratched. My shoulder was dislocated." He still takes medications for headaches. "I was still in a daze one full day. I didn't know if I was going or coming." There was no RA. "The next day I was in a state of shock and excruciating pain. I didn't know what to do. I was not in my right mind for a week. I was frightened all the time. I thought I would be an invalid for the rest of my life." He thinks about the accident almost every day. "Everytime I cross the street I get into a panic. I'm scared of cars." He formerly had nightmares. "I saw myself in a wheelchair without my left arm."

The worst effect of the accident was that he must stay home most of the time like "a prisoner in the house." He wanted to go back to school; it was never to late to learn. Now he feels useless. "I don't see the light at the end of the tunnel." He doesn't feel enjoyment. He feels messed up in his head. He spends most of his time laying down. Religion is a solution.

Asked if he saw himself as different, or not his real self, he asserted that he "doesn't feel right, and doesn't know how to explain it. I used to talk to everybody, now I feel worthless." He hides his feelings. His condition has not improved, although he takes occupational therapy for his arm. Asked how he feels about the future, he asserted: "After 5 months I don't know what to think." He has contemplated suicide, but doesn't think he will do it.

Case 31: Intrusive Anxiety After a Ceiling Fell on a Woman's Head

She tries not to think of the accident, but thoughts come back unexpectedly once or twice a week. Nightmares occur almost every night, fear of which prevents sleep and also wake her up. "I feel cold blood running down my neck and arm. I feel like my eyes are closed and I feel I'm going to die and I wake up."

Nervousness causes her to avoid being around people since she feels watched. Although her feelings are weaker, she tries to hide them, but she has difficulty with her temper: "I start to yell at every little thing. I am constantly screaming. I find I can't control my temper."

She cannot work due to pain and restricted movement. "It looks like my future will be different. I want to go back to work and enjoy my life. I just feel I can't do it because of the pain. I lost my sexual drive. I have no sex desire. My lover is getting annoyed. I don't have energy or desire."

Case 32: Identity Change

A middle-aged woman whose vehicle was struck from behind while stopped waiting for a light perhaps did not strike her head, although her arms were bruised. She went to the ER and was kept for 4–5 hours. She had a few drinks prior to the accident, which "may significantly compound the effects of head injury in various ways" (Bakay et al., 1980, p 357). "I feel I'm encapsulated. Something is around me. I'm not part of the world. Most people don't realize I have a problem. I have this space, this personal little fog that separates me from everybody else." On the Rorschach she perceived "chicken face," "skin hung up to dry." Her figure drawings had only a line for eyes, i.e., no pupils.

16
Expressive Deficits: Inability to Describe Impairment

Overview

It is often impossible to obtain a comprehensive and accurate statement from the brain-damaged person. It requires effort by the interviewer to *attempt* to obtain information concerning their adaptive status and their mood. All of the various components of the Taxonomy of Neuropsychological Deficits conspire to hamper communication. "Expressive deficits" is a term I proposed to describe brain-damaged victims' inability to describe the accident, or its adaptive and emotional after-effects.

Brain-damaged victims' communications affect the kind and quality of information available to an examiner or therapist, perhaps drawing attention to less significant problems that exist. This may occur due to embarrassment concerning a troublesome condition, or even embarrassment concerning the inability to express oneself clearly.

Emotional blandness and various forms of depression, common after brain damage, make it difficult for the observer to recognize the deep distress experienced because of impairment and disorganization of life. The depressed person's dull mood can be misunderstood as indifference, since many do not communicate their intense emotional pain and hopelessness.

Reduced expression or experience of anxiety also prevents the victim from calling attention to other forms of impairment. Perhaps a lack of foresight or judgment will cause the person not to realize that they have created acts damaging to themselves, or are likely to do so in the future.

Even when there is concern with injury and impairment, eliciting information is not always easy or straightforward. Expressive deficits may represent a symptom in every area of the Neuropsychological Taxonomy. Reasons why information in the record may be inaccurate are discussed in Chapter 1. Problems of interviewing are noted in Chapter 21.

Expressive deficits lead to various consequences:

1. *The examiner reaches an incorrect conclusion* concerning the presence or the extent of brain damage (Parker, 1987, 1988).

2. *Compensation for injuries is inadequate* (see Chapter 14 on Adaptability).
3. *Treatment planning is inadequate.*
4. *The extent of brain damage is underreported.*

Clinical Examples

Case 33: Expressive Deficits in a Child Knocked Down by a Car

This is an example of an 11-year-old child who appeared clinically very pleasant, and without apparent distress. Only through her mother's statement, and the comprehensive neuropsychological examination, was it possible to determine the after-effects of an automobile accident in which she was knocked down.

Emotional Behavior

She was motivated to do well, and expressed herself spontaneously. Her mood was pleasant and appropriate. *She did not appear clinically depressed, angry, or anxious.*

Child's Statement

She remembers being hit by the car, and what she was doing. When the EMS arrived, they picked her up. They taped something to her face and chin to stop the bleeding. Her cheek was scraped. She was frightened. She does not claim bad dreams at the time of the accident or later. She does not claim unconsciousness. She is sad when things do not go her way. She denies headaches or dizziness. She had a pain in her right leg when she fell to the ground.

Neuropsychological Implications

There is no claim of loss of consciousness. This is a frightening experience for anyone, but Natasha does not claim intrusive anxiety. If anything, she seems to minimize any after-effects.

Mother's Statement

Her daughter was on the street and was hit by a car. She saw her about an hour later, and she remained in the hospital for a couple of hours. Seizures are denied.

Concern

She complains of stomach pain, but she is not sure how often. She sleeps a lot, some days all day. She stays in bed on days she complains about her stomach. Although the amount of liquid imbibed is normal, she gets up every night two times to urinate. On some days after a normal night's sleep she stays in bed and may sleep for a while. (Apparently, this is not necessarily school days.) She describes her as more emotional since the accident. She is very touchy and complains that her brother bothers her. She acts as though she is depressed.

Anxiety

Her mother believes that while her daughter was in the hospital she was nervous. She acted like she was calm, but was looking around and did not seem to be at ease. She is afraid of crossing the street. She does not want to do anything, just wants to play with her toys. She complains about household chores. She describes her as tending to hold her feelings back, which is similar to her effort to deny anxiety immediately after the accident. After the accident she cried a lot in school. She told the teacher she might be hit by a car. Despite the description of holding back her feelings, she loses her temper and hits her younger brother. She is described also as being frightened, and crying too easily. She does not want to go outside, which surprises her since they live in a hot, stuffy apartment, and she still stays in. She goes out only if her mother has an appointment to take her somewhere.

School and Learning

She is about to enter the sixth grade. She does not concentrate normally. The teacher told her that she daydreams. However, she had some counselling for this condition, even before the accident, which continued after the accident. She gives up too easily since she does not have patience. When she is asked to do things, she forgets. Her math grades have gone down since the accident.

Social

When she is with other children she behaves normally, but this is not very often. She does not start conversations with strangers. If a child she knows speaks to her, she avoids the child.

Worst Effect of the Accident

The worst effect of the accident is the child's fear.

Personality (Rorschach Inkblot Test and Drawings)

There is a discrepancy between her demeanor and what she experiences. Overtly, she is a pleasant child, cooperative, and denies to the examiner any emotional distress. This is reflected in a Rorschach drawing of two dancers, poorly constructed, who are "happy." Poorly perceived human figures are suggestive of discomfort with one's self-image, i.e., a lack of comfort in the way one's self is experienced. She would like to be assertive and outgoing, and this figures in her fantasies, but there is a forced quality in its expression. Her tendency to conceal her feelings is revealed by a "mask of a cat," and the denial of anxiety by "a costume . . . [representing] a bat." There are specific signs of anxiety: "snake;

bat; crawling bug; spiders; monster." She tries very hard to exercise emotional control (all of her Rorschach responses were precise, with no vagueness permitted). This is unusual for a child, i.e., a denial of the normal emotionality and spontaneity expected in an 11-year-old. Moreover, she projected no color responses, which would be noteworthy at any age, but, in the context of an accident, indicates depression together with a repressive style to conceal anxiety. Her mother's description of her as withdrawn was confirmed by the total lack of human figures and the presence of only three Popular responses (frequently perceived), which measure thinking in conformity with others.

Case 34: Apparent Indifference

A 25-year-old man was examined several years after an auto accident in which he was rendered unconscious. A normal EEG and CT scan of the brain were reported although he was diagnosed as having a "concussion." He described his feelings as weaker, could not find words to express himself, and does not remember what he does not remember. Clinically, his mood was in the pleasant to dull range. He expressed depression, and wept when he was led to discuss his situation, but did not show anxiety. He asserted that others do not understand him. (His unhappy mood and subclinical aphasia would have been difficult to detect without a thorough interview and/or examination.)

Case 35: Denial at the Time of the Accident

A 13-year-old boy was in the front seat of a car next to his father when another car drove in front of them. Their car smashed into it. The boy's head struck the dashboard, creating a considerable laceration. His father stated: "He just looked at me, he was very dazed. He said 'yeah'. His eyes were glazed over. I asked him again, 'Did you hit your head?' and he said 'No, I'm fine.'" Actually, he was holding his head up and blood was dripping down the back. At the hospital, 20–30 minutes later, he was sitting, and his eyes started to clear. (At the time of the accident, he was unable to report the extent of his confusion, and might have been permitted to proceed without treatment.)

Requirements for Accurate Self-Report

To offer an accurate self-report requires quite complex cognitive functioning, indeed an intact brain. Therefore, the greater the damage, the harder it is to communicate problems.

- *Awareness* that a change has taken place. Lack of awareness of illness itself is called anosognosia (Bisiach et al., 1986). Memory problems also exist (Levin, 1987). Various kinds of agnosia and neglect imply lack of awareness of the nature of the injury.

- *Experiencing distress*. Cerebral damage, leading to reduced intensity of affect, by its nature would prevent the patient from total reactivity to the impaired state.
- *Remembering* that some dysfunctioning has occurred.
- *Sufficient intelligence and judgment* to evaluate consequences of one's actions. With certain kinds of injury, e.g., dementia, or the frontal lobe syndrome, poor adaptation is not realized.
- *Motivation* to communicate distress. The victim must feel that it is useful and proper to tell the examiner about adaptive problems.
- *Emotional credibility* of self-expression. Depression or loss of prosody may give the false impression of indifference or lack of suffering.
- *Clarity of consciousness*. Reduced arousal or activation will hamper communication.

Taxonomy of Expressive Deficits

Preexisting Conditions

- *Alexythymia:* A condition not necessarily caused by brain damage, in which the person does not identify or label feelings, fantasies, or physiological reactions (Acklin & Bernat, 1987; Taylor, 1984). Alexythymia may not be a single personality characteristic (Norton, 1989).
- *Preexisting low intelligence:* The postinjury ability to express problems would be an extension of a prior communication and comprehension problem, in any event, further hampering any effort to communicate the circumstances and result of an injury. The unintelligent or illiterate subject would have particular difficulty (even preinjury difficulty) in self-description of significant functions (Lecours et al., 1987).

  - The inability to judge the poor quality of performance, change of behavior, or maladaptive reactions and their implications; maladaptive behavior.
  - The inability to grasp the facts describing an accident.

Deliberate Concealment of Legitimate Symptoms

- *Religious beliefs:* One woman engaged in litigation against her religious belief, only because of her husband's insistence. It was as though God had visited this affliction on her for His own reasons.
- *Fear of loss of employment:* Inability to work may be concealed by an injured worker. Perhaps the deficiency is attributed to personal stress. The employee is afraid that if the employer knew the extent of the inability to function due to headaches, and loss of concentration, problem solving ability, and memory, etc., employment could be terminated (Parker, 1987). He or she may succeed temporarily in concealing reduced effectiveness since other workers help in covering up.

• *Reduced social acceptability:* People fear loss of friendship should their limitations be known. One man did not want to discuss his loss of sexual ability with his friends, because bragging about sex with their wives was a source of prestige. A boy would not acknowledge in a psychometric test (true/false responses) any significant degree of anxiety. On the Rorschach Inkblot Test, which makes it harder to conceal basic feelings, he revealed a gross level of anxiety and feelings of bodily damage.

• *Embarrassment* is caused by the conspicuousness of impaired verbal expression, e.g., word-finding difficulties or other receptive and expressive problems. The brain-damaged victim stays away from any topic requiring detailed use of language. Perhaps they state that "everything is fine" or use nonverbal communication, express generalities, refuse to talk, or remain isolated.

One woman's seizures were concealed since she was reluctant to tell her neurologist that she lost bladder control.

A child did not tell his parents of a serious fall resulting in unconsciousness.

A woman may be fearful of revealing a beating by her husband (Hales & Yudofsky, 1987, p. 180).

• A *"Spartan mentality"*: Some people are trained not to express emotional pain. Perhaps they give themselves reasons not to ask for what is coming to them, or to assert their rights, etc. (Parker, 1981).

• *Pride:* The wish to overcome affliction by oneself leads people not to state the extent of impairment.

• *Avoidance:* Individuals avoid facing situations in which they are unable to succeed, or that will create anxiety. They may take a less demanding job or avoid challenging situations. Unless one asks about reduced efforts, the individual may appear to be stable and uncomplaining.

Inability to Express Dysfunctions

Neuropsychological

• *Impaired consciousness:* The patient is neither alert to his own condition, nor to the examiner's questions, and cannot relate significant problems, due to confusion, poor alertness, dizziness, etc.

• *Lack of insight:* Some people do not realize the extent of their intellectual impairment. Factors such as these should be considered: impaired memory, reduced comprehension of current condition, and inability to process complex information. Professional level individuals return to work unaware of IQ deficiencies of 20–30 points that produce gross deficits of ability.

• Right hemisphere-damaged patients may state that they are now "okay" or "much better"—even with a physical disability—when, in fact, they may behave childishly or without expression.

• *The victim may not associate injury with the symptom:* One automobile accident victim, himself a physician, described his condition: "I didn't see the change in myself. I didn't know that was wrong." His psychotherapist pointed out that he was once better able to concentrate. "I thought that's the way its always been. How else could it have been. I was unaware that my symptoms were related to the accident. I denied I was ill and acted as if nothing was wrong. I went to a conference, received 35 hours of credit, and I don't remember anything. I thought everybody else was strange. I was seeing them differently. I thought that my therapist was asking strange questions!"

Temporomandibular joint syndrome (see Chapter 4 on Trauma) can cause headaches that are not associated with a blow.

Brain damage, which is not properly diagnosed at the time of trauma, may be forgotten and therefore not associated with subsequent problems of personality and cognitive effectiveness.

- *Sensory neglect or agnosias:* The injury prevents the individual from realizing that sensory stimulation is not registering. Lack of sensory input may be general (anosognosia) or specific (agnosia). Damage to particular areas of the brain (e.g., parietal, frontal, limbic, and central, Livingston, 1984, p. 1152) makes the victim unaware of incoming information from the contralateral side, disinclined to move in that contralateral space, or inattentive (see also Chapter 6 on Consciousness, e.g., Neglect).
- *Communication deficits:* Aphasia describes an inability to understand others, find appropriate self-descriptive words, or express otherwise understood thoughts coherently. The patient may avoid embarrassment by remaining silent or evasive.
- *Impaired intelligence or comprehension:* This refers to an inability to understand the deficit and its effects. With reduced judgment the patient cannot evaluate what is wrong. Reduced standards of performance, foresight, and planning ability may not be recognized.
- *Poor memory:* Confusion and dizziness contribute to poor memory immediately after an impact. The victim feels light-headed, is unable to comprehend what has happened or where he is, does not think clearly, etc. They may refuse to undergo examination (see above). A deficit cannot be reported if it is not remembered. Anterograde and retrograde amnesia prevent a person from describing the circumstances surrounding an accident, particularly if accompanied by seizures, confusion, and altered states of consciousness. "I don't even remember what I don't remember!" During a period considered to be recovery, the patient's poor memory may not be realized by the onlooker (posttraumatic amnesia) because overtly the behavior seems normal. Subsequently, at the time of an examination or interview for some other purpose, the patient may not remember dysfunctions or their consequences.

A patient told the writer that she had no problems with cooking. Only 2 days afterward she realized that she could not remember many recipes, which hampered her.

An alcoholic may be amnestic for a fall while inebriated (Hales & Yudofsky, 1987, p. 180).

One victim, pressed at an Examination Before Trial (part of a precourt procedure), was asked why he did not go in an ambulance; he said: "I must have spoken to the police, but I can't remember talking to a policeman . . . I have no memory. I don't remember whether I said to the policeman that I was hurt. Somebody should have taken me to a hospital."

- *Compensation for deficits:* The client may not be completely aware of deficits that are coped with by using various strategies. Of course, successful use of coping strategies may conceal dysfunctioning from an examiner. Examples include memory problems that are solved through the use of lists, and a man with a poor sense of direction who takes a compass and a map with him wherever he goes.
- *Organic mood dysfunctions:* The very damage makes it difficult for the onlooker to form an accurate assessment of the condition (see Chapter 13 on Cerebral Personality Disorders).
- Emotional blandness or endogenous depression is one of the primary signs of brain damage (see Chapter 13 on Cerebral Personality Disorders). The brain-damaged person often expresses himself with a flat affect, a seeming lack of concern, even when describing the most painful kind of impairment, despair, or damage to life-style. Thus, the patient may be assessed as unimpaired; dysfunctioning is not taken seriously, or it remains unrecognized because of the lack of complaints.
- Brain damage can mimic emotional disorders, i.e., create bizarre thinking and gross disorders of affect (crying, laughter, rage).
- *Poor judgment gives the impression of indifference:* The patient appears as though psychopathic (behavior that is socially self-destructive is expressed as though it were actually satisfactory). Inability to monitor behavior, and to learn from experience, gives the observer the impression of indifference or immaturity ("frontal lobe syndrome").

Psychodynamic

- *Reluctance to relive the trauma:* The individual may be reluctant to express a complaint to avoid the pain. Perhaps crying would make the patient feel conspicuous when discussing the trauma and its after-effects. Moreover, repetitive or intrusive memories and reminders of impairment, pain, and loss of the quality of life lead to active attempts to avoid discussion of the experience. One woman who was knocked down by a car said that she "pretended that there was no accident."
- *Psychogenic depression* and a suppressive or constrictive reaction style can be misconstrued as indifference. The depressed person is very aware of mental pain and is self-preoccupied. Their dysphoria can be missed unless the observer is astute or motivated to probe deeply.
- *The defense of denial:* It is difficult to accept that brain damage is highly impairing and generally permanent. The loss of ability to enjoy life, and assets that are valued, is so painful that self-concealment is common. This is to be distinguished from "agnosias" and inability to express emotional pain (Parker, 1981).

- *Avoidance:* Individuals avoid facing situation in which they are unable to succeed, or that will create anxiety. They may take a less demanding job or avoid challenging situations. Unless one asks about reduced efforts, the individual appears stable and uncomplaining.

Special Effects of Pain *(see Chapter 15 on Stress)*

- *Chronic pain can give the impression of exaggeration* for the purpose of obtaining compensation (Adams & Victor, 1989, pp. 1193, 1196). However, chronic pain may be related to a withdrawal effect from endogenous opioids (Beutler et al., 1986), which in turn may be depleted after the long-lasting stress of an accident, injury, and impairment. This could be a reason why pain is experienced long after an apparent injury seems healed (see Chapter 15 on Stress).
- *Pain has a complex interaction* with many other experiences and personality characteristics, affecting and relating to ability to express other feelings, expectation of assistance, etc. It can be a substitute for anger and depression.

Conclusion

The assessment of a known or potential brain-damaged victim requires both an intimate knowledge of the range of potential deficits, active probing to aid the patient express himself, and also a comprehensive examination to detect impairment since self-description is likely to be an insufficient guide to the patient's functioning.

17
Environmental Neurotoxins

This chapter will alert the practitioner to the hazards of manufactured and natural substances that cause TBI. Exposure can be through the lungs, skin, water, and food. A few common neurotoxins are discussed in some detail to enhance familiarity with neurotoxic symptoms. For detailed information the reader is referred to Bondy and Prasad (1988) on toxicity of metals, Gosselin, Smith, and Hodge (1984), a comprehensive source of industrially based substances, with their trade names and toxicity, Hartman (1988) on neuropsychological effects, Guthrie (1986) and R. Levin (1987) lead poisoning, and Tilson and Sparber (1987) on metals in combination with organic compounds, e.g., tin, lead, mercury.

Exposure

Our industrial society constantly exposes individuals at work and play to toxic substances. Great tragedies include Minimata Bay, Japan (mercury, see below) and Bhopal (12/3/84, methylisocyanate, described by the 1988 World Almanac, p. 685, "as history's worst industrial accident," i.e., 2500 deaths. Hartman (1988, p. 17) asserts that human beings are exposed to over 53,000 different substances, for which safety standards have been set for only 588, and only 1667 are regulated for neurotoxic effects. R. Levin (1987, p. I-3) lists 24 synthetic organic chemicals and 10 inorganic chemicals found in drinking water for which maximum contaminant level goals should be reached.

Estimates of individuals exposed to toxic substances in their jobs vary from 7.7 to 20 million. In 1982 it was estimated that 100,000 chemicals were in use in American industry, of which 575 were deemed dangerous in large doses, exposing 20,000,000 American workers to known neurotoxins (Anderson, 1982). Occupations considered at risk include agricultural workers, chemical workers, degreasers, dentists, dry cleaners, electronics workers, hospital personnel, laboratory workers, painters, plastics workers, printers, rayon workers, steel workers, transportation workers, and hobbyists (Hartman, 1988, p. 22). A list of occupations at risk for particular organic substances used in industry is offered by the National Institute for Occupational Safety and Health (NIOSH) (1977).

Prenatal exposure is serious since the placenta does not act as a barrier to protect the fetus against most drugs consumed by the mother (Szeto, 1989). Not all prenatal exposure has been proven to have detectable neuropsychological effects, and the reader is referred to the volume concerning prenatal use of drugs edited by Hutchings (1989) for studies of alcohol, caffeine, methadone, heroin, marijuana, nicotine, tobacco, amphetamine, etc.

Toxic Effects

Neurotoxic effects vary from subtle to fatal. Intermediate levels of toxicity, at least acutely, result in confusional states and/or impaired learning and memory. The level of impairment may vary with the neuropsychological system. I examined a man exposed to mercury at work, whose mind was clear, but whose body was bent due to spasticity. Particular pathological lesions are associated with given organometals in the central nervous system (Chang, 1987). Not all toxins cross the blood–brain barrier (Cooper, Bloom, & Roth, 1986, p. 211). One should differentiate between anoxia (simple lack of oxygen, e.g., drowning), and carbon monoxide poisoning (Laplane et al., 1989 offers some cases), wherein carbon monoxide binds to hemoglobin and competes with oxygen for a considerable period of time. This prevents sufficient oxygen from being absorbed by hemoglobin and thus oxygenating the brain and other tissues. The large demands of the brain for oxygen have already been noted in Chapter 2 on Neuroanatomy. Both anoxia and carbon monoxide poisoning could ensue from a fire in a confined space.

Norton (1986) classifies nervous system toxicants according to whether they cause anoxia, damage myelin, cause peripheral axonopathies, affect the neuromuscular junction, or cause localized CNS lesions. Solvents may accumulate in fatty tissue in the body, and lipids of the myelin sheath of the axons. Neurological effects include disturbance to gray matter, disruption of neurotransmitter metabolism (Hartman, 1988, p. 6) and of the myelin sheath of the central CNS axons, depletion of particular neurotransmitters centrally or peripherally (Cooper et al., 1986, p. 211), demyelinization of peripheral neurons and axonal degeneration, disturbance of synaptic junctions of the neuromuscular system, damage to specialized CNS nuclei, including the cerebellum and limbic system (hippocampus), and damage to the peripheral nervous system (Chang, 1987; Norton, 1986).

Vulnerable physiological systems include sensory and motor pathways, complex and lower level cognitive functions, life support systems based on the hypothalamus and medulla, voluntary and involuntary movement (pyramidal motor system, basal ganglia, cerebellum), and emotional components (limbic system, i.e., hippocampus, amygdala, pyriform cortex; Messing, 1987).

The pattern of damage varies with the level of maturity of the nervous system. In younger organisms, the brainstem, sensory relay nuclei of the thalamus, and hippocampus are more likely to be affected, while in mature individuals, it is the cerebral cortex (Norton, 1986). I have examined one child, exposed in utero to toxic fumes from a printing plant used by his mother, who did not develop hands or feet (thalidomide-like syndrome). There was evidence of defective neuropsychological development. Strub and Black (1988; p. 350) report on a case of an artist stricken with brain damage when cleaning brushes, as well as workers exposed to hydrocarbon solvents.

Metal exposure in general, and lead in particular, can impair the immune system, and alter host resistance to infectious agents and tumors. Lead toxicity impairs the two major types of immune response: (1) Cell mediated immunity, and (2) humoral immunity, or production of antibodies. It increases susceptibility to bacterial and viral infections. This is confirmed by laboratory and clinical studies. The dose, route of exposure, and genetic constitution may influence the adverse effects of lead in immunity.

Toxic Substances

Neurotoxic Substances (Man-Made and Natural)

By Substance

Neurotoxic substances include addicting drugs (opiates and synthetic analgesics, barbiturates and alcohol), anesthetic gases (which affect operating room personnel, Anderson, 1982); sedative-hypnotic drugs (barbiturates), (mercurial) antifungal seed coatings, antidepression drugs, stimulants, psychoactive drugs, bacterial toxins, plant poisons, venoms (bites and stings), thallium, carbon monoxide, cyanide, lead, fuels (volatile compounds including leaded gasoline), hexachlorophene, acrylamide, bromophenylacetylurea, carbon disulfide, hexanedione, organomercury compounds, antineoplastic agents, toluene (glue sniffing) and other solvents (Hartman, 1987), isoniazid, triethylene, tricyclo and trimethyl compounds, organophosphorus compounds, insecticides (DDT, pyrethrins), organic insect sprays, heavy metals such as mercury, alcohol, cocaine, marijuana, hallucinogens, amphetamines, PCP, "Designer Drugs" (Hartman, 1987, 1988; Norton, 1986; Victor & Adams, 1985, p. 826), carbon disulfide, graphite, inorganic lead, organic lead, trichloroethylene, vinyl chloride, xylene, kerosene, naphtha, and manganese (NIOSH, 1977).

Sample Household and Consumer Neurotoxic Substances

Household and consumer neurotoxic substance include typewriter correction fluids, room deodorizers, liquid waxes, brake fluid, windshield wiper fluid, transmission fluid, lighter fluid, hair spray, and dry-cleaning fluid, aerosol pain relievers, fly sprays, antiperspirants, paint strippers, model and household cements, finger polish (Hartman, 1988, p. 135), organic compounds used as plastics stabilizers and catalysts, antipsychotic drugs, insecticides, paints and glazes, plastics, polyurethane, vinyl compounds, and drugs of abuse.

Neuropsychological Symptoms

This section will offer examples of symptoms, not associate particular symptoms with given neurotoxins. The reader can be alert to them so that in the course of professional contacts, as one interviews and receives information about occupational, recreational, and domestic exposure, potential victims may be recognized and referred for further examination.

Early Behavioral Effect

Industrial studies show that behavioral effects of exposure to neurotoxins are detected at low levels of exposure before neurological effects (Thatcher, Lester, McAlaster, & Horst, 1982; Valciukas & Lilis, 1980). There is a question as to whether there is any safe or "threshold" level of exposure. Even levels of lead considered safe cause workers to be at risk for brain dysfunction (Valciukas, Lilis, Singer, Fischbein, Anderson, & Glickman, 1980).

Typical early symptoms include tremors, loss of coordination, paralysis, impotence, numbness, pain, damage to senses (vision, hearing, touch, smell), reduced alertness, reduced IQ and other cognitive deficits, lethargy, irritability, hallucination, psychosis, headaches, depression, anxiety, loss of libido, loss of memory, loss of manual dexterity, loss of visuomotor tracing, loss of mental flexibility, inability to detect figure-ground relationships, and decreased word fluency (Anderson, 1982).

Characteristic Dysfunctions After Chronic Exposure Are Highly Varied

Acute industrial level exposure may lead to dizziness, convulsions, and coma. Other neuropsychological dysfunctions include decreased general intelligence (including attention, concentration, abstract reasoning, efficiency, learned skills), motor impairments (including speed, coordination, and strength), memory and learning impairments (short-term, new learning, and long-term memory), visuospatial impairments, personality impairments, vision and other sensory functioning impairments, and conditioned response deficits. Anosmia due to cadmium exposure has been reported. Autonomic symptoms involve size of pupil, tachycardia, blushes, cold hands, sexual dysfunction and anxiety (Lecture by J. A. Valciukas, to New York Neuropsychology Group, April 16, 1986; reduced grip strength and wrist drop, Hartman, 1988, p. 24; Hasting & Sun, 1987; NIOSH, 1977, p. 363).

Expressive Deficits

Inability to express dysfunctioning (see Chapter 16 on Expressive Deficits) was observed by Hartman (1987). Low levels of exposure to led to complaints about fatigue, sleepiness, depression, and apathy. Higher levels accompanied symptoms of forgetfulness and sensorimotor complaints. With still higher levels the complaints were somatic or emotional, rather than cognitive. It was hypothesized that the patients had deficits of attention, abstraction, and also impaired introspective abilities, so they did not realize the extent of their cognitive losses.

Personality Considerations

Lindberg, Basch-Kahre, and Lindberg (1982) offered psychoanalytically oriented psychotherapy to house painters and industrial painters whose symptoms included memory loss, attributed to psychological causation (e.g., trauma in the proverbial first year of life, alexithymia, or inability to express feelings with consequent somatization; see Chapter 15 on Stress), compensation neurosis, or unconscious conflicts. Psychotherapy offered some benefits, and motivation to return to work had some effect on the outcome. The conclusion attributing the deficits to personality factors is doubtful, since effectiveness of treatment, neuropsychological dysfunctions, or the proportion of workers that returned to work were not followed up or specified. Rather, the difficulties of psychotherapy were observed. This should not be surprising in view of the probability that genuine neuropsychological deficits seem not to be a focus of attention.

A group of individuals exposed to formaldehyde for 37 months (Cripe & Dodrill, 1988) with initial complaints involving concentration, memory, fatigue, and emotional control, and subtle complaints continuing 21 months after removal from the substance, could not be differentiated from controls by neuropsychological tests. Neither IQ tests nor other measures of complex cognitive functioning were administered. On the Minnesota Multiphasic Personality Inventory (MMPI) they did express emotional and somatic concerns. A study of workers using phenol formaldehyde (aerospace aircraft assembly) demonstrated an organic brain syndrome, which may persist indefinitely, i.e., dementia, headaches, irritability, fatigue, personality change, depression, and memory lapse (Adler, 1989).

Sample Neurotoxic Effects

Methyl Mercury-Minimata Disease

Symptoms include constriction of visual field and other sensory disturbance (100%), ataxia, impairment of speech, hearing, and gait, tremor, mental disturbance, exaggerated tendon reflexes, hypersalivation and hyperhydrosis, muscular rigidity, ballism, chorea, pathological reflexes athetoxis, and contractures (Tilson & Sperber, 1987, p. 83).

Organic Mercury

This is the "mad hatter's disease" involving motor and sensory deficits, cerebellar ataxia, slurred speech, paresthesia, visual field constriction, tremor, pyramidal signs, and recognition time (Mercury Exposure, 1980).

Metallic Mercury

Symptoms include irritability, excitability, loss of control, withdrawal, headaches, weakness, loss of memory, tremors, melancholia, delirium with hallucinations, and manic depressive psychosis (NIOSH, 1977, p. 371; Strub & Black, 1988, pp. 354–355).

Lead Poisoning

The public is exposed to a variety of sources of lead, i.e., gasoline, industrial processes, and drinking water (natural levels, corrosion of plumbing, glazes, batteries, housepaints) (Hartman, 1988, p. 72; R. Levin, 1987, Chapter 2). Airborne lead falls on food and water (Marshall, 1983). Children (see Chapter 19, Children's Brain Damage) and adults are at risk, with different types of exposure.

Lead interferes with heme synthesis, a process important for oxygen transport and detoxification of toxic substances. Inability to break down tryptophan in the liver leads to excess levels of tryptophan and serotonin in the brain, and neurotoxic effects, including inhibiting and slowing certain kinds of neurotransmission, decreased nerve conduction velocity, decreased reaction time, and altered brainstem and auditory evoked potentials. Lead also interferes with the ability of brain cells to use oxygen and calcium, interfering with a variety of neuronal and other physiological processes. Cerebellar effects impair coordination.

The higher the degree of lead absorption, the higher the degree of risk (Valciukas et al., 1980). After initial exposure, there may be a long period of progressive dysfunctioning due to the gradual death of brain tissue. Then release of the neurotoxin stored in body fat or other sites may occur, or the brain may be affected by release of toxic metabolites as they are cleared from the body (Singer & Scott, 1987). Different pathological effects occur, with the same level of blood lead, when children with chronic exposure and continuous release are compared to children with single acute exposure (Hartman, 1987).

Specifically psychological symptoms include psychosis with hallucinations, tiredness, restlessness, sleep disturbance, nightmares, impotence, irritability, loss of appetite, depression, confusion, anger, fatigue, and tension. In higher concentrations, organic lead can produce delirium, convulsions, and coma. Lead intoxication can be mistaken for a major affective disorder (Hartman, 1988, pp. 77–82).

I have examined a professional man after exposure to leaded gasoline who had an estimated loss of 25 IQ points, and other processing and sensorimotor deficits. Some children recently examined at least 3 years after exposure showed no evidence of cognitive loss (using school and IQ percentiles as a baseline), but did manifest brainstem disorders (coordination, balance). These could create significant adaptive problems. The children showed significant Rorschach signs of emotional distress, related to a concurrent family breakup.

Lead Poisoning in Children

Children are considered to be at greater risk than adults since they absorb more lead per unit of body weight than adults and release more lead due to higher mineral turnover in bone (Hartman, 1988, p. 75). Lead toxicity has been defined for children as 25 µg of lead per dl of blood and 35 µg/dl of free erythrocyte protoporphyrin (FEP, an associated physiological measure). According to Menkes (1985, p. 509), there may be convulsions, or depression of consciousness, followed by hemiplegia or other neurologic sequelae. Eventually, these children have a lowered global IQ, and impaired associative abilities, visual-motor performance, and fine motor coordination. When compared to matched nonexposed children, they lack self-confidence, and exhibit distractibility with a shortened attention span and a tendency to impulsive behavior.

Low level lead exposure (blood leg of 30–50 micrograms/dl) affects CNS function. It is reflected in EEG patterns and CNS evoked potentials in children with neuropsychological deficits (Goyer, 1986).

However, other studies have failed to find an adverse effect on mental functions, and some believe that the former observations can be explained on the following basis: if a child has one sign of emotional disturbance, namely pica, other signs of emotional and cognitive disturbances are likely.

Increasing levels of exposure to lead (as measured by the level of lead in the dentine of shed teeth) have a variety of deleterious effects (Needleman, Gunnoe, Leviton, Reed, Peresie, Mahjer, & Barrett, 1979). Teachers rated them as more distractible, not persistent, more dependent, and unable to follow simple directions or sequences of directions. They had longer reaction times for complex verbal tasks, auditory discrimination, and reaction time after a delay.

The following information concerning the origin and outcome of lead poisoning is from R. Levin (1987), in an official report of the U.S. Environmental Protection Agency.

Prenatal

Prenatal lead levels, which can be significant, are associated with reduced gestational age and reduced birth weight, which in turn are significantly associated with reduced neurobehavioral performance at three months.

Neonatal Observations

Prenatal lead exposure correlated with jitteriness and hypersensitivity. This effect seems related to psychomotor ability at age 6–7 (R. Levin, 1987, p. III-38).

Postnatal

Lead blood levels are predictive of children's height, weight, and chest circumference. The effects of lead poisoning are described as similar to traumatic or cerebral infectious injury, i.e., permanent damage from cortical atrophy, hydrocephalus, convulsive seizures, and severe mental retardation. Reexposure leads to seizures, nervous disorders, blindness, hemiparesis, sensory motor deficits, short attention span, behavioral disorders, mental retardation, cerebral palsy, optic atrophy, and visual–perceptual problems. They may show gross or lesser mental retardation, or clumsiness and balance problems that are impairing or conspicuous in a growing child (midbrain or cerebellar dysfunctions).

Neurological effects (after given blood levels, measured in μg/dl):

80–100: encephalopathic signs and symptoms;
60: peripheral neuropathies;
> 50: seven times more likely to have repeated grades in school or be referred to the school psychologist;
30–50: abnormal EEG patterns and slow wave voltages;
40: CNS cognitive deficits, e.g., IQ deficits;
15: altered CNS electrophysiological responses. Estimated IQ losses have been determined for children described as asymptomatic.

Changes in CNS Functioning

Changes involve slow wave EEG patterns, increased latencies in brainstem auditory evoked potentials, beginning to appear at 15 μg/dl, and negative correlation between blood lead and nerve conduction velocity in children at levels of 15–90 μg/dl.

IQ loss and exposure (R. Levin, 1987, p. III-40):

Lead level	Mean IQ loss
15–30	1 to 2
30–50	4
> 50	5
> 80	16

R. Levin (1987, p. III–40) observes that "permanent IQ effects may result only from fairly long periods of exposure, and a child who has a certain blood level for a relatively short period of time (perhaps, a few months) may not suffer the full effect."

Thirteen Children with Plumbism Examined by the Author

I examined a number of children who were referred because of learning and behavioral problems severe enough to result in litigation. The etiology was ingesting lead-based paint, and in two cases (including a prenatal exposure) ingesting lead from improperly glazed houseware ceramics. Lead poisoning had been medically documented, but the data did not permit association of particular levels with IQ. Characteristically, the children had received chelation therapy to remove the lead from the body. A variety of standard intelligence tests were utilized, and the results were averaged (Full Scale WAIC-R; Stanford Binet, IV Ed. and Kaufman Assessment Battery for Children Composite).

Number of cases: 13
Ages: 5-1 to 14-6
Exposure: Most 2–4 years, one prenatal
Median age: 8-3
Range of Full Scale IQs: 60–108 (Only exam or latest exam)
Mean Full Scale IQ: 79.9
Reexamination after a mean interval of 39 months (1-7 to 6-1 years)
Number of children re-examined: 8
Mean IQ difference: − 2.75 points
Range: +6 to −5

This sample of lead poisoned children exhibited mean intellectual functioning in the Borderline range, with a wide range of cognitive ability from Average to Mentally Retarded. With no preinjury baseline estimated, it is possible that there were cognitive deficits among the three children with average range functioning (90–109). After an appreciable length of time, the average IQ loss was not large. Only in a single instance (− 13 point) was there a very large loss of Full Scale IQ.

From these results one may speculate that cognitive loss resulting from lead toxicity is highly variable. One child with an IQ in the mentally retarded range had been exposed to methadone in utero. There is evidence that deleterious effects seem synergized by poor environmental circumstances (Hans, 1989), and one group of drug-dependent mothers gave birth to children of average level IQ (Kaltenbach & Finnegan, 1989).

In addition to cognitive deficits, sensorimotor symptoms are common, e.g., subcortical deficits of balance and oculomotor function. These have implications for difficulties in performing sports by generally reducing agility, a capability important in growing children. It leads to reduced social acceptability. Moreover, subtle deficits, e.g., problems of coordination, can create the feeling of being impaired, causing considerable loss of self-esteem and problems of identity.

Solvents

An estimated 2 million American workers utilize solvents in painting, roofing, printing, drycleaning, degreasing, and glazing (White, 1987). Inhalants create intoxication lasting a few minutes to 1–2 hours. Side effects include headaches, pain in the extremities, photophobia, diplopia, tinnitus, menstrual disorders, depression, anxiety, difficulty in concentrating, tiredness or weakness, and a variety of autonomic effects (see "solvents" above). Clinical manifestations of intoxication are similar to the early phase of alcohol and the second stage of anesthesia, i.e., progressive, generalized CNS depression and cortical disinhibition. Accident proneness, antisocial behavior, and self-destructive acts are observed. The psychological state is typical of delirium, with a variety of cognitive, motor, and emotional symptoms (Young & Lawson, 1988).

Subsequent neuropsychological symptoms include dementia, deficits in immediate memory span, short-term memory, learning, mental tracking, attention/concentration, visuospatial ability, and anterograde memory deficits, slightly greater impairment for delayed recall (Wechsler Memory Scale—Revised), inebriation, giddiness, confusion, dizziness, nausea, and vomiting (Crossen & Wiens, 1988a; White, 1987). Although recovery from an acute episode is expected, these substances concentrate in the lipids (fats) of the CNS white matter, to be released later (Strub & Black, 1988, p. 353).

Illegal Drugs

- *"Synthetic heroin" or MPTP* produces permanent Parkinsonian symptoms by selectively destroying nigrostriatal dopamine neurons (Cooper et al., 1986, p. 211). This can be inadvertently created by excessive heat in the manufacture of synthetic heroin (Lewis & Lawson, 1988).
- *PCP* (Young, Lawson, & Gacano, 1980): CNS effects related to dosage: blank stare, nystagmus, ataxia, dysarthria, coma, rigidity, prolonged coma, EEG effects, impaired thought, hallucinations, and combativeness.
- *Opiates* (Lewis & Lawson, 1988): Opium-like drugs are heroin, morphine, codeine, methadone, and meperidine. None of these substances has superior analgesic qualities to morphine, and tolerance develops rapidly.
- *Marijuana* (McCaig & Lawson, 1988): The psychoactive compound of *Cannabis* is tetrahydrocannabinol (THC), which may be present from 1 to 10%, but up to 15% in hashish, produced from its resins and flowers. THC's locus is believed to be the hypothalamus, where it blocks ACTH production (see Chapters 2 on Neuroanatomy and 15 on Stress). ACTH controls the metabolism of fats and carbohydrates, accounting for the sluggishness associated with marijuana usage. There is still no evidence that *Cannabis* causes permanent neuronal damage.

Medically Prescribed Psychoactive Drugs (Lawson, 1988)

These affect the CNS (motor symptoms, e.g., Parkinsonian syndrome, dystonia, akathisia, dyskinesia, and drowsiness) and ANS (blurred vision, constipation, diarrhea, dizziness, fainting, and urinary retention).

Assessment

EEG, CT scan, and MRI often offer normal findings. This could lead to misinterpretation of symptoms of moderate encephalopathy to be considered "functional," hysterical, or malingering. This error can be avoided with careful mental status and neuropsychological testing (Strub & Black, 1988, p. 351). Subclinical central nervous system dysfunction can be revealed by neuropsychological tests, signaling an unsafe environment, and lead to the study of exposed workers (Valciukas, Lilis, Eisinger, Blumberg, Fischbein, & Selikoff, 1978; Valciukas, 1985).

Neurotoxicity does not create a unique pattern of neuropsychological dysfunctioning. Even gross cognitive deficits may not appear (Messing, 1987). Hartman (1988, p. 37) observes that the Full Scale IQ derived from the Wechsler Adult Intelligence Scale—Revised is not particularly sensitive to neurotoxins, although subtests may be. The writer recommends a broad-based examination to document objective and subjective deficits (see Chapter 21, Assessment). A list of procedures and batteries to assess neurotoxicity is offered by Hartman (1988, Chapter 2), and a brief battery by Valciukas et al. (1980).

White (1987) offers these principles of differential diagnosis between neurotoxic poisoning and conditions such as Alzheimer's disease (AD):

1. IQ should be monitored for progressive cognitive loss.
2. Aphasic errors should be studied to determine whether they are characteristic of the patient's history, e.g., stroke, childhood dyslexia.
3. Do retrograde memory problems date to toxin exposure or more extensively?
4. Extent of attention and visuospatial deficits should be determined, though both are common to AD and exposure to solvents.
5. Rate of decline can differentiate between toxins (rapid) and AD.

Useful neuropsychological procedures include visual intelligence, visual-motor functions, general intelligence, memory, scanning, psychomotor speed and dexterity, attention, concentration, and abstract thought. A cognitive and personality baseline estimate should be obtained (with exploration of preexposure depression, anxiety, distraction, thought disorder, and malingering). Emotional stress, sleeplessness, withdrawal from caffeine or tobacco, illness, prior head injury, and poor nutrition can all affect assessment (Hartman, 1987).

Other Neurotoxic Effects in Children

Lead poisoning in children is common, but poisoning by thallium, arsenic, mercury (Menkes, 1985), and cadmium (Thatcher et al., 1982) is less well known. For example, cadmium has a significantly stronger effect on verbal IQ than does lead and lead has a stronger effect on performance IQ than does cadmium (Thatcher et al., 1982).

Organometals have a relatively specific pattern of pathological lesions in the CNS: mercury-cerebellum and calcarine (visual) cortex; tin-limbic system, primarily the hippocampal formation; lead-diffuse damage to cerebral cortex, brainstem, and spinal cord (Chang, 1987, p. 103). Symptoms of methylmercury poisoning (Minimata disease) illustrate the vulnerability of the developing nervous system to neurotoxins. They appeared weeks to months after birth: lethargy, delayed movement, and deficits of vision, sucking, swallowing. Additional symptoms include retardation, deficits of gait, vision, etc. (Chang, 1987, pp. 83–84).

Toxic-Related Seizures

Lead, insecticide, carbon monoxide, and other agents caused hypoxia; withdrawal from alcohol or barbiturates and antipsychotic drugs such as phenothizines or butyrophenone can cause seizures (Herskowitz & Rosman, 1982, p. 333).

18
Recovery from Brain Damage

Overview

The most significant consequence of TBI is reduced adaptive ability, i.e., inability to perform one's usual tasks and to enjoy life. Deficits are extremely persistent, and one study showed that patients continued to seek help for an average of 7.3 years after an accident, and perhaps for decades later (Karol, 1989). The term recovery has several meanings, e.g., return to a premorbid level of competence (Pirozzolo & Papanicolaou, 1986), and the patient's status after reaching a plateau. I will use the term *recovery* for the process of healing, and *outcome* to signify the status of the TBI victim after a plateau has been reached. Outcome is an interaction between deficits, morale, social support, and the demands made on the person.

This chapter will emphasize conditions affecting outcome and prognosis. The initial stages of recovery after severe TBI include delirium, mania, depression, disorientation, PTA, agitation, and combativeness (Klauber & Ward-McKinley, 1986). Degrees of impairment found in hospitals or rehabilitation centers are described by Grant and Alves (1987). Refer also to Coma Data Bank findings in Chapter 13 on Cerebral Personality Disorders.

Criteria of Recovery

What does it mean when we read that "head-injured patients who recover to a normal level of orientation, and are no longer confused or grossly amnestic by 2 weeks after injury, can be expected to attain a good recovery in most cases, although moderate disability may persist in some patients" (H. S. Levin, 1987)? Some accident victims, though ambulatory and able to get around, are really not functional. The patient who is impaired, and a burden to himself and to the community, would not agree that his life had been without loss. Levin himself observes that recovery to an average IQ is not sufficient when there are problems of flexibility in handling problems, guiding one's own behavior, initiative, planning, scheduling, etc.

There Is No Single Criterion Measuring Outcome

There is no universally accepted criterion concerning the severity of damage or of recovery. No doubt, each profession uses its own standards. To the neurosurgeon who has just saved a life threatened by intracranial hemorrhage, walking is a successful outcome. To a disturbed family, interpersonal factors and ability to earn a living are salient. Accuracy of assessment of outcome would be increased by including posttraumatic emotional reactions and their neurophysiological concomitants and health.

Recovery can be measured in terms of relatively narrow systems (memory, sensorimotor, cognitive, physical rehabilitation or classical neurological signs). However, practical adaptive recovery requires cognitive abilities or other higher functions. Intellectual sequelae may impede subsequent occupational and social adaption more than physical disabilities (Tabaddor et al., 1984). For practical purposes return to work is a significant criterion of outcome, which integrates effective functioning in many areas (Bond, 1983a).

The true criterion of recovery is reachieving or exceeding baseline measurements for adaptive functions. Recovery plainly means that the person has resumed the ability to perform at the preinjury level. I have occasionally observed individuals who seemed to have exceeded preaccident levels after the injury, although I do not recommend trauma as a corrective measure for improving life-style.

Baseline

Since impaired individuals may have average-range functioning although being inefficient or seriously impaired, recovery cannot be assessed without a baseline. This baseline essentially has two components:

Adaptive Functioning

This includes descriptions from teachers, employers, family, friends, military records, etc., of preinjury effectiveness and personality.

Psychological Test Scores

School and military records will serve as an example of cognitive and achievement scores that indicate the preinjury level of effectiveness.

Level of Recovery Is Unpredictable

Recovery is a complex process, varying with many personal and environmental factors, and the criterion that is used. I know of one case in which a neurologist complained that a neurosurgeon claimed excellent recovery after surgery for brain trauma. On examination, the patient was completely aphasic! Many professional reports exaggerate the extent of recovery because the examination procedures did not explore or detect deficits over a sufficiently wide range of functions, particularly affect and "higher" cognitive functions. In addition, easy tasks were administered that did not challenge the patient.

Severe brain damage usually has a poor outcome. Further, there is an imperfect correlation between measures of trauma [e.g., length of coma, length of post-traumamatic amnesia, presence of hematoma, skull fracture, and the Glasgow Coma Scale (see Glossary)] and the ultimate outcome. People with severe injury, i.e., long coma, may resume life with some kind of success. I was embarrassed in court, when, after describing a man's brain damage, and predicting reduced employability, the defendant's attorney pointed out how much money he was earning (more than the examiner!). On the other hand, Alves (1989) observes that even so selected a group as college football players violated expectations that there would be uneventful recoveries following mild head injury. Rather, concussion injuries often resulted in disruption of cognitive functioning, with problems of attention, concentration, and memory.

Probability of Return to Work, and Effects on Employability

The expectation of returning to work will depend on the extent of the injury and general motivation, which includes the type of position to which the patient will return (see below). Kreutzer et al. (1988) estimate that return to employment of persons with moderate to severe injuries, as determined by duration and depth of coma, is less than 50%. During the first 7 years the unemployment rate may be 70%. Emotional and neuropsychological changes are the greatest causes of reduced employability. These include loss of sensory, motor, intellectual, and insight capacities, unrealistic expectations, sensitivity to heat and noise, and propensity to be distracted, confused, or irritable. Feedback is essential to maintain relationships with other workers and the employer.

Variables Affecting Recovery

Outcome varies with the nature of the injury, the support received by the victim, the promptness and efficiency of rehabilitation, the passage of time, and the supportive functions detailed in Chapter 11 on Efficiency and Control.

The Nature of the Traumatic Brain Injury

Some of the variables include the *locus of the injury, volume of tissue loss, anatomical extent of the damage* (*focal* versus *diffuse*), and *laterality* (Grafman et al., 1988). There is a low correlation between these variables and outcome, except at the extreme end of brain damage, i.e., generalized deficits and poor prognosis.

Passage of Time

The rate of recovery varies for different neuropsychological functions, as well interactions with many other factors (see below). Ability to perform practical tasks, of course, is also determined by support of, or interference by, the functions described as "Efficiency and Control" (Chapter 11). There is evidence that whatever recovery takes places is likely to occur by 1–3 months after injury (Stuss et al., 1989), with which I concur.

A survey of neurobehavioral problems most often reported by relatives showed relatively little change over time. Slowness decreased from 86% after 3 months to 67% after 1 year. Other symptoms, listed in decreasing order of frequency, were tiredness, irritability, poor memory, impatience, tension and anxiety, bad temper, personality change, depressed mood, and headaches (54 versus 53%). Over a (longer) period of time, the relation between the severity of injury and outcome diminishes (Thomsen, 1989), i.e., there is some variability that is introduced by unknown causes.

Level of Intelligence

Higher premorbid intelligence is positively correlated to percentage of postinjury employment (Mayes, Pelco, & Campbell, 1989), although this trend is related to preinjury occupational level (see below) and motivation to return to work. The demands of the job at the time of injury can determine whether a person can return to employment. If they are high relative to the preinjury performance, then even minimal deficits can impair employability. Even a minor loss causes ineffective salable skills (Adamovich, Henderson & Auderbach, 1985, pp. 12–13).

Preinjury Personality Characteristics

The patient's attitude toward adversity (see Chapter 15 on stress resistance) and ability to obtain others' cooperation will certainly contribute to adaptation after TBI. Since the predicted change after TBI is in the direction of withdrawal, dependency, and inability to maintain former obligations, a higher baseline of social adaptiveness is very advantageous. Resumption of relationships with family and friends and willingness to meet strangers are criteria of recovery. It may indicate ability to overcome fear of rejection.

Preinjury motivation, education, and persistence in learning can have a positive effect on outcome. Brain-damaged Vietnam veterans, whose preinjury score's on the AFQT were below the 50th percentile, but had a relatively higher preinjury education (some college) actually showed some postinjury gains on this test. This effect was not observed by those who were in the higher preinjury score distribution. On the basis of a more direct study of the relationship between education and outcome it was concluded that the relationship is equivocal (Mayes et al., 1989).

Preinjury emotional disturbance of behavioral problems: Individuals who have sustained head injuries have a disproportionately high incidence of premorbid personality or behavioral disturbances and family pathology (Mayes et al., 1989).

Social and Family Support

After brain damage, the victim is confused, impaired, and suffering. Therefore, the quality of life, as a minimum, and the healing quality of environmental support as an optimum, will have considerable impact on outcome. The victim's family can be critical of the inability to resume a normal life, due to incomprehension of the severity of brain damage. This is counterproductive, since premature reentry into the work force can create unnecessary failure.

At the negative end, I know of one case in which an injured woman was taken from an ER because of her companion's impatience. Then her family told her to wait for medical attention until she could find a lawyer, who would then recommend a physician.

Positively, the degree of final recovery is considerably enhanced by the extent and sophistication of rehabilitation services. Social support is vital at the earliest possible moment after TBI. Some individuals with severe brain damage who received good rehabilitation services as soon as they were able to participate in a program, with personal support, made a surprising recovery.

Motivation

The significance of ego strength for recovery (see above) is consistent with my experience with the Freedom from Distractibility Factor on WAIS-R and WISC-R: TBI victims with high motivation tend to do relatively well on measures of short-term memory and concentration. Sometimes this measure was paradoxically the highest, i.e., with other evidence of impairment, including cognitive functioning, they showed great efforts to perform.

Willingness to rehabilitate oneself, e.g., to resume former employment, varies with attitude toward independence, self-image, social support, etc. Stress-related symptoms affect morale and self-esteem (see Chapter 15 on Stress). Motivation varies between determination and apathy. There can be problems of initiating action in the frontal lobe-injured patient. Even a formerly ambitious individual may become content to spend time watching television (Thickman & Ranseden, 1986).

Motivation cannot be separated from the question "To what is the victim expected to return?" This will be affected by employment, i.e., salary, working conditions, the value of a career, other job-related or family-related satisfactions, etc. (see occupation, below). *The idea that litigation influences unwillingness to return to work is not supported by the evidence* (Uzzell et al., 1987).

Reaction to the event affects motivation to resume a normal life. This includes feelings of revenge and hostility against the party considered responsible for the accident (Barton, 1985). However, anxiety, embarrassment about scarring, etc., can also affect a person's ability to enter into former pursuits.

Communications Skills

Communications skills, e.g., carrying on and understanding a conversation, are considered excellent predictors for a successful return to work (Ehrlich & Barry, 1989). The degree of recovery should be assessed by using the patient's premorbid level of functioning as a baseline, not the maximal disability after injury. A number of rating scales assessing a variety of adaptive functions are offered by Grant and Alves (1987).

Professional Support

Professional caregivers play a significant role in affecting motivation. Inadequate diagnosis or communication of disability may hamper return to work. One common deficiency is the brief physical examination, which is obviously inadequate to establish deficiencies (Hoffman, 1986) in so profound and complex a condition as brain damage and related trauma. The patient is perplexed over his or her deficiencies, and is not referred to appropriate psychotherapeutic or rehabilitative services. Nevertheless, it is believed that victims of mild and traumatic brain damage, who receive appropriate evaluation and treatment, can expect a good prognosis (Alves, 1989).

Hoffman (1986) also notes a passive "fix me" role on the part of the patient, i.e., lack of assumption of any responsibility for assisting in the recovery process. Of course, a psychodynamic explanation, or malingering, may not suffice, if the true condition is the organic personality syndrome with its affect on purposeful behavior.

Careless handling by physicians or lawyers can affect reactions to a trauma (Barton, 1985). Attorneys used to tell a client not to return to work since that would "jeopardize your case." This is being challenged more often by defense attorneys. When treatment was recommended, e.g., psychotherapy, the patient may be asked in court whether he followed this suggestion. Any health care professional has had contact with individuals who could benefit from treatment but found some reason not to try it.

Private physicians, as well as those retained by plaintiff or defendant, may offer an opinion concerning the victim's condition before all of the information pertaining to a case is available, ignoring subjective complaints, or not giving thorough examinations. This arouses considerable resentment. Physicians retained by the defense sometimes take an aggressive stance toward the patient, which arouses the feeling that legitimate complaints are ignored.

Level of Brain and Somatic Injuries

Major somatic injuries delay return to work because of problems with health, mobility, scarring, stamina, etc. Longer coma and PTA are associated with worse outcome. Oddy, Humphrey, and Uttley (1978) report for a sample of relatively young adults, with a posttraumatic amnesia of 24 hours or more, subjective symptoms often did not interfere with resumption of employment. Nevertheless, only 22 of 45 who were working at the time of the injury were employed 6 months later. Those with PTA longer than 7 days were more likely to suffer from boredom and reduced social life (making and receiving visits, maintaining close friendships).

Preexisting Condition

Outcome can be affected by preexisting personality conditions and cognitive level. Premorbid language capacity and cerebral asymmetries may account for variabilities in recovery potential (Naeser & Palumbo, 1987) as revealed after a detailed study associating subcortical lesions with speech and language deficits.

A trauma ordinarily does not totally impair techniques of coping with stress (see stress resistance in Chapter 15 on Stress). Shapiro (1984, p. 120) has stated it well: "It was not the pre-existing character structure that caused psychic pain, rather the accident and its psychological sequelae had rendered that former level of adjustment inadequate to cope with the current anxieties, depressions, or other symptomatologies." The difference between making a significant recovery or not may be that the victim could not adequately handle the stress of the injury (Barton, 1985, p. 5). Perhaps there were other recent stresses, and the latest was "the straw that broke the camel's back."

Age

The effect of age on outcome is controversial. Adamovich et al. (1985) believe that higher age may be a poor prognostic indicator. On the other hand, Uzzell et al. (1987) showed that more older individuals than younger workers with minor injury returned to work. This "may relate to the more established work history of an older person, or to differences in the kind of brain damage incurred" (relatively more focal contusions than diffuse injuries). Unemployment increased to 55% in the younger group (excluding premorbid unemployed persons). Thomsen (1989) divided victims of blunt head trauma into those who were aged 15–21 and 22–44 when injured. They had PTA from 1 to 3 months or more. There was a correlation between length of PTA and the number of problems at a second follow-up 10–15 years after the injury. There was a highly significant negative correlation between the number of problems at that time and the age when injured. The types of problems that increased were aspontaneity, restlessness, disturbed behavior, lack of sexual inhibition, irritability, emotional blunting, and emotional lability. Younger victims had an increased risk of sensitivity to distress. This seems related to a frontal lobe disorder, which is consistent with the age of the victim, i.e., lack of development revealing itself in particular symptoms.

Occupation

One study of minor head injury 3 months after an accident (Rimel et al., 1981) determined that executives and business managers returned to work 100% of the time, minor professionals 83%, clerical sales, 79%, machine operators, 63%, and unskilled laborers, 57%. These results are attributable to motivation and retained resources. The most frequent subjective complaint was persistent headaches varying greatly in intensity and frequency (78%). Other complaints were memory deficit (59%), difficulty with household chores (14%) and use of transportation (15%). The particular cognitive and personality characteristics hampering return to work are probably in the areas of efficiency and control (Chapter 11), reduction of cognitive level (Chapter 9), and poor morale and anxiety (Chapter 15). Low intelligence is a poor prognostic indicator, as is a job requiring speed, safety and efficiency (Adamovich et al., 1985).

Litigation and Malingering

There is a stereotypical belief that emotional disturbance and inability to perform precede the outcome of court trial, and then disability and distress rapidly disappear. Cytowic et al., (1988) note that inability to return to work and dependence on public assistance are observed in persons of varied personality structure.

Malingering may be defined as making a claim of injury or dysfunctioning that is exaggerated or does not exist. Although the neuropsychological examination can identify a potential malingerer or an exaggerated claim, I have observed (and occasionally been deceived by) the following: a greater recovery than acknowledged, concealing preexisting conditions (hospital record indicating a drug addiction; hospitalization for psychosis), making a false claim, and exaggerating discomfort.

It has been suggested by Leigh (cited by Grant & Alves, 1987, with consistent evidence) that when one differentiates between posttraumatic and postconcussional syndromes (PCS), the PCS is related to heretofore poorly documented neural injuries. In fact, such symptoms, including endogenous depression, persisted after a claim was settled.

Nevertheless, malingering is rare. Physical signs attributed to a "functional overlay" in noninjury cases, i.e., apparently competent limbs and nerves that misbehave according to the examiner's beliefs, are apt to be attributed to deception in legal matters (Cartlidge & Shaw, 1981, p. 153). Livingston (1985, p. 1155) observes that when a physician interprets a patient's difficulties in terms of what is predetermined to be reasonable, or current physiological knowledge, it leads to overestimating the number of malingerers. Lack of information concerning toxic effects (in this case memory and behavioral changes after exposure to organic solvents, Strub & Black, 1988, p. 353) can lead to the assumption of malingering.

I believe that the impression of widespread malingering stems from the high proportion of false-negative statements made by superficial or biased examiners. The chief defense against malingering is the wide-range examination including detailed interview (see Chapter 21 on Assessment).

Litigation probably does affect return to work, although not merely in the form of increased delay (Kelly, 1981, cited by Cytowic et al., 1988). Length of time between injury and trial is correlated with the size of the claim for damages, making an insurance company and defendant reluctant to settle. They delay going to trial since injuries may produce sympathy for a badly injured person, and they try to wear down the plaintiff and find evidence for recovery (malingering).

Residual Deficits

Emotional Problems

Persistent personality changes have been observed in one-half to two-thirds of head injury victims in studies up to 10 years (Grant & Alves, 1987). These authors differentiate between *social competence* (skills needed to negotiate one's social environment) and *psychosocial distress* (awareness of inability to meet social expectations). Neurophysical complaints (e.g., ambulation and self-care) are less affected than work and family relations.

The family may suffer considerably from the TBI victim's behavioral problems, e.g., irritability, anger, poor motivation, problems of assuming responsibility. Behavioral maladjustment is considered to be a major cause of chronic disability after severe head injury, posing an enormous burden on families (H. S. Levin, 1987). Spouses complain that their husbands or wives had changed dramatically, i.e., loss of spontaneity, childishness, irritability, and emotional lability (alternating apathy and aggressiveness). Families were soon broken up. A child's relationship to his or her parents was difficult, with father–son relationships being particularly vulnerable. Sometimes the patient dominated the parents. The family tended to become isolated since visits by friends, neighbors, and siblings ceased. Although marital relationships need not be hampered, single individuals are more likely to become dependent on their parents. After 6 months, poor memory, loss of temper, and fatigue were the most common symptoms. Only 23% claimed to be symptom free (Oddy et al., 1978).

Thomsen (1989) produces evidence and cites other studies to show that the *emotional condition by and large deteriorates over time.* This could be due to a pathological process, or to the results of continued frustration secondary to impairing neuropsychological deficits.

Levin (1985) reports that a chronic group of brain-damaged patients showed more depression, anxiety, and confused thinking than a group evaluated during the first 6 months. Further, cohabiting relatives view the psychopathology of head-injured patients as intensifying over time.

Cognitive Impairment

Mayes et al. (1989) review the literature concerning cognitive recovery, and state that prior evidence showed that the greatest degree of recovery occurs in the first 6 months after brain injury. This is consistent with my findings (see Chapter 9 on Intellectual Functioning), which offered evidence that average cognitive loss, as measured by IQ, reaches an early plateau after TBI.

Different results were obtained from a younger group studied by Mayes et al. (1989), with a mean age of 16.6 years, a mean duration of 57 days of coma, and using only the Verbal Scale of the WISC-R and WAIS-R; they found that 44%

plateaued in 6 months, 82% in 12 months, and 97% by 18 months. The greater the degree of earlier intellectual recovery the better the final outcome. It was claimed that Performance IQs are "spuriously low" secondary to physical impairments. (However, since Performance IQ is typically more impaired than Verbal IQ and since the speed effect can be taken into account in assessing the results, a major gap in available information exists in assessing recovery rates with a group of this type. Moreover, the somewhat different task required for Performance IQ, with the assumptions of holistic, nonverbal reasoning, and fluid intelligence applied to new problems, is ignored by this explanation.)

The level of injury incurred by this group, using coma (with its implied greater primary damage, and the presence of secondary damage), was greater than the group I reported (see Chapter 9 on Intellectual Functioning). It may be that reaching a plateau takes longer because of long-lasting effects of secondary injuries, which take longer to heal or to be accommodated to. The greater the length of coma, the greater the loss of VIS points. The estimated preinjury IQ was 102.5 (approximately the 56th percentile) and was based on a variety of group and individual intelligence tests, while the final Verbal IQ was about 86 (18th percentile) regardless of pre-injury IQ, controverting the usual view that the higher the baseline, the better the outcome. There was no significant relationship between preinjury intellectual level and Outcome Verbal IQ, with the Verbal IQ loss being proportional to the preinjury estimated intelligence level. There were no significant differences in Verbal IQ when groups were compared according to preinjury intellectual level. Indeed, the greater the premorbid intellectual level, the greater the Verbal IQ loss. It is implied that there is a greater degree of adjustment and coping required by the patient and family.

Cognitive impairment may persist in the absence of significant focal motor and sensory deficits, interfering with resumption of daily activities. Examination of sensorimotor functions will often reveal marginal signs of dysfunctioning ("soft"), which can indicate that some deviation from a baseline exists. Some TBI victims manifest considerable recovery with only latent covert deficits.

Grafman et al. (1988) present surprising results using a paper-and-pencil test of intelligence, i.e., the Armed Forces Qualification Test (AFQT). There was a "regression to the mean effect" after brain damage, i.e., those below the mean before injury tended to raise their scores, and those above the mean tended to drop. This pattern held whether the lesion was right, left, or bilateral. Although these findings seem different from those obtained with an individual test of intelligence (see Chapter 9 on Intellectual Functioning), with complex overt psychomotor verbal expression required, it is consistent with other findings that one may not detect a deficit in all cases of intellectual level per se, and adaptive dysfunctioning may be due to other areas. It also indicates that *findings are influenced by the nature of the task assigned to the patient.*

Memory

Complaints of memory loss for ongoing tasks, word-seeking, and other long-term retrieval deficits are very common after TBI. Recovery is inversely related to the degree of neuropathological damage. Memory recovery was positively correlated with the ego strength scale of the MMPI. Recovery of neuropsychological functions was correlated with absence of significant personality disturbance (Trexler & Zappala, 1988). The question of morale is discussed below.

Language

One may take a pessimistic attitude toward recovery of language after considerable damage to the dominant hemisphere, regardless of some transfer or residual functioning by the nondamaged right hemisphere (Van Lancker, 1985).

Sexual Behavior

The stages of the recovery process for sexuality illustrate the complexity of the recovery process after serious brain damage (National Head Injury Association, 1987).

- Acute: Exposure, fondling, public masturbation, deviant ideas.
- Post acute: Confabulation, inappropriate joking, repeated references, disturbance of drive.
- Reentry: Insensitivity, distractibility, role change, and various symptoms from different systems.

Sexuality was systematically studied by Kreutzer and Zasler (1989) in a group of male TBI victims: 57% reported a decrease in sexual drive and 14% reported an increase. A majority reported declines in self-confidence, sex appeal, and depression. One-fifth reported no change in these areas, although about one-tenth reported an increase in personal sex appeal. Single patients had no steady heterosexual relationships: 40% reported good relationships compared to preinjury, and none described their current relationship as excellent. It was concluded that head injury alters sexual functioning and desire mostly for the worse. A majority of respondents reported decreased erectile function, libido, and frequency of intercourse.

Posttraumatic Syndromes

"Minor" Head Injury (MHI)

This has been called a problem of "national public health importance" (Alves & Jane, 1985) that is difficult to define. Minor head injuries are one of the most common reasons for hospital admission, and can result in "potentially lethal complications. Even minor trauma is now recognized to cause nerve fiber degeneration. Pathological change occurs even with PTA of 10–15 minutes or less requiring urgent neurosurgical management."

MHI is sometimes used for injuries with loss of consciousness of less than 5 minutes, scores on the Glasgow Coma Scale of 13–15 (considerable responsiveness), and hospitalization for less than 48 hours (Dacey & Dikmen, 1987). *It is a gross error to assume that a minor head injury (postconcussion syndrome) or a whiplash (no contact between the head and a hard object) does not cause permanent or serious consequences.* Dacey and Dikman (1987), after summarizing the literature on the complications of apparently minor head injury, assert that "despite an initially normal neurological examination or mild alteration of the level of consciousness, 1–3% of patients who have sustained a minor head injury will require a neurosurgical operative procedure." These patients complain for a longer period of time than was once suspected. Patients are deemed to have minor brain damage at the time of hospital discharge but are still disabled (Rimel et al., 1982). The symptoms of victims of minor and severe head injured groups are reported to be similar, i.e., memory loss and headaches (Uzzell et al., 1987).

Severe symptoms produced by relatively minor injuries, i.e., headaches, giddiness, memory defects, impaired ability to concentrate, personality changes, vertigo, fatigue, sensitivity to noise, etc. are characteristic of genuine brain damage, and frequently persist. *Very few of these patients have focal neurological deficits but "their relatively less disabling symptoms may significantly affect their ability to resume normal lives."*

Miller (1986) states that subtle neurobehavioral consequences of seemingly "mild" head injuries may have been grossly underestimated, i.e., headaches, memory problems, and emotional stress, which interfere with personal, social, and vocational adjustment.

A certain pattern is common: problems of balance, dizziness, memory, and headaches, sensitivity to noise, sleep problems, loss of temper, etc. It has been observed that the PTS is uncommon with severe head injury for some obscure reason (Strub & Black, 1988, p. 332). Probably their ability to comprehend and respond to their situation (expressive deficits, or bed-ridden status) prevents adequate assessment.

Concussion

Severe symptoms may be produced by relatively minor injuries, although very few of these patients have objective focal neurological deficits. Nevertheless, "their relatively less disabling symptoms may significantly affect their ability to resume normal lives."

Concussion refers to a common pattern of deficits occurring after brain damage, often in the absence of demonstrable or focal neurological deficits, and is evidence that some brain damage has occurred. Concussion has been defined as referring to a "temporary" dysfunction. Therefore, by definition, the patient is expected to recover, but, as observed, frequently does not. Constant features include a mechanical impact to the head, or an abrupt acceleration–deceleration impact of the brain within the skull, with immediate impairment of neural functioning. Concussion is considered to end when the patient has full consciousness and orientation is achieved (Strub & Black, 1988, p. 315).

A major site of physiological impairment is likely to be in the brainstem. When injury includes rotational and acceleration–deceleration injuries, shearing will occur throughout the cerebral hemispheres (Dacey & Dikmen, 1987). Neurological impairment is usually transient, and there are no macroscopic or microscopic abnormalities. Minor concussion (with momentary unconsciousness and other neurological signs) is followed by confusion before achieving normal awareness. Prolonged cerebral circulation time may be associated with headache, dizziness, poor effort tolerance, irritability, and problems of concentration and memory (Lishman, 1987, p. 170).

The following pattern is evidence that some brain damage has occurred: problems of balance, dizziness, memory, headaches, sensitivity to noise, sleep problems, loss of temper, giddiness, fatigue, impaired ability to concentrate, personality changes, etc.

Moderate Head Injury

There is a group of patients with damage intermediate between the "minor" and severe groups. This can be defined in terms of the Glasgow Coma score (e.g., 9–12, Rimel et al., 1982). They are likely to be older, of a lower socioeconomic class, have a higher incidence of alcohol abuse, and previous trauma. The incidence of focal lesions is higher than with minor injuries. There are more complaints of headaches and memory problems. About one in six people have a disability on discharge following acute care (Kraus & Arzemanian, 1989).

Severe Head Injury

Seven days of amnesia is sometimes used as a criterion for severe head injury. The effect is attributable to torsional and shearing forces directed at the white matter of the cerebral hemisphere and the upper brainstem, primarily the midbrain. During impact, the head moves violently, and the brain twists and turns. Damage occurs to the brainstem reticular substance, along with other midbrain structures. After prolonged coma, dysarthria, imbalance, ataxia, limb tremor with dysmetria, and pseudobulbar syndrome are observed (see Chapter 13 on Cerebral Personality Disorder). During the period of recovery oculomotor nerve (III) and motor dysfunctions ("extrapyramidal tract") may be observed (Strub & Black, 1988, p. 330).

Brain Damage and Social Use of Alcohol

Social factors increase the risk of head injury (Hartman, 1988, p. 183). A family history of alcoholism doubles the likelihood of having a significant head trauma. Alcohol intoxication (incidence and level of intoxication) is greater in moderate than minor head injuries (Rimel et al., 1982), or is associated with hospital admission rather than being sent home from the emergency room. It is associated more with being a pedestrian knocked down by a car, or being assaulted and falling, than being a motorist (Bond, 1986). In one series of cases of minor head injury, some alcohol was present in the blood of 43% of the patients (Rimel et al., 1981). In a study controlling the conditions of an automobile accident, e.g., use of seatbelt, deformation of the car, accident type, "the proportion of alcohol-involved drivers killed was 3.85 times the proportion killed who were not alcohol involved. The relative differences . . . were greatest in the less damaging crashes." The intoxicated passenger may also be at risk (Waller, Stewart, Hansen, Stutts, Popkin, & Rodgman, 1986).

Combative behavior may be more likely when a brain-damaged person becomes intoxicated. Brain damage may increase the likelihood of causing pathological intoxication, with increased likelihood of illegal activity (Lishman, 1987, p. 509). Alcohol itself is toxic, as well as the congeners that accompany it in alcoholic beverages. Head injuries in alcoholics can be mistaken for an abstinence reaction (Loberg, 1986).

Repeated Mild Brain Damage

The effects of trauma are cumulative (Strub & Black, 1988, p. 326). Recovery is slower, and eventually there is unquestioned permanence. Eventually, the cumulative deficits equal major injury, with motor, cognitive, and emotional symptoms.

Behavioral disinhibition characteristic of frontal lobe injury is common, although the temporal lobe and hippocampus are also vulnerable. A variety of cortical and subcortical signs are observable. Each injury reduces reserves (ability to deal with complexity higher than the usual adaptive demands) and daily competence (the ceiling beyond which the person is unable to perform).

Typical examples of multiple injuries come from sports, i.e., boxing, steeplechase riders, football, wrestlers, etc. Recovery is slower, and eventually there is unquestioned permanence. Deficits are motor, cognitive, and emotional. Behavioral disinhibition characteristic of frontal lobe injury is common.

An example was offered of a single blow having a disproportionate affect in a previously undiagnosed AIDS victim, as well as viral encephalitis and dementia of the Alzheimer's type (Naugle, 1987). It was inferred that prior trauma or diffuse pathology renders the person subject to gross impairment.

Clinical Examples of "Mild" Brain Damage

The following reports illustrate interviews (see Intake Procedures), neuropsychological examination findings, abstracts of neurological reports, and use of an interview with a youth's mother to obtain a baseline and changes in personality. The hospital course of a severely injured youth is included to give an idea of the brain-damaged person's experience after injury causes hospitalization.

Case 36: Auto Accident

A middle-aged woman, a college graduate, whose employment required verbal and conceptual skills, was driving a car, when another vehicle appeared in front of her. Her car struck it, and she did not suffer LOC. When the other woman drove away, she chased and cornered her. The other driver then tried to assault her and prevent her from calling the police. She did not go to the hospital.

Afterward, she complained of inability to think clearly, confusion, and various somatic signs of anxiety. She had visual problems with the left eye and could not see to the side, i.e., she bumps into things. She makes mistakes, thinks more slowly, and cannot communicate as well. She felt sad, anxious, and her feelings were out of control. She experienced social withdrawal and feels damaged. Her current WAIS-R IQ of 99 (47th percentile) was an estimated loss of 19 points (Matarazzo & Herman, 1984). Verbal and Freedom from Distractibility Factors were measured around the 70th percentile, but Perceptual Organization (holistic and nonverbal reasoning) was in the 22nd percentile. On the Wide Range Achievement Test—Revised (WRAT-R) a spelling percentile of 81 confirmed a higher preinjury level. In contrast, arithmetic was achieved at the 23rd percentile. A low arithmetic score on WRAT-R (visually presented problems), relative to WAIS-R arithmetic (orally presented), is common in the presence of visual–perceptual problems.

Interview

Do you still think about, or dream about the accident? She thinks about the accident every time her back hurts (several times per day), but has not had any dreams about the accident.

What is the worst effect of the accident? She is frightened by driving, will not use a cab, and has severe anxiety about unrelated activities. She is depressed and nervous.

What is the effect of the accident on your life and goals? She had to cancel a variety of plans, and could not make a business presentation.

Do you see yourself as different, or not your real self? "Yes. I was at a business meeting but I really was not there. The words had no meaning. I couldn't make a decision when asked. I was someplace else. I wasn't functioning. I couldn't think. It was important and I couldn't be part of it. In another professional matter I could not come to a decision."

Are there any changes in your feelings since the accident? "I feel terrible. I can't drive home across the country with my daughter. I also have to break a plan with a friend."

How do you feel about the future? "I hope I'll be all right emotionally. Its more than the pain. I hope I'll get over my fear of driving. I feel out of control of my life. I'm doing stupid things."

Case 37: Falling Object

A middle-aged woman was injured by a falling object in a store. After 1 year she was still unable to return to her job as a skilled office worker.

Were you dazed or unconscious? I was unconscious for a few seconds. When I came to they were applying ice to my head. There was a big bump on my head (left occiput).

Memory for events before and after the accident? She had no loss of memory for events before the accident but experienced loss of memory for 5–10 seconds after the accident. "As soon as I felt the pain I sat down."

Statement about injury: She went to the ER for a few hours. She felt dizzy. There was a further delay, so she went home. She reported for work 2 days later, then went to her own doctor.

Statement about disability: She still feels disabled and has never returned to work because she feels dizzy. She takes medication for headaches and dizziness. She cannot do any house chores in this condition. "I can't do anything that needs concentration."

Effects of anxiety: She thinks about the accident sometimes, but does not dream about it. She does not have intrusive thoughts or avoid any activities because of anxiety.

Other aspects of emotional life: Her feelings seem weaker than before the accident, and sometimes she hides them. She has a problem with temper.

Life-style: She spends most of her time at home. She cannot read, watch TV, or do household chores. "I just sit or lie down. Now I have no friends. I can't look after my son. I get angry at him for little things."

Do you see yourself as different or not your real self? "Yes. I was very outgoing. Now my life has been changed totally. I used to play sports, badminton. I tell myself I'm not sick. I tell myself its not happening to me. I have to live for my son. I feel like a handicapped person. I have my hands and legs but cannot function as a normal person. I have to depend on people to take me shopping. I can't stand on line. I have a floating sensation. I don't want to choose among products. I don't have patience to sit with my son."

Social life: "I can't date, go out mostly with friends. I get nervous because I have to search for words and I forget what they are talking to me about. The accident has made me depend on people. I was a very self-reliant person."

Treatment: Medication and biofeedback.

Morale and attitude toward the future: "I can't work. I had to borrow money."

Case 38: Clinical Course After Cerebral Contusion: Adolescent

The accident occurred to a 16-year-old boy, who, while riding a bicycle, was struck by an automobile, knocked into the air, struck the automobile hard enough to break the windshield, and then struck his head on the curb. He was momentarily conscious, remembers people gathering around, and then lapsed into unconsciousness. He was able to respond momentarily to his mother in the ambulance and the hospital by pressing her hand. He was examined when he was 20.

Abstract of Medical Reports

He was found by the Emergency Medical Squad lying in the street unconscious. Arrived in ER in a lethargic, obtunded condition. Nonresponsive to verbal stimuli but responsive to deep pain . . . bilateral Babinski. (Nursing): Pupils pinpoint . . .

vomiting. 8/27: Hard to arouse but can be aroused with persistence. 8/28: Lethargic, responsive to painful stimuli and can be easily aroused though sleeping most of the day. 8/29: Continues to be very restless. Mental status changing frequently from alertness to stupor. 8/30: Arousable on verbal stimulation but lethargic. Remains incontinent of urine. Must be fed. 9/1: Patient progressively gets better. He is more awake. Oriented to the time, person, and space, but remains sleepy. 9/2: Assisted out of bed . . . Instructed not to get out of bed alone, unsteady gait . . . Disoriented, moving from bed to bed, wandering out of his room. Incontinent of urine. 9/3: Stated he "just came from . . . which was a confabulation." (He was otherwise) oriented to place and time. 9/3: Knows he is in a hospital. 9/5: Does not respond to all questions. 9/7: Alert but still confused. Constantly asked for his doctor. States that he is supposed to go home today and that he will meet his mother downstairs . . . Ambulating in room, very agitated. 9/9: Alert, oriented, out of bed to chair and bathroom. Gait steady . . . very anxious to go home. 9/9: No complaints . . . Repeat CT. No subdural hematomas. MD stated: He did not manifest any hard localization or lateralization.

Audiological evaluation: Normal hearing left ear, and severe to profound loss right ear (4/8).

Discharge record: 9/10: Cerebral contusion . . . limitations to physical activity.

X-Ray: 8/25: Negative for skull and C1–C5.

CT scan:

8/25: There is evidence of soft tissue swelling in relation to the left temporoparietal region. The third and lateral ventricles are rather small in size, which is probably normal for the patient's age.

8/28: No interval change. (Comment repeated about small ventricles.)

10/2: The third and lateral ventricles are somewhat prominent but unchanged from the previous examination.

MD (11 months later): Examination reveals subjective complaints referable to the neck and lumbar area and to the musculoskeletal system; he is not disabled and requires no further care.

Physiotherapist

Physical examination reveals a posttraumatic sluggish gait and lack of coordination. Physiotherapy was started to alleviate pain, prevent muscular atrophy, prevent range of motion limitation, and restore function. The patient reacted poorly to physical therapy. Treatment is ongoing and the prognosis is guarded.

MD

"He does not have much memory for the events immediately preceding this accident. Since the hearing in the right ear was so profoundly reduced, as was its speech discrimination . . . the patient was fitted with a hearing aid which shifts sound from the right side of the head to the left ear . . . Helped him considerably in localizing sounds coming from his right side."

Diagnosis

1. Posttraumatic clinical manifestation of a cervical disc lesion with secondary radiculopathy;
2. Posttraumatic concussion;
3. Posttraumatic headaches, and disordered sleeping.

Neuropsychological Implications

The history of unconsciousness, lethargy, confusion, sleepiness, disorientation, fabulation as to events, agitation, etc. is characteristic of subcortical brain damage, and is usually accompanied by measurable neuropsychological deficits. One may wonder whether the last brain scan detected a neurological deficit, i.e., prominent rather than small third and lateral ventricles. Perhaps there has been loss of cerebral tissue. There are conflicting statements about any residual orthopedic deficits. Loss of hearing on the right side would be impairing generally, and socially conspicuous. This would create social problems in a developing adolescent boy.

Baseline: His mother denied illness during pregnancy or birth injuries. Early in life the patient was hospitalized for a high fever, and they kept him there for 4 days. She cannot tell the examiner his temperature at that time. He began kindergarten at 5. He was retained in the fourth grade. He did not pass the reading test. She insisted he be retained, although the school wanted to promote him. He was also retained later on. He might have been retained in Junior High School for remedial reading, but apparently the accident intervened. He went to a parochial school where she felt he had a good education and good discipline. He started JHS in the sixth grade. He was to enter the ninth grade.

Before the accident: "He was cooperative and neat; he wasn't that good in school, but I always helped him. He just came out of Junior High School, and was planning to go to a printing school. He went to this school over the summer. He studied how to be a printer."

Accident: She believes that he fell on the car, slid down, hit his head on the car, and then on the curb.

Since the accident: "He does not want anybody to turn the light on. He curses his mother and sister, bothers them, calls them names, and bothers people on the street. He talks to himself. He cannot remember the next day or the next hour. He is constantly eating. He takes medication for emotional problems and goes to weekly psychotherapy. The tranquilizers helped him considerably. He is no longer getting into arguments or fights. Before, he would be up all night long. He went back to school but was not doing anything. He would sit in the lunchroom. His mother encouraged him to get a job. He does not want to hear any suggestions. When he gets paid, he cannot use the money well. If he buys something, it is too small. Then he is too ashamed to take it back. Now his mother buys clothes that fit him. He has to be supervised to make decisions. He has to be told what to wear when he looks for a job. However, he can travel by subway and knows his directions. Previously, he worked for 2 weeks in a noisy factory. He was bothered by noises and she told him to quit. He is in the first week of a new job. He works as a night guard in an apartment house. Socially he is different. Before he took medication, he had a chip on his shoulder. Now he seems not to have friends. Basically he is in contact only with his mother and sister. If girls call, he says he is not here. He goes to the Y to play basketball; sometimes he goes to the movies, or window shopping, or to ball games. "If we ask him to join us he won't go."

This youth was marginally effective, if school performance is the criterion. There are indications both of a recovery process and of the impairing effects of severe brain damage. His persistence in finding a job he can handle illustrates a healthy motivation. Apparently, the damage to his brain has reduced his ability to screen out intruding auditory stimuli that impaired his ability to function at that job. His judgment is poor, and he requires medication to prevent himself from bothering people, and acting out his temper. He lacks self-assertion, i.e., cannot return to a store, and is too ashamed to respond to girls. Discrepancies between his statement and his mother's may be due to his filling in facts missing because of anterograde amnesia.

Conclusion

Potential for recovery varies with the preexisting intelligence, occupation, intellectual level, personality, etc. With severe injury, the likelihood of return to work may be less than half. Factors influencing employability are very numerous. Apparent recovery, using a focal neurological examination as the criterion, may conceal disabling deficits. It is questionable as to whether there is ever complete recovery after significant evidence of more than minor brain damage.

19
General Principles of Children's Brain Damage

Overview

Trauma is the primary cause of mortality in childhood, accounting for half of all deaths (Fenichel, 1988, p. 260). It is the most common neurologic condition resulting in hospitalization of children under 19 years of age (Hynd & Willis, 1988, p. 257). This chapter will discuss childhood TBI, and its effect on the ability to function in areas such as education, employment, and social relationships. In addition to all of the dysfunctions of the various systems, there are special developmental considerations.

It is a misconception that there is generally complete and quick recovery, except in the most severe cases, and that existing special education and developmental disabilities programs adequately serve those who need long-term services (Ylvisaker, 1989). I have observed that impairment after TBI is often not recognized in school or the medical office: children often do not receive medical follow-up; careful and appropriate neuropsychological studies are rare; in general, professionals in the school system are not appropriately trained to rehabilitate or recognize the brain-injured child; and, there may be a reluctance to "stigmatize" a child as brain damaged if this condition is assessed. For information concerning related areas, such as learning disability and attentional deficit disorders, see Begali (1987, Introduction) and Hynd, Connor, and Nieves (1988) for an overview.

Definition of the System

A normal child grows up with the ability to think, solve problems, learn, enjoy life, and get along with others in the family and community. Intellectual standing relative to others is maintained over the years. Nonintellectual functions such as feelings, motivation, and concentration maintain goal-directed behavior. Psychomotor functioning is well developed and contributes to skills and social acceptability. Self-esteem provides an impetus for learning and social integration. Development involves both losing irrelevant old functions to increase control over cognitive and sensory and motor functions (Dennis, 1988), and also developing new learning.

Neuropsychological Dysfunctioning

Brain damage, which affects the very organ of action, adaptability, and acquisition of knowledge and judgment, grossly impairs the development of a child. Thus, differences exist in patterns of recovery and compensation between adults and the developing child. The effect of brain damage depends on the time since the injury, since there are recovery and impaired developmental effects operating in opposite directions. After brain damage, children have less accumulated knowledge and established skills on which to rely. Brain injury may predominantly affect the acquisition of new skills. As children grow older, the intellectual demands on them, and the need for cognitive flexibility and for autonomy, are greater. There is an interaction between impaired development, organic personality damage, social consequences of failure and poor adaptation, deficient morale due to a damaged sense of identity, and emotional distress. Inability to learn leads to depression and further deficits in school achievement.

Development of Normal and Impaired Children Is a Complex Process

In normal development functions evolve and develop in an integrated and/or synchronous fashion, i.e., there is an "orchestration" of development. Therefore, delayed development in one function can have a cumulative effect on many subsequently developing functions. For example, what appears to be a relatively unitary function, e.g., verbal ability, becomes appreciably more complex between the ages of 5 and 15 (Crockett et al., 1981), i.e., many aspects of verbal and nonverbal ability are utilized in language and communication.

Etiology

Comparison with Adult Injuries

The Maturing Brain Responds Differently to Trauma

Although, after 2 years of age, the brain, skull base, and calvarium resemble those of the adult, trauma to the nervous system of children affects an organ still in the process of maturing and acquiring new information (Shapiro, 1987). The immature brain is more susceptible to the effects of infection, seizure disorders, and malnutrition. In the adult head injury victim, the maturational processes of the brain and its coverings have essentially (though not completely) halted.

Children Are Less Likely to Be in High-Speed Motor Vehicle Accidents than Adults

Children are injured on bicycles, or are pedestrians struck by an automobile that is either moving slowly or trying to stop. They develop elevated ICP more frequently and earlier than adults (Luerrsen, 1985). Falls, a common cause of accident, causes less trauma than high-speed vehicular accidents to which adolescents and adults are prone.

The Injury Occurs in an Undeveloped Brain

Cognitive and emotional maturity is impaired; children have more to learn than adults.

Brain Damage May Not Be Recognized in Children

Head injuries are easily incurred in children, but are underdiagnosed for many reasons. The general neglect by the community is discussed in Chapter 1. Expressive Deficits are discussed in Chapter 16. A review of "children at risk" lists "physical harm" among life stress, but nowhere mentions traumatic brain injury as contributing to emotional disorders (Lewis, Dlugokinski, Caputo, and Griffin, 1988). Even among neuropsychologists there is a question about whether mild head injury may have persistent effects (Ylvisaker, 1989). Since cognitive effects may take some time to be conspicuous, as a rule after accidents I recommend an examination or reexamination after the first grade in preschool children, and after 3 years for older children. This offers an opportunity for deficits of development, including learning, to be displayed, and for the children to be given substantially greater challenges to overcome.

Overemphasis on Physiological Functioning

After brain trauma, there can be considerable improvement of sensory and motor deficits and development, which can lead one astray, i.e., ignoring cognitive impairment. Evaluation based on resolution of acute deficits and focal neurological signs is likely to underestimate the disability.

Ignoring Future Development

Brain injury may predominantly affect the acquisition of new skills. Assessment at a given age does not assess functions that are ordinarily not developed at that age. Negative findings can be incorrect. Skills that are in a rapid stage of development, such as writing, may be more affected by cerebral injury than well-consolidated skills. However, if the injury takes place at a time that writing is not expected, then one must wait until a developmental milestone is not successfully achieved before one is aware that the child is impaired.

Documenting Only Overt Deficits

Because of expressive deficits, or the lack of a thorough examination, the parent or school system may have an incomplete picture of the range of neuropsychological deficits. The recovery of motor-speech and simple auditory comprehension and linguistic structure can give the false impression of normal communication

(Jaffe, 1986), creating the illusion that development is normal while academic achievement is very poor. Thus, a test battery based on complaints is likely to be incomplete and miss significant dysfunctioning (Berg, 1986). Subtle and delayed after-effects are ignored.

Insensitivity to Aphasia

Communication and comprehension deficits are easily missed by the professional. It requires very little mental ability to carry on a simple conversation, such as "How are you feeling," or "What did you do today?" Although children's aphasic problems seem to show more rapid improvement than adults, one must be alert to other significant cognitive deficits. Even after apparent recovery, communications problems can be serious. Subtle problems in using words for problem solving, or communication, can lead to abandonment of verbal activities. In turn, development of normal social relationships is impaired at the cost of concealing the inability to speak properly. These problems can be detected on examination years later (Woods, 1987).

Some Characteristic Causes of TBI in Children

Perinatal trauma (Hovind, 1986) is likely to be extracranial hemorrhage, cranial fractures, intracranial hemorrhage, cerebral contusion, cerebellar contusion, medullary injury, and peripheral nerve injury. Characteristic injuries are trauma and infections, anoxia, vascular diseases, toxic and metabolic diseases, chromosomal anomalies, congenital neoplasms, and intracranial hematoma as a result of falls (the most frequent cause) and also in abused children. Accidents comprise 16% of hospital admissions for children, and 41% of mortality. Under the age of 2 (Di Rocco & Velardi, 1986) *falls, road accidents, and child abuse* are common. Child abuse is associated with neurological injury (see below) from shaking the head. Adolescent *suicidal attempts* include guns, overdosing with insulin, hanging, electrocution, falls, carbon monoxide poisoning, and driving into an oncoming truck. These youths may have a long period of preinjury behavioral problems, and the neurological consequences are severe: blindness, psychosis, memory and other cognitive deficits, loss of motivation, spastic quadraparesis, suicidal, violent ranges, global intellectual impairment, hemiplegia, anhedonia, sleep disturbance, etc.

Child Abuse

This has been called the "shaken-baby syndrome." Head injury is the leading cause of death from child abuse, and half of survivors are left with permanent neurological handicaps (Fenichel, 1988, p. 260). The shake-whiplash injury involves forceful shaking of the infant, creating an acceleration–deceleration of the brain within the skull. The infant is vulnerable since the poorly developed neck musculature cannot support the relatively large head. There is high mortality and residual damage. The setting creating the suspicion of child abuse is the presence of retinal and subdural hemorrhage, and intracerebral hematoma (Shapiro, 1987). Subdural hematoma is characterized by failure to thrive, pallor, irritability, jitteriness, hypertonia and hyperreflexia, etc. (Herskowitz & Rosman, 1982, p. 576). Hadley, Sonntag, Rekate, and Murphy (1989) report that of 13 infants with nonaccidental trauma, all presented with profound neurological impairment, seizures, retinal hemorrhages, and intracranial hemorrhage. Autopsies on eight who died revealed that none had a skull fracture. The pathology was at the cervicomedullary junction, which impairs vegetative functions necessary for life. In addition, shaking injuries can create hypopituitary conditions (see Endocrine Disorders, below, and Chapter 8 on Neurophysiological Functions).

Anatomical Development

Brain Weight

The brain is the fastest growing organ, with a metabolic rate double that of an adult. Though body weight in the newborn is only 5% that of the adult, the brain comprises 15% of total body weight, compared to 3% in the adult. At birth, the brain weighs 350–400 grams, 24% of the adult value. It reaches 1000 grams at 1 year and 75% of adult brain weight at the end of the second year of life. During the first 2 years of life there is approximately a 350% increase, followed by a 35% increase during the next 10 years; over 90% of adult brain weight is reached by the sixth year. The brain increases in size during the first year through increasing size and branching of neural processes, increasing glial cells, and growth of myelin. Although brain weight is 95% complete by age 10, bodily weight is only 50% complete (Peacock, 1986). By age 14 the brain has reached adult weight. Brain growth continues at a slow pace until age 12–15, when there is an average weight of 1230–1275 grams in females and 1350–1410 grams in males (Adams & Victor, 1985, pp. 420–422; Katzman and Pappius, 1973; Livingston, 1985, p. 1169; Martin, 1985; Wethcrby, 1985; Willis and Widerstrom, 1986).

Myelinization

Functional adequacy is dependent on development of the myelin sheath around the neuronal axon. A trauma occurring before maturity may not be immediately apparent, because undeveloped aspects of brain function are not challenged by tasks. Only when a developmental schedule is not met does it become apparent that permanent compromise of functioning has occurred.

Corticospinal tracts are not myelinated until around 1–1½ years. Myelinization is mostly complete by the end of the second year, but continues until after age 20. Myelin exists in posterior frontal and parietal lobes at birth, and the occipital lobes (geniculocalcarine system) myelinate soon after. Myelinization of the frontal and temporal lobes proceeds during the first year of postnatal life.

Most of the myelinization of the cerebrum is completed by the end of the second year. The prefrontal cortex is relatively late to mature. Myelinization continues to the end of the second decade (Katzman & Pappius, 1973).

Simultaneously, synaptic and dendritic changes occur. There are also more subtle changes in neuronal development, and biochemical alterations linked to maturation (Norton, 1972). There is an increasing complexity of fiber systems through late childhood and adolescence and perhaps even into middle adult life. Until around 20 (and perhaps later), the brain continues to mature anatomically and/or physiologically. The effect of trauma on these processes and the resumption of this orderly progression after physical injury are unknown. (There is a detailed chart on p. 461 of Adams & Victor, 1989, based on Yakovlev and Lecours, on specific areas of myelinization and their dates.)

The Skull

The immature brain is encased in a skull that is designed to allow the head to pass through the relatively restricted birth canal and to enable the maturing brain to grow. At birth, the sutures between the bones are not completely formed, i.e., the brain is protected only by soft membranes and skin. The bones forming the sides and roof of the skull are united by membranes. Some of those at the base of the skull are united by cartilage. Somehow, this type of development contributes to potential depressed skull fracture in utero and during delivery (see Yamamoto and Sato, 1986, for a complete description; Hynd and Willis, 1988, p. 41 for a diagram). Certain skull bones are in several pieces (Lewis, 1936, p. 141); of greatest relevance are the frontal, occipital, temporal, and sphenoid bones. Gaps between bone are called fontanels. These close at different ages, ranging from posterior at 2 months after birth, to 26 months in late cases for the anterior fontanel (Peacock, 1986).

The orbital roof and floor of the middle fossa are smooth and offer little resistance to the shifting brain during the first years of life. The subarachnoid space is smaller, and the growing brain is closer to the dura mater than in the adult. Since immature skull is soft, thin, and pliant, due to unfused suture lines, it is more easily deformed by external trauma (Shapiro, 1987). This increases vulnerability and affects the nature of traumatic injury. A somewhat different interpretation of the physical vulnerability of young children is offered by Lishman (1987, p. 171). The pressure of the blow is better absorbed, vessels are less readily ruptured, and transient rises of intracranial pressure are accommodated. It is more easily deformed by external trauma than the rigid skull of older children and adults. Lishman cited three references, more than 18 years earlier, asserting that "there is general agreement that the overall incidence of sequelae is lower in children than adults." It is more likely that brain damaged children, followed for a number of years, and examined with measures of complex functions and personality, would show significant dysfunctions.

Childhood status may be categorized as follows: (1) hard neurological signs, (2) soft neurological signs (also called minimal brain dysfunction or MBD, or borderline), (3) learning disabled with no positive neurological signs, (4) normal, and (5) psychiatric, emotionally disturbed, or a behavior problem (Gaddes, 1981).

Loss of Sensory and Motor Functions

Sensory and motor functions often seem normal at neurological examination, although subsequently there are signs of cognitive impairment. On the other hand, sensory and motor deficits can exist in the presence of a high level of intellectual achievement.

Szatmari and Taylor (1984) observe the difficulty of making differential diagnoses among brain damage, neurological disease, behavioral disorder, psychiatric conditions, learning problems, and hyperactivity. They make useful distinctions between different signs, and offer certain generalizations:

Neurological Signs

These are always qualitatively abnormal, reflecting some form of structural brain damage.

Major Signs. These can be validated neuropathologically.

Minor Signs. These are major signs expressed in a muted form (see Soft Signs, below).

Functional or Developmental Signs

Acquisition of a Certain Skill

Examples are coordination of finger movements and recognition of directions.

Extinction of Primitive Responses

Examples are overflow movements and extinction of primitive responses.

General Principles

- Performance depends on both maturation and integrity of the CNS.
- One type of brain dysfunction may not be associated with another.
- Neurological signs need not correlate with behavioral manifestations of poorly defined conditions such as minimal cerebral dysfunction.
- Disordered behavior may be more associated with developmental than neurological signs.
- Poor motor coordination and overflow are more associated with behavioral and learning difficulties than other minor signs.
- Children with clear-cut brain damage may not have major, minor, or developmental signs. The presence of developmental signs alone is not evidence for brain damage.

- There is no evidence that children with developmental signs or immaturity will catch up.

Soft Signs of Sensory and Motor Deficits

Examples of neurological soft signs are offered by Nichols (1987): poor coordination, abnormal gait, impaired position sense, nystagmus, strabismus, astereognosis, abnormal reflexes, mirror movements, other abnormal movements, and abnormal tactile finger recognition. Their incidence was from 0.8 to 14.2% of their sample.

When a factor analysis was performed, which included achievement measurements and IQ, the following factors were elicited:

   I. Reading, spelling and arithmetic (with no significant sensorimotor loading);
  II. Hyperactivity, impulsivity, short attention span, and emotional lability;
 III. Socioemotional immaturity, withdrawal, and hypoactivity;
 IV. Poor coordination and abnormal gait.

These findings are neuropsychologically reasonable, i.e., reflecting cognitive functioning, hyperarousal and poor control, reduced affect, and brainstem deficits of motor control. The number of soft signs was associated with maternal illness and smoking, and pregnancy complications.

Sensory and motor deficits are common among children with head injuries whose impairment may not be obvious. Soft signs can be aspects of normal development that become abnormal only if they persist beyond the age at which they are usually outgrown (Tupper, 1986), or borderline deficits in which the presence of impairment is not clear.

Motor

Motor problems may impair a child directly, e.g., slowness in learning to use a pencil, poor handwriting that slows performance time and antagonizes the teacher. They may reflect perceptual problems in which copying and visually creative tasks are impaired due to deficits of holistic organization preventing creation of a model for the child to express. Even if the inner image of desirable performance is adequate, motor problems will offer the impression of reduced mental ability.

Symptoms include (Tupper, 1886) clumsiness, difficulty in constructional and coordination tasks, immature grasp of a pencil, inability to catch a ball, lateness in developmental milestones, primitive reflexes, motor impersistence, poor gait and posture, poor fine motor coordination, speech articulation problems, and tactile extinction on double simultaneous stimulation.

Clumsiness and vestibular dysfunction (balance) are severe handicaps for a growing child. Deficits affect social relationships and self-esteem through the inability to engage in skillful activities such as competitive sports, riding a bicycle, etc. Children bitterly complain about loss of coordination and balance.

Sensory

Brain injury may cause loss of vision and hearing, impairing the ability to learn and communicate. These are frequently ignored after trauma, and may be detected only years after the accident.

Unsteadiness of gait is the most prominent postconcussive symptom in infants and small children, which may clear in 1–6 months. Older children may complain of headaches, and not appear ataxic, although they complain of dizziness for which they have compensated (Fenichel, 1988, p. 229).

Loss of Speed

Brain-damaged children react more slowly on tests of visuomotor, spatial dexterity, copying, visuospatial and informational processing both verbal and visual (Stroop Color and Word Test, Golden, 1978). These difficulties disrupt their classroom performance. Slowness may not be detected if it is assumed that certain skills are performed automatically such as writing. The child copes with the mechanics, not concentrating on the teacher's presentation, and finishing only a portion of the task (Berg, 1986; Fay and Janesbeski, 1986; Golden, 1978).

Cognitive Deficits

Cognitive effects probably vary with the nature of the function measured, and the way one measures it. For example, Aram and Ekelman (1988) determined that age of lesion was not related to performance level for right or left lesioned children when the Woodcock–Johnson Psycho-Educational Battery was the criterion, although considerable IQ effects were detected (see below).

The same measure of relative rank is used for IQ and academic scores, i.e., percentile or relative rank. Uninjured children are able to solve more difficult problems, remember more, etc. The brain-damaged victim has increasing deficits of ability to solve problems and learn.

Site and Lateralization of Injury

Lateralization of function (as opposed to impairment) is difficult to establish with certainty (Berg, 1986; Crockett et al., 1981). Cognitive deficits after lateralized brain injuries seem less specific in children than in adults (Chadwick & Rutter, 1983). However, there is a tendency for all tests of scholastic attainment to show greater impairment with left-hemisphere lesions, somewhat more marked in the children who were under 5 years of age at the time of injury. *Warning*: Deficits in one area can impair learning and other achievements in another.

Diffuse, left-sided, and early brain injuries are generally more impairing than focal lesions (see above, and Chapter 3 on Principles of Neurobehavioral Functioning). Although children may often show complete recovery after focal lesions, diffuse lesions often show devastating effects on follow-up. Right-sided lesions hamper spatial simultaneous and nonverbal thinking, but these may be less critical for academic success than sequential and verbal processing (usually more dependent on left cerebral lobe functioning). Frontal lobe lesions may hamper efficiency, but be undetectable until puberty because associated deficits may be confused with immaturity (see Chapter 13 on the Frontal Lobe).

Language and Verbal Skills

Left hemisphere rather than right hemisphere lesions, and anterior rather than posterior injuries are more likely to impair language. Earlier life subcortical lesions are more disruptive than cortical ones (Aram & Ekelman, 1988). Within the right hemisphere, vulnerability increases from subcortical to cortical lesions (Dennis, 1988). Tests of scholastic achievement and cognitive scores show greater impairment with left hemisphere lesions, particularly in children who were under 5 at age of injury. The locus tends to be less specific in children than adults (Berg, 1986).

Verbal ability may be more highly related to academic achievement than any other measured, limited ability. It is also a key factor in general adaptability. The left hemisphere is primary in contributing to verbal processing and comprehension. It is further hypothesized that there is a greater functional commitment of the left hemisphere to language as the child approaches puberty. With increasing age, there is a trend for damage to a particular hemisphere to produce a more focal and less generalized deficit, i.e., lateralization increases (Berg, 1986). Nevertheless, measurement of left hemisphere damage, with deficits of verbal ability, becomes confounded with measurement of the accomplishments of verbal ability, i.e., a primary repository for learned information of all kinds. This led to the somewhat fallacious differentiation between tests that "hold" after TBI, as a measure of former ability, versus those that are more susceptible to brain damage. Consequently for most people, left hemisphere damage affects to some extent current verbal ability (i.e., "fluid" intelligence) and also verbal memory ("crystallized" intelligence"). It appears to be almost universal that the average Verbal−Performance (nonverbal) IQ in almost all TBI research studies (laterality studies of right brain damage excluded) indicates a verbal advantage, consistent with the idea that new learning is more susceptible (in general) to TBI than retention of previously learned material. This is (again, in general) consistent with clinical experience.

Academic Achievement

Aram and Ekelman's study (1988) indicated that brain-damaged children had lower percentile scores across a variety of measures, and those with lesions anterior to the Rolandic fissure had higher IQ scores; there was no significant effect of anterior or posterior lesions, whether they occurred in the left or right hemisphere, on academic achievement. There was some evidence that left subcortical lesions create significant learning deficits. Small perceptual speed and memory effects were created by lesions of either side. Reading seemed to be the most generally affected function, with right lesioned children showing deficits for mathematics. Left subcortical lesions had the most pronounced effects on reasoning, perceptual speed, reading achievement, and written language. Reorganization and recovery of function seemed less here than for cortical lesions alone. Right cortical lesions created greater deficits than subcortical lesions, particularly with mathematics and written language. These findings were not related to IQ differences, when the groups were categorized by age of or site of lesion. This is consistent with the earlier discussion concerning interaction of multiple brain areas in complex functions.

Grades

The author has repeatedly observed that shortly after TBI the child may initially achieve their former IQ scores and rank on nationally standardized objective tests of academic achievement. Therefore, performance level immediately after an accident may actually be a baseline for studying future performance. There is so little difference in demands made from one grade to the next that the child coasts along on previous achievement and somewhat lesser mental abilities. It may require several years before there is a significant decline. Probably this is due to the use of prior learning, i.e., relatively similar demands are made on the child from one grade to the next. Only after a considerable length of time do the demands to learn new material expose deficits in comprehension and learning. Therefore, the writer recommends reexamination 3 years after an accident in cases in which the child seems to have no measurable cognitive deficits.

Impaired Memory

Problems of memory and new learning are the most common cognitive sequelae of closed-head injury according to Ylvisaker (1989), creating a significant barrier to school achievement. The effect of memory loss depends on which function is deficient, e.g., the sensory channel, or whether short-term or retrieval from long-term storage, etc. Analysis of whether the problem lies primarily in visual or auditory processing and storage can help in developing new learning strategies (see also Chapter 9).

Difficulties in Dealing with Complexity

Shapiro (1987) observes that although physical abilities seem normal, deficits still exist. Increasing difficulty in processing larger amounts of information creates problems as the complexity of learning required increases, so that the child may fall considerably behind his peers on intelligence and academic testing (Ylvisaker, 1989). Teachers estimate that head-injured children have the following rates of difficulties: 25%, reading vocabulary; 50%, rate of reading; 70%, higher levels of comprehension; 90%, comprehension of passages of substantial length. This is in accord with my suggestion that *assessment should always use complex tasks with a high ceiling to detect possible deficits.*

Concentration Problems

Learning deficits are partially attributed to distractibility, lack of persistence, and impulsivity (Ewing-Cobbs, Fletcher, Landry, & Levin, 1985). This is an example of deficits of mental efficiency leading to ineffective performance in the presence of higher intellectual potential.

Language and Communication Disorders

Verbal dysfunction and lack of development are characteristic signs of childhood brain damage. Deficits may reflect a combination of basic verbal dysfunction, loss of ability to memorize and learn, and concentration problems. Language deficits contribute to later academic problems. Verbal IQ seems to be the best predictor of academic success, although IQ scores are usually not very reliable until age 6. It has been claimed that the Kaufman Assessment Battery for Children overcomes this deficit (Smith, 1989).

Before the Age of 2 Years

Language development can be delayed with damage to either the left or right hemisphere.

Preschool

The first symptom of an underlying neurological dysfunction can be a delay in, or a failure to develop language. Communication difficulties can be a sensitive indicator of neurodevelopmental disorders. Children with preschool language disorder are at high risk for academic difficulties (Swisher, 1985).

Older Children

After head injury, initial aphasic problems are likely to be nonfluent (Ewing-Cobbs et al., 1985; Wetherby, 1985). When overall language performance and ability to name familiar objects were assessed a minimum of 1 year after closed head injury, increasing deficits appeared. The pattern of deficits was considered similar to that of adults (Jordan, Ozanne & Murdoch, 1988).

Nonverbal Reasoning and Information Processing

These are overlapping functions that integrate holististic, nonverbal, and simultaneous mental processing. These are very sensitive to trauma and neurotoxins (see Chapter 17). Functions involved include: learning letters or combining them into words; drawing from imagination; copying materials from the blackboard into notes; ability to read a map, understand geometry, prepare and decipher technical drawings, recognize faces, orient oneself in space, reading arithmetic problems, and calculations generally.

For example, a child (or an adult) may have a far higher level on the orally administered Arithmetic section of the Wechsler Intelligence Scale for Children (WISC-R) than on the geometrically arranged and visually presented Wide Range Achievement Test—Revised (WRAT-R). The person must grasp the nature of the problem, then perform the usual numerical operations, while keeping vertical and horizontal relationships correctly aligned.

Occupations that require these functions include engineering, drafting, physical sciences, mechanic, and fine arts.

Developmental Problems

Missed Developmental Milestones

The effects of TBI depend on the stage of development at which it occurs, and the extent to which the slope of development is reduced. Children develop "chronological age" but not "mental age." They deviate more and more from their peers as learning milestones are missed or reached late. An example is a delay in or a failure to develop language, which is often the first symptom of an underlying neurologic dysfunction.

Reduced Mental Efficiency

The pattern of cognitive functioning following head injury provides no useful guide to the locus of the brain lesion in the individual child. However, there is a tendency for all tests of scholastic attainment to show greater impairment with left-hemisphere lesions, somewhat more marked in the children who were under 5 years of age at the time of injury. Deficits in one area can impair learning and other achievements in another.

Although IQ is a familiar measure of cognitive ability (though not the only component of effectiveness), below the age of 6 the unreliability of IQ measures makes it an uncertain indicator of long-term mental ability (Swisher, 1985).

Brain injury in young children may predominantly affect the acquisition of new skills. *This is attributable to the TBI itself, and also to disturbed behavior.* The latter prevents learning at the expected rate, i.e., reduced problem-solving ability and creates problems of attention, memory, organizing assignments (Cohen, 1986). The child slows down the class being unable to do what teachers take for granted in terms of performance, which creates irritation with him or her by teacher and classmates.

Delayed and Subtle Expression of Impairment

Deficits are more likely to be immediately detectable in adults since, as noted, inability by the child to perform may take years to be manifested. Although it is frequently stated that the child has a greater capacity for recovery, follow-up studies indicate that their deficits are as great as adults (Ewing-Cobbs et al., 1985). Thus, *life-long subtle deficits, which perplex the patient, originate in childhood.*

I have had numerous experiences of interviewing adults for their health history, and hearing reports of accidents with personality or cognitive changes, which the patient did not previously connect with an earlier injury. Examples include dyslexia, clumsiness, difficulties in using language properly, cognitive efficiency (e.g., IQ), and academic achievement.

Vulnerable to Further Damage

Reduced judgment exposes the child or adolescent to risks of further injury, i.e., including use of alcohol (with likelihood of greater effects of subsequent brain damage), reckless driving, other dangerous acts that are self-motivated due to poor judgment, or may occur because of the inability to withstand social pressure, dangerous actions in sports, combativeness, etc., to which children and youths are prone. The child's predisposition to further injury through impulsive risk-taking behavior may be poorly controlled by their family (Green, 1985).

Timing of Related Functions Is Not Synchronized

Cognitive functioning depends on coordinated maturation of various functions (e.g., learning to read involves perception and sequencing). School tasks and other problem-solving situations become relatively more difficult for the brain-damaged child. Variations in the synchronous development of these skills leads to different patterns of linguistic, cognitive, and social development (Wetherby, 1985).

Later functions are dependent on the presence of earlier functions when academic and social demands are made. A delay in functioning impairs higher functions maturing later that would integrate or rely on them. One dysfunction becomes added to another causing secondary disruptive effects so that integration, synchrony, and sequencing of subsequent development do not occur. For example, learning calculations involves visual perception to acquire and organize information about digits and their visual presentation; numerical concepts such as more or less, multiply or divide; verbal ability to understand the teacher; memory; psychomotor skills to reproduce the assignment, etc.

Unusual Compensatory Strategies

Children may compensate for an inability to compete through using maladaptive or socially conspicuous techniques. Such strategies, or deviant linguistic rules, vary from the usual mode of acquiring language skills, creating inadequate problem-solving styles and social skills. Deviant communication and understanding further interfere with social relationships.

Emotional and Social Problems

Behavior disturbances are extremely disruptive consequences of head injury. They are related to the severity of injury, and are frequent when 1-year follow-up studies are performed. A higher proportion of children show emotional after-effects and increased psychiatric risk after moderate to severe brain trauma than mild injury (Rutter, Chadwick, & Shaffer, 1983). Although childhood brain damage is not clearly associated with any particular diagnosis (with the probable exception of depression), having brain damage reduces one's adaptability and therefore capacity to deal with the ordinary demands of life. Associated fright, scars, etc., add to problems of adaptation (see also Chapters 13 on Cerebral Personality Disorders and 15 on Anxiety).

Preinjury personality, behavioral and cognitive level, and psychosocial circumstances, including family setting, affect the outcome (Lishman, 1987, pp. 172–173). Personality changes are greater in children than adults. Psychiatric disorders are more persistent than cognitive disorders, which may be compensated for. Inability to succeed and to be accepted contributes to depression, which in turn hampers ability to function competently in school. Rutter et al. (1983) concluded that cognitive deficits may become much attenuated after 2 ¼ years postaccident, but psychiatric disorders continued as a persistent problem.

Noncognitive Contributions to School Failure

Noncognitive deficits such as poor social skills, anxiety, and inferiority feelings such as being unattractive, incompetent and rejected, hamper the ability to compete. Emotional regression, or immaturity, prevents the child from meeting social expectations, antagonizing teachers and peers.

The children feel inadequate and are easily upset. They exhibit uncontrolled activity, tiredness, short temper, depression, agitation, confusion, and discouragement. TBI children are susceptible to stress, sensitive to noise, and easily fatigued. Therefore, they should be gradually reintroduced to a school program, and school personnel should coordinate with rehabilitation professionals. These behavioral problems may occur a number of years after the injury, and appear to be permanent in some children (Begali, 1987, p. 71; McGuire and Rothenberg, 1986).

Stress Reactions Characteristic of Childhood

As in the case of adults, posttraumatic stress disorder is not contingent on any preexisting condition. The sequence of dynamic experiences in childhood stress has been summarized by Green (1985), using child abuse as a model: (1) The event causes ego disorganization, (2) there is a narcissistic injury, i.e., a sense of being devalued, (3) primitive defense mechanisms, (4) a compulsion to repeat the trauma, and (5) hypervigilance to avoid recurrence.

Childhood stress differs from that of adults (Terr, 1985; Chapter 15, Stress). It is asserted that children are less prone to denial, intrusive flashbacks, and psychic numbing (although these do occur). In their place are greater use of posttraumatic play (reenactment) and a foreshortened view of the future (belief that one will not live one's life as long or fully).

Children vary in their reaction to trauma: Some complain severely if they think that anyone will listen to them. Others try to be brave and to pretend that nothing has happened. Frederick (1985) lists a variety of diagnoses associated with disaster, molestation, and physical abuse. Depressive reaction is also common, which can conceal other symptoms such as anxiety. *The clinician should not assume that the child is indifferent to some serious trauma without careful exploration* (see Stress Reactions, Chapter 15 on Stress).

Temperamental Changes

Temperament has been defined as the nonverbal expression of energy and emotion (Parker, 1981, Chapter 5), and behavioral traits that appear early and consistently (Lewis et al., 1988). "Difficult" patterns of temperamental characteristics play a significant role in the development of behavioral disorders (Thomas and Chess, 1977, p. 46). Temperamental problems can lead to adaptive deficits in school, and problems with social acceptability. Brain damage enhances poor impulse control by reducing social inhibitions and impairing cognitive and adaptive functions, and defenses of the ego (see vulnerability to further damage, above).

Problems of control are conspicuous, e.g., "disinhibition and socially inappropriate behavior reminiscent of the adult frontal lobe syndrome" (Lishman, 1987, p. 173). Temperamental problems frequently observed after brain damage include overactivity, restlessness, impulsive disobedience, explosive outbursts of anger and irritability, lying, stealing, destructiveness, aggression, increased tantrums, impulsiveness, socially uninhibited behavior, poor goal orientation (distractibility and lack of persistence), low frustration tolerance, and poor motivation.

Apparent Academic Indifference

Children pretend indifference because of the pain of failure, leading to antagonism by teachers and peers. They are forgetful, experience "absence" attacks, and concentrate poorly.

Social Rejection

Inability to develop and succeed at the same rate as one's peers, scars, and various disorders result in ridicule, peer impatience, etc. The child becomes fearful of rejection and is socially isolated. This in turn results in poor learning, social reinforcement as an inadequate person, identity problems, etc. The "difficult" child further irritates the people around him, does not meet the values and expectations of parents and teachers, and does not fit in well with a peer group.

Impaired Sense of Identity and Acceptance

Physical disability, illness, and varied kinds of incompetence create fears of rejection, abandonment, or loss of love. These are compounded by school failure, criticism, and sensory and motor deficits. Scorn and frustration result from being impaired, unable to keep up with one's peers, and then rejection. The brain-damaged child feels incompetent, scarred, unattractive, unliked, and damaged, and experiences pain, loss of mobility, loss of balance, etc.

Further negative feedback actively adds to the already low sense of self-esteem, social isolation, and belief in a bleak and unfriendly future.The lack of positive feedback, i.e., absence of reinforcement, causes poor morale for meeting tomorrow's tasks.

The child's sense of identity, and awareness of his body, and development of a normal sense of self are grossly impaired by brain damage. Impaired bodily image results directly from brain damage, and from the somatic and psychic effects of trauma. The sense of self remains primitive, although overt behavior may seem to be relatively mature (see Chapter 7 on parietal lobe and bodily image). They continue to experience themselves at the pre-injury level of development, or even more regressed, than before. The injured child, particularly one who has undergone hospitalization and has scars from the accident or surgical procedures, experiences restraint due to casts, pain, and loss of mobility, is anxious about competing with peers, angry at the pain and loss of progress, may blame himself for the disaster, and fears disfigurement.

The kind of ego distortion will vary with the age at which the damage occurs (Pfeffer, 1985). During the first 2 years of life, the child has insufficient self-other differentiation. Illness is perceived in terms of terror and total dissolution of their world. The school age child, who does not fully understand how the body functions, may perceive the after-effects of the trauma idiosyncratically, i.e., their relationship to the parents and their own bodily functions are interrelated. In adolescents, body image and self-esteem are interwoven, and there are fantasies of bodily disintegration, loss of control, and shame.

Development of Autonomy Is Impaired

The child more than the adult experiences being overwhelmed by helplessness after brain damage. They do not have the memory of, and therefore the hope of returning to, independence and achievement. The parents' protectiveness becomes increased, further impairing the child's ability to learn autonomy, and to enjoy self-reliance.

Perception of Being Vulnerable in a Dangerous World

The author has observed that adults who were overwhelmed as children frequently have impaired stimulus barriers. The most casual events, e.g., passing people on the street, or continued exposure to a noxious but not necessarily dangerous person, is experienced by them as though they were defenseless against some great threat. It can be inferred that the developing child who has been struck down by a major force will experience himself as vulnerable, i.e., believing that he may be damaged more easily than other people.

Characteristic Emotional Changes *(Benedek, 1985; Pynoos and Eth, 1985)*

Chronic High Level of Anxiety

See Chapter 15 on Stress. Children develop low self-confidence, reluctance to attempt new activities, impaired social relationships, and vulnerability to neurotic problems.

Chronic Defenses Against Anxiety

Defenses include reversing the outcome (denial-in-fantasy), inhibition of thought to avoid reminders, journalistic recounting of the event, and substitution of new fears.

Withdrawal

After traumatic stress, children experience a decreased interest in play and other enjoyable activities, feel more distant from their parents or friends, experience themselves as being alone, and seem to avoid awareness of their feelings (Pynoos, Frederick, Nader, Arroyo, Steinberg, Eth, Nunez, and Fairbanks, 1987).

Emotional Constriction

Reduced experience and expression of affect and pathological denial are found in children as well as adults. Numbing of responsiveness or reduced involvement is shown through reduced interest in significant activities, feelings of detachment or estrangement, and constricted affect. These give the impression of uninvolvement or disinterest, but the numbing is considered to be defensive (Benedek, 1985).

Regression

Traumatized children climb into bed with their parents, suck their thumbs, become enuretic, etc.

Propensity to Pain

Anxiety contributes to a pain-prone emotional response to stress. Initially, the child's autonomic nervous system is under relatively poor control, in comparison to adult levels of function, so that anxiety may be transformed into colic. Subsequently, when regression occurs, pain is part of the affective response (Krystal, 1984).

Depression

Depression seems to be associated with lesions in the right frontal and left posterior regions (Rutteret et al., 1983). Depression can also follow from the child's awareness of deficiencies, social rejection, and subtle problems that are not understood by himself or others. As noted in Chapters 13 and 15 Cerebral Personality Disorders and Anxiety, depression is extremely common after TBI.

Ongoing Neurological and Medical Dysfunctioning

Posttraumatic Seizures

Febrile Seizures

Prior exposure can predispose children to posttraumatic seizures. They may result from infection of the nervous system (e.g., meningitis), or the reflection of an underlying seizure disorder. Only 2% of such children have epilepsy by age 7 (Fenichel, 1988, pp. 18–19). Consequently, seizures subsequent to trauma are likely to be an injury-related phenomenon.

Basilar Migraine

This is brainstem or cerebellar dysfunction, which in turn serves as a trigger for a seizure (Fenichel, 1988, pp. 229–230). The seizure is preceded by ataxia of gait, visual loss, vertigo, tinnitus, hemiparesis, and paresthesias.

Incidence

Children experience seizures at each level of severity of injury. Late seizures are reported in 32% of patients having immediate seizures. They may occur at night without awareness by the child or parent. Posttraumatic seizures occur more frequently within the first year following head injury than in subsequent years.

Overall, the risk, of seizures is variously estimated as 5–13 times the general population in the first year, and 3–4 times that expected in the subsequent 4–5 years. No clear increase in risk could be demonstrated beyond 5 years after injury.

The risk of late epilepsy in children is less than 2% when consciousness is preserved or impaired for less than 1 hour. The incidence rises to 5–10% with prolonged unconsciousness. Laceration of the brain by bone fragments or foreign bodies, resulting in cortical scarring, causes a rise to 25–30% (Shapiro, 1985). There may be a recurrence of, or increase in seizures around puberty, when hormonal changes may inhibit the brain's ability to restrict abnormal neuronal activity (Wolraich, 1984).

Neurobehavioral Consequences

Early onset epilepsy is associated with the greatest intellectual impairment (Hart-lage & Hartlage, 1989). There is evidence of progressive loss of existing language in children after continued epileptic seizures (Dennis, 1988). An epileptic child may give the impression of being absent-minded, e.g., due to partial seizures or other motor or sensory dysfunctions, without loss of consciousness, and considered inattentive.

Attentional deficits seem to be associated with measures of abnormality from EEG. Although epilepsy is poorly correlated with intelligence and other cognitive functions, the IQ of children with epilepsy tends to be skewed toward the lower end of the range (probably due to the injury itself), although epilepsy has some secondary and impairing effects. A disproportionate number of children are at a below-average level of educational achievement.

Parents may foster dependency and have lower standards, which lead to reduced self-esteem for these children (Bolter, 1986). Grand mal and other seizures cause the child's activities to be restricted due to overprotectiveness. Epileptic children are poorly accepted, and may experience cruelty and abuse from peers and teachers alike. They have a relatively high proportion of emotional problems, though not a unique syndrome.

Cognitive Effects of Anticonvulsants

Single or multiple drug uses can create neuropsychological deficits: learning ability, visuospatial performance, behavioral problems, nystagmus, ataxia, cerebellar signs (coordination and balance, presumably), memory impairment, decreased attention span, personality change, deficits of psychomotor performance, concentration, problem solving, possible induction of encephalopathy, hyperactivity, drowsiness, headache, dizziness, drooling, confusion, abnormal behavior, and diplopia (Bennett and Krein, 1989; Corbett and Trimble, 1983; Fenichel, 1988, p. 36).

Hyperactivity and Attention Deficits

These conditions are defined as motor activity excessive for the child's age, with inattention, and hyperactivity, with onset before age 7. "Absence attacks" from seizures also impair continued attention in school.

Endocrine Disorders

Brain damage may cause hypothalamic and pituitary disturbances, which could be manifested immediately or only at puberty (see Pituitary Gland, Chapters in chapters 2 and 8). Hypopituitarism, a possible consequence of parental assault (head shaking in cases of child abuse), or other head trauma, may become evident through growth retardation, or lack of secondary sexual development at puberty (Epstein et al., 1987; Jaffe and Hayes, 1986). Head trauma is often overlooked as a cause of anterior pituitary insufficiency leading to diabetes insipidus (Findling and Tyrell, 1986). Chronic psychological stress may also induce shutoff of growth hormone secretion, with psychosocial dwarfism (Reus and Collu, 1988). In older boys it may cause delayed onset of secondary sexual characteristics. Trauma-caused injury to the pituitary and hypothalamic systems can also cause thyroid failure, delayed or precocious puberty, myxedema, amenorrhea, impotence, diminution of sexual hair, loss of libido, growth retardation, absence of secondary sexual development evident at puberty, diabetes insipidus. It is suspected that stress can delay puberty in women, but the evidence is not clear for males (Reus and Collu, 1988). Precocious puberty may be linked to a CNS lesion (Ducharme, 1988).

Lead poisoning causes a biotoxic interaction of lead with calcium messengers (needed for intracellular functioning and transport) and neuroendocrine function.

Migraine Attacks

Head trauma, including trivial blows to the head, provokes migraine attacks through stretching or other distortion of cranial arteries (Fenichel, 1988, p. 75). A severe migraine attack, with headache, vomiting, and transitory neurologic deficit (including cerebral blindness), suggests intracranial hemorrhage (see basilar migraine under Seizures, above).

Recovery

The extent of recovery will depend on the criterion being used. For example, one author felt that the findings were encouraging when, of 21 individuals who had sustained head trauma 9–10 years earlier at approximately 11 years of age, only 3 were seriously impaired as adults (Vignolo, 1980, cited by Berg, 1986).

Sequence of Recovery After Severe TBI

McGuire and Rothenberg (1986) offer this progression of recovery for serious cases. Early: The child has decreased ability to process information, and may include language problems, agitation, and regression of social functioning. Middle: Increased comprehension deficits are under- or overestimated, with decreased compliance and motivation. Late: In the context of apparent recovery, there is decreased attention span and capability of using abstract concepts, impulsiveness, and poor judgment, with increasing awareness leading to depression.

Plasticity

This is a hypothesis concerning altered function in the remaining areas when a portion of the brain is injured. It is believed that neuronal patterns may be reorganized or new neurons proliferate.

Alternate Brain Areas

Transfer of functions can contribute to recovery, leading to considerable improvement (sometimes even clinical recovery). The recovered function utilizes other brain areas, e.g., the opposite hemisphere. For example, Rey et al. (1988), studying individuals with intractable early epilepsy, showed an increased proportion of left handers in a sample of individuals with a high percentage of left hemisphere epilepsy. Altered behavioral strategies, such as compensation, may assist adaptability. The extent of damage to the original tissue, and long-distance effects, is concealed by behavior using other parts of the brain and/or functions.

Smith, Walker, and Meyers (1988) notes that removal of pathological tissue results in enhancement of capacities (verbal, nonverbal, sensory, and motor) of the residual intact hemisphere and other structures once they are freed from disruptive pathologic influences. He offers an example of a child suffering from left spastic hemiplegia from birth, who developed seizures, and right ventricular enlargement reflecting atrophy of cerebral substance. Mental ability regressed from, being advanced one year in verbal capacity at age 2 1/2, down to a WISC-R IQ of 54 (Verbal IQ = 66; Performance IQ = 49) at age 5–8. After right hemispherectomy, 19 months later the Full Scale IQ was 90 (Verbal IQ = 96; Performance IQ = 87). Substantial recovery of function is considered evidence for plasticity of brain function, in contrast to the theory that it is relatively fixed.

Recovery Is at the Expense of Other Functions

Brain tissue that is used to replace damaged areas is not available for normal development of the functions they ordinarily serve. This has been called the "cognitive crowding" model (Lewis and Harris, 1988). In the damaged brain, bilateral representation of both verbal and spatial functioning in a site usually emphasizing one or the other hampers the alternate function. Should sprouting of new axons occur, the ensuing pattern into which they reach after reorganization would differ significantly from the ordinary neural organization. Although aphasia may not occur after left hemisphere damage prior to the attainment of language, sparing might be achieved by sacrificing some functions primarily subserved by the right hemisphere. Aphasia acquired after age 10 is more permanent.

Limit of Plasticity

It is controversial how plastic cerebral function is and the age beyond which the brain cannot compensate for loss. Some authors suggest that after a very early age, lateralized brain damage leads to some permanent deficit. However, Smith's case (1988) discussed above suggests that some improvement can occur after damage and recovery, in this instance after damaged tissue is removed. Brain plasticity may depend on the degree of commitment to its usual functioning of those parts of the remaining brain areas at the time of injury. Freedom to change probably decreases with age.

A Spectrum of Plasticity

The potential for assuming new functions seems variable. For example, the damage to visual tracts from the retina to occipital cortex is not compensated for after TBI (although some sensitivity to light may remain). The higher mental abilities are probably less dependent on particular loci, and, therefore, relatively focal damage will have less effect than diffuse damage.

Length of the Recovery Period

Most intellectual recovery occurs during the first 6 to 18 months, depending on the study. Intellectual gains may continue slowly in more severe injuries. Verbal skills recover more quickly than visuospatial skills. The latter may continue to improve for 2 years, and sometimes a late recovery is reported. There may be a later fall-off in verbal skills. Intellectual ability can improve for up to 5 years, and perhaps over a longer period if it were measured (Begali, 1987, pp. 28–29).

Age of Injury

There is considerable controversy about whether the age at which a child incurs an injury affects the outcome, when the range from childhood through adolescence is included. Opposing findings concerning age, as well as nonsignificant relationships between the age of injury and outcome have been reported (Mayes et al., 1989). TBI in younger children can create more profound neuropsychological deficits with more generalized effects.

The recovery of function and residual deficit can vary with age at which TBI was incurred. For example, evidence is presented below that an earlier injury can cause greater cognitive deficits than a later one. The alternate (right) hemisphere may substitute for the left to a varying extent, and there can be reduced levels of both verbal and nonverbal abilities. In an older individual, left brain damage is more likely to result in a balance in favor of nonverbal performance over the verbal functioning and less global and more focal deficits (Pirozzolo and Papanicolaou, 1986). This is not supported by the evidence from several other studies reported. It has been asserted that after a certain age, plasticity is far less, and a left brain injury causes a deficit that is not compensated for by the right hemisphere. However, Table 19.1 suggests that plasticity, i.e., substitution of the alternate hemisphere, is relatively greater when the injury occurs later rather than earlier. Younger children seem to have less ability to cope with the residual effects of brain damage (Crockett et al. 1981).

Skills that are in a rapid state of development may be more impaired than those that have already been consolidated. For example, written language was more affected by trauma in children than adolescents (Ewing-Cobbset et al., 1985). However, if the injury takes place at a time that writing is not expected, one may not be aware that the child is impaired until a developmental milestone is reached.

TABLE 19.1. Age and lateralization of lesion and WISC IQ.

	Verbal	Performance	Mean IQ	V–P
Early right	94.7	89.1	91.9	+5.6
Early left	93.8	90.9	92.4	+2.9
Late right	104.6	90.5	97.6	+14.1
Late left	102.2	102.8	102.5	−0.6
Mean	98.8	93.3	96.0	+5.0

I have reviewed three studies of the effects of injuries according to age, lateralization, and effect on Verbal and Performance IQ (different revisions of the
Wechsler Intelligence Scale for Children) (Arem and Ekelman, 1988; Riva and
Cazzaniga, 1986; Woods, 1987). Because of the contradictions and differences
between studies based on slight deviations of age of lesion, I decided to cut the
Gordian Knot and simply present the average findings, in the hope that there
might be a generalization, always remembering that averages conceal individual
cases that reveal significant principles if studied in detail. Subtest findings were
not available to calculate the various factors, which would have offered more precise findings (Verbal, Perceptual-Organizational, Freedom from Distractibility).

What to make of it all?

• Many children with brain damage are functioning in the average range. In fact
left late lesioned children in the Aram and Ekelman group had a mean Full
Scale IQ of 117 (SD ± 17.8) in the high average range.
• Early right lesions are the most impairing and late left the least impairing, if
Full Scale IQ is the criterion.
• Early lesions have a general impairing effect, more so on nonverbal processing
than verbal processing.
• Nonverbal processing is generally vulnerable, except for relatively late left
lesions.
• Late right lesions have a larger effect on Performance than Verbal IQ.
• Nonverbal, holistic intelligence develops laterality later than Verbal.
• Verbal processing is more vulnerable earlier, regardless of laterality.

Ogden (1988) studied two individuals with left hemisphere injuries in infancy
and 18 months, followed by extensive surgical removal in the teens of the left
hemisphere. Both individuals married and were employed. One person's IQ
increased from 64 to 87, while the other declined from 80 to 71. Verbal IQ was
almost always higher than Performance IQ during repeated measurements over
12 and 18 years. Thus, the right hemisphere did compensate for verbal ability in
place of the left hemisphere.

Withal, there are great deviations within each group, and each child merits
careful study, with every effort made to establish some baseline to determine
whether deficits or lack of development ensue from TBI.

The Role of the Family

A surprising degree of recovery of capacity to cope with academic and social demands can be achieved with support, training, and supervision posttrauma. Unfortunately, parental incompetence, e.g., lack of supervision, permits actions by children leading to injury (falling out of a window, getting hit by a vehicle, etc.). Thus, the seriously injured child may not receive intelligent support within the home, nor will efforts be made to recruit community facilities.

Prognosis

Slight deficits can anticipate subtle, or major ones, later impairment. Because of the complex interaction of lateralization and age of injury (see above), and family support, ultimate status with regard to intellectual level and/or pattern of cognitive deficits cannot be predicted with certainty from initial test findings, or documented location of brain damage. An exception would be gross damage accompanied by serious cognitive deficit, which is likely to produce permanent impairment. Otherwise, the level of recovery of ability cannot be accurately predicted (IQ, or academic ability). Effectiveness will involve a summation of effects ranging from recovery (positive) to inability to keep pace (negative).

Intellectual Recovery

Most intellectual recovery takes place during the first 6 months, though intellectual gains may continue slowly in more severe injuries. Verbal skills recover more quickly than visuospatial skills, though they may fall off later. Spatial skills may continue to improve for 2 years, and sometimes a late recovery is reported.

Limb Paralyses and Deficits

Left hemiplegics are less likely to develop speech problems (right hemisphere), while right hemiplegics have increased proportions of speech problems. Change of handedness after an accident is evidence for damage to the dominant cerebral hemisphere.

Coma

See Chapter 6 on Consciousness. Although length of coma is considered the best single criterion of degree of permanent impairment, in practice, the correlation is low. Some children may be unconscious for weeks, and make a good adaptive recovery (with detectable suffering and impairment), and other children may seem to be hardly injured and their cognitive abilities are severely impaired.

Coma lasting longer than 3 days is associated with a drop of IQ, and coma of less than 6 weeks is associated with independent functioning in different proportions depending on the study. Coma of 3 months duration is associated with "moderate disability or good recovery" in 90%, i.e., independent functioning. Such claims ignore actual neuropsychological deficits, i.e., do not indicate full recovery. Although postconcussive cognitive effects are relatively rare in children, subsequent mental and emotional deficits are overlooked (Shapiro, 1987).

Posttraumatic Amnesia

PTA of at least 1 week is associated with cognitive and behavioral sequelae. The majority of children with 3 weeks PTA show persistent cognitive impairment.

Case 39: Clinical Example of Severe Childhood TBI

This cases illustrates the complexity of neuropsychological findings after severe TBI, i.e., different patterns of efficiency on different functions, and also how a good impression from a cooperative child can conceal communication and cognitive deficits. Only parts of the author's findings are presented.

An 11-year-old child was struck by a car, and was in a coma for at least 12 days. There was verified bilateral damage to the frontal, temporal, and bilateral lobes, cerebral edema, displacement of the ventricles, parietal skull fracture, thoracic and abdominal injuries, and orthopedic and skull fractures. Experience indicates that children with gross illness have deficiencies in maturation, i.e., their sense of self remains vulnerable to further injury and often remains undeveloped.

Review of the educational records revealed that in general her conceptual abilities and social development were highly undeveloped. Verbal deficits are frequently referred to, with mathematics adequate (if visually, not verbally presented, according to some evidence). She was seen as making inadequate academic progress (despite prior retention in grade, resource room, etc.). At the time of initial hospitalization, her achievements scores (Wide Range Achievement Test—Revised) were above average, although her IQ was 69.

Her mother made the following statement: Since the accident she fell three times. She doesn't have strength in her left arm. Once she fell out of a bunk bed while playing with her sister. She couldn't hold herself. She bumped her head, but there was no loss of consciousness. She complains of visual problems, but the hospital hasn't found anything. There are no scars, but her arm is bent from a subsequent break. She has not had seizures. She complains of headaches almost every day. They are in the occiput and temples. She tires easily when walking. She also complains of leg pains. There are no complaints of nightmares or bad dreams.

She first became concerned at age 9. She forgets a lot. She trips over people a lot. I have to be careful on the street. She falls. She bumps into somebody. From the way she laughed in the hospital, I thought she was nervous. She said she did not remember what happened to her.

School and Learning

She is in special education. Before she would cry because it took a long time to do her homework. She could not understand it. Mrs. X gave a mixed message about her effectiveness: She gives up too easily, but her concentration is normal. She forgets too easily at school and at home. Her grades have improved since the accident. Asked about her current vocabulary it is described as small. Asked for an example of a sentence spoken in the last day, she stated: "Mom, do I have to go to the doctor?"

Personality

The worst effect of the accident is temper. She was quiet; now for any little thing she screams a lot. She is described as more emotional than before the accident. At times she does not express her feelings when she might be expected to. At other times she loses her temper or cries too easily. She is not easily frightened. At times Mrs. X considers her reaction strange.

Social

Social relations with family and friends are adequate. She does not associate with strangers. Previously, but not this year, a teacher told her that "she was on another planet."

Worst Effect of the Accident

The worst effect of the accident is temper.

Other Problems

She is losing a lot of hair, but lab tests were normal. She clears her throat constantly. She has pains in her legs that cause her to cry.

Neuropsychological Implications

There is no evidence for a preexisting condition. After the accident, she suffered from aphasia, from which she has not completely recovered, on the basis of her simple speech. Temper, headaches, bumping into things, and fatigue are frequent symptoms after head injuries. Weakness causes her to remain vulnerable to further injury. Leg pains are also an uncomfortable symptom, that could further affect gait, athletics, games, etc.

Clinical Impression

A. was an Hispanic appearing child of average height for her age, who weighed 96 pounds by report. She was accompanied by her mother. She was pretty, slender, and well dressed and groomed. There were no visible scars, but her mother called the examiner's attention to a curve in her arm, allegedly related to a break.

Social quality: She initiated no conversation, but cooperated well without exception.

Alertness: When she was oriented to a task, there was no problem. However, at the beginning, it was revealed that she continues to have a problem with verbal expression. She was perplexed at requests to further explain a response, even when it later became apparent that she knew the answer. She could not answer such questions as what she had for lunch. Finally she replied: "Ham, cheese, and whipped cream." When the examiner asked her about the latter, she realized that it was an error, but she could not correct herself. She was asked to turn around, and take a box from a shelf marked "beads." She needed a great deal of direction to find this right in front of her, an unusual deficit.

Problem-solving style: When oriented, she worked independently and paced herself appropriately. She seemed careless, but able to improve her responses when she realized they were wrong. She used preplanning only for easy items, and trial-and-error, a relatively immature approach for midrange items.

Emotional behavior: She was motivated to do well, but seemed largely unexpressive, i.e., no anxiety, depression, anger, reaction to success or failure, or other personal reaction.

Morale: Adequate, i.e., she did not complain in advance about anticipated difficulties.

Communication: She worked with no comment, had difficulties comprehending instructions occasionally (noted above), and had a slight problem with enunciation.

Coordination problems: She used an immature way of holding the pencil, i.e., somewhat in the palm of her hand.

Physiological/stamina: She did not need excessive interruptions for rest.

Neuropsychological Implications

The examination is a suitable sample of her performance. Evidence for impairment includes difficulties in following instructions and finding things around her, deficits of verbal expression when her response is wrong or inadequate, immature problem-solving style, lack of emotional response, and inability to initiate social contact.

Review of Psychological Records

The following tests scores were taken from the records, with the examination of 1989 administered by the author. Observe that the slight deviation in IQ over the years is within normal fluctuation. However, the percentile ranks of overlearned materials, i.e., from the WRAT-R, drifts downward over 4 years from above average to below average, while the IQ remains at the borderline level. Moreover,

TABLE 19.2. Wechsler Intelligence Scale for Children—Revised.

Scale	6/85	2/87	8/87	6/88	8/89	Deviation since 6/85
Verbal	60	72	77	60	60	0
Performance	80	84	96*	78	78	−2
Full Scale	69	76		68	66	−3

*Prorated from two subtests.

this child's difficulties would not have been detected from casual observation, since she was pleasant, pretty, well-taken care of, made no demands, and did not exhibit any dysphoria. That point alone makes one consider a cerebral personality disorder. The cognitive test findings are summarized in Tables 19.2 and 19.3.

Personality (Rorschach Inkblot Test and Drawings)

The mask-like representation of the faces in the drawings is consistent with the clinical impression, i.e., a girl who tries to be conforming to make a good impression, but does not let the outsider know what she is really experiencing. The imperfect limbs (lacking hands, fingers, feet) point to feelings of gross inadequacy, which is consistent with her problems of performance (verbal and sensorimotor). The effort to conform to what is expected of her is reflected in the forced use of color in an inaccurately perceived goldfish. Although she is capable of pleasant feelings ("two ladies dancing"), a credit to the care she has experienced since her injury, these are outweighed by signs of depression and anxiety ("skeleton," "rat," "monster").

Neuropsychological Implications

Although her demeanor is conforming and pleasant, she experiences considerable distress, whose nature is consistent with the kind of trauma and consequent impairment she has experienced.

TABLE 19.3. Wide Range Achievement Test—Revised.

	6/85	2/87 (percentile)	8/89
Spelling	79	23	
Reading	92	21	9
Arithmetic	66	32	16

Conclusions

Traumatic brain injury in a developing child requires extensive exploration, as well as patience in many instances, to permit it to enfold. All of the neuropsychological systems can be affected, creating complex deficits in cognitive, sensorimotor, and personality development. Maximum recovery requires extensive family and educational support.

20
Principles of the Wide-Range Neuropsychological Examination

This chapter will discuss general principles of assessing adaptive functioning in the suspected or known case of TBI, for outpatient assessment of both children and adults. The information elicited is relevant for diagnosis of traumatic brain injury and emotional reactions to the stressful event and impaired condition, psychotherapy and other forms of rehabilitation, employability, academic performance, and compensation (litigation, social security disability, workers compensation, etc.). Some specific procedures are listed and described in Chapter 21 and the Appendix. A recommended report form is described in Chapter 22.

For readers who are not neuropsychological examiners the information will offer guidelines enabling them to judge whether the range and focus of information available in a report is sufficient to meet the needs of their client.

The writer emphasizes a wide range of information gathering to assess as broad a spectrum of deficits (refer to Taxonomy) as feasible. Since every assessment procedure is limited, the examiner is encouraged to integrate information from many sources, and to make referrals where appropriate for further examination, e.g., with neurological procedures (including imaging).

A complete neuropsychological examination is time consuming, and therefore may be costly. I have adults come in for a full-day examination (8 hours). Analysis and report writing take at least another 8 hours for adults. Other neuropsychologists perform even more comprehensive examinations. One may conclude that a "screening" examination is just that, and in no way substitutes for a wide-range and comprehensive exploration by competent personnel.

Further, assessment of the personality, mood, and morale of the TBI victim is an essential component of the neuropsychological examination that is often neglected. I am in accord with the observation made by Allen, Lewis, Peebles, and Pruyser (1986): "Neuropsychologists at times attempt to rule out psychodynamic factors (e.g., affective states, conflicts and character patterns) as contributors to test findings, seeking to reduce the patient's responses to an illusory 'pure gold' of unalloyed brain-based behaviors."

Therefore, the concepts and tools of clinical psychology used for diagnosis and assessment of psychodynamics are a valuable contribution to assessment of TBI.

Yet, the clinical psychological examination alone is insufficient, leading to such an error as misattributing emotional changes to dynamic factors.

Overview

Traumatic Brain Injury and Emotional Stress

The technical background and clinical requirements for examination of these conditions led to the recommended procedures. This is not primarily designed to answer questions of localization, although it contributes to this. Nor is it designed to aid in the diagnosis of medical conditions such as senile dementia of the Alzheimer .Type, Parkinsonism, Korsakov's amnesia, etc., although these patients' adaptive functioning could be assessed.

Examination of a Broad Range of Functions Is Encouraged

Detection of brain damage, and assessment of its effects on adaptation combine (1) assessment over as wide a range of functioning as possible, and (2) recognition of the characteristic symptoms, patterns, and deficits after traumatic brain injury.

A comprehensive battery offers more information than only cognitive, sensorimotor, or emotional functioning (see preferably exploring the entire Taxonomy of neuropsychological systems). Tupper (1986) asserts that a 2-hour screening battery is a waste of money, when the same information could be gained from a 1-hour screening test administered by a school psychologist right in the child's school. I do not agree. I have seen numerous incompetent and incomplete "full" examinations administered by presumably competent and licensed psychologists who did not understand the complexity of traumatic brain injury. By not exploring the emotional and personal aspects of impairment they did a profound disservice to their clients.

Awareness of the Limitations of a Set of Procedures

Awareness of the range of functioning satisfactorily explored sets limits to conclusions that may be supported by the examination, and encourages referral for further exploration.

What Is the Prognosis?

The examiner attempts to indicate whether recovery will take place, and how long a time is required.

Impairment

After a diagnosis is established, the examiner is concerned with the effect of the patient's condition on daily adaptive functioning, i.e., work, school, family, enjoyment of life.

What Kind of Treatment Is Needed?

Is the patient suitable for psychotherapy, cognitive rehabilitation, vocational retraining, etc. What will it cost?

Attribution

In forensic cases, if an injury is demonstrated, can it be attributed to a particular accident or set of conditions (e.g., lead poisoning or other neurotoxin), i.e., what is the "proximal cause."

Training of the Examiner

The clinical neuropsychologist is both a clinician (interested in how people live and suffer) and a specialist in neural functioning (facts, procedures, and principles of how the brain works and is damaged). The psychologist interested in assessing brain trauma victims should have either formal neuropsychological training or supervised experience. Some thoughts about training are offered by Bornstein (1988). Board Certification in Clinical Neuropsychology by the American Board of Professional Psychology is a measure of proficiency.

To understand the details of how a particular patient is injured, and implications of medical diagnosis and treatment, training in biology, chemistry, and some physics is important. The clinical neuropsychological examination and report uses specific psychological principles and procedures, knowledge of neuroanatomy, pathology, and physiology, and access to medical information concerning injury during the trauma and illnesses consequent to it. Texts and journals in neuropsychology, general anatomy, neurology, neuroanatomy, endocrinology, Merck's Manual, and an up-to-date medical dictionary are useful.

Neuropsychology is more than brain–behavioral relationships. The examiner and rehabilitation specialist should understand occupational principles, i.e., how people earn a living and why a given pattern of impairment would prevent return to, or retraining in, a prior occupation, or set limits to the kind of rehabilitation that would be successful. Understanding of personality dynamics, educational principles, experience as a psychotherapist, etc., all make a contribution to interviewing, record review, assessment, and responding to questions such as those listed above.

Some Principles of Interpretation

Relates Findings to Brain Dysfunctioning and Pathophysiology

The history of the patient, i.e., background and manner of injury, is integrated into clinical findings. There are differences in whether there has been a penetrating head wound or blunt trauma, whether or not there are serious secondary pathological complications (see Chapter 4 on Trauma), the work and social pattern preinjury, etc. The pattern of deficits, pre- and postinjury history, medically documented brain damage, etc., shape interpretations and determine the necessity for further exploration.

Scientific Basis

A thorough neuropsychological assessment requires understanding current knowledge in areas such as neurology, endocrinology, toxicology, and physics. Special study, including the possibility of a data base search, is needed when a relatively unfamiliar symptom or trauma is involved. Electronic data bases offer a body of knowledge concerning trauma, toxins, disease, relationship between injury site and symptoms, etc. In addition, the neuropsychological examiner should have access to a medical library and/or basic medical texts referring to the kinds of patients likely to be referred for examination.

A Question Is Addressed and a Formulation Is Reached

A comprehensive examination addresses specified questions or problems, and is based on some preorganized structure or concept of how neuropsychological functions are organized. This contributes to a more meaningful and economical organization of the report, including an organized summary and/or formulation of the manifold findings.

Does Not Overemphasize Test Findings

Psychological conclusions should not ordinarily be based solely on psychometric considerations, e.g., cut-off scores or regression equations. Conclusions follow from the medical and historical data, pattern of psychological performance, comparison with an estimated baseline, the style by which a patient approach a task, etc. To assess an individual exclusively on the basis of psychological test findings is merely to describe functioning. Research does not encourage drawing too specific conclusions concerning etiology or location of an injury from individual tests.

Utilizes Style or Process of Performance

The approach recommended by the writer emphasizes understanding the way a person functions, from which other conclusions may be drawn, e.g., adaptive ability and presence and/or location of brain damage. Clinical observation contributes to understanding how different processes may contribute to adequate functioning or dysfunctioning. *Both the score, and how it was achieved, are significant.* Conclusions based almost exclusively on objective score, percentile, etc., can be erroneous. The brain-damaged person may not be impaired if one looks only for reduced ability (e.g., dementia). Inability to monitor performance, or to stay on task, can be impairing in the presence of a relatively high IQ. Examples of analysis of how the patient approaches tasks are offered by Kaufman (1979) and Kaplan (1988).

A brain-damaged person may be a contributing member of the community, and even enjoy many aspects of his life, provided the approach to tasks is relatively efficient, and strategies are used that compensate for, or by-pass deficits. Counseling evolves from awareness of how the TBI victim approaches tasks, problems, emotionally stressful events, etc.

Accepts the Limitations of Neuropsychological Testing Alone

A fine example of assessing the limitations of a single, well-regarded test is offered by Bigler (1988). The WISC-R does not directly assess motor or sensory abilities, it assesses language only incompletely, and provides no in-depth assessment of memory. Similar deficits exists for all other measures. Since precise predictions cannot be made from neuropsychological instruments, the test results should be integrated with information from nontest materials, e.g., records, self-descriptions, interviews with collaterals, observations, and baseline estimate.

To Assess Impairment, Function Is More Significant than Localization

For purposes of therapy, litigation, rehabilitation, compensation, etc., impairment is the critical issue. With the probability of diffuse injury, and in view of the limitations of any psychological procedure, determination of localization should be attempted cautiously, and only with integration of wide-ranging procedures, including sensorimotor functions, available imaging data, etc.

Understands Statistical and Psychometric Limitations of Test Findings

Many assumptions concerning the significance of particular deviations between scales or subtests are statistically incorrect. For example, relatively large deviations between Performance and Verbal IQs, or between subtest standard scores, are necessary for reliable conclusions to be drawn. Use of appropriate tables precludes attributing a deviation to TBI (or other dysfunction) when it is within normal limits.

A few examples are offered: intersubtest scatter on the WAIS-R (Matarazzo, Daniel, Prifitera, and Herman, 1988; frequencies of difference between Verbal and Performance IQs on the WAIS-R, including deviations by IQ level and size of deviation (Matarazzo and Herman, 1985); and V–P IQ differences for different levels of education, including sex differences (Bornstein, Suga, and Prifitera, 1987; Matarazzo, Bornstein, McDermott, and Noonon, 1986); and, the percentage of children offering a particular range of WISC-R scaled scores (Kaufman, 1979, pp. 197–199).

The use of these data may be illustrated. Assume that a person of estimated baseline IQ 115 and an education including some college has a 0 or slightly negative Verbal–Performance IQ. Although this deviation is statistically within the normal range, the trend for somebody with a higher than average education is to have a positive V–P IQ score (with the reverse for lower than average education). Consequently, the examiner should be alert to the possibility of a disorder that lowered the Verbal IQ, even if the obtained result is within expected limits.

In selecting procedures, and/or using particular rules that have evolved concerning cut-off scores or patterns, two considerations are in order: (1) their effectiveness in reaching correct diagnoses. This is sometimes approached through the comparison of "hit" rate contrasted to population "base rates." Statistical considerations are offered by Willis (1988). (2) The desirability of having norms such as age, education, and preinjury IQ estimate, as opposed to merely a score reflecting the average of a group of brain-damaged victims available for a particular study.

Pathognomonic Signs Are Less Useful for Diagnosis than Baseline Deviations

I recommend that a pattern contributes to hypotheses concerning the location of damage (e.g., common left-sided cerebral hemisphere association between verbal deficits and right visual field deficit). This is necessary, since pathognomonic or relatively narrowly defined "signs" of brain damage are infrequent in outpatient victims of TBI. Examples include perseveration of response, rotation in visuospatial tasks, and reversal of angle direction in reproducing geometric figures (Bender Gestalt).

Caution is recommended in using a "sign" approach for diagnosing brain damage, e.g., the number of errors in performing a test. Typically this ignores baseline considerations (expected pre-injury performance). An example is the manual for the Wisconsin Card Sorting Test (Heaton, 1981). Various cut-off scores are offered for perseverative responses (18, 19), and perseverative errors (13 for brain damage and 16+ for frontal lobe involvement). The standardization group (by age) involved IQs ranging from 110 to 114. Is one to conclude that a person with a current or preinjury IQ of 90 can be appropriately by assessed using these findings? My opinion is no. Rather one must use what is called on the firing range "Kentucky Windage." Just as the marksman aims at a target depending on the direction and velocity of the wind, the psychological examiner, without precise educational, age, and IQ norms (which is usually the case!), must evaluate the likely significance of a score or deviation within the context of the entire performance. This was described by a master clinician (Piotrowski, 1957, Chapter 12) as *the principle of the interdependence of components*.

A more applicable procedure (for psychological as opposed to sensorimotor functions) is *assessment of deviations from an estimated baseline,* in particular for "higher" cognitive functions. One must also be sensitive to the emotional effects of stress accompanying the accident, and caused by being impaired.

Principles for Selecting a Neuropsychological Battery

I offer an approach to selecting a neuropsychological assessment battery, using as a basic principle that no one group of procedures will suffice for all persons of a given age. Thus, one's clinical population, experience, preferences, etc., could lead different examiners or institutions to somewhat different approaches to assessment of TBI victims. The key integrating concepts are, however, the need for a wide range of exploration, recognition of the deficits found in diffuse brain injury, and attempt to use up-to-date procedures, concepts, and scientific findings.

The guiding principle evolves from the findings of Zygmunt A. Piotrowski (1937)· *The victim of brain damage displays both cognitive deficit and emotional distress*. This contrasts with the observation made by Kaplan (1988), that "clinical neuropsychologists . . . rely on [approaches using standardized and flexible batteries] designed to assess cognitive functioning [that] are predicated on the idea that the final solution to a problem, arrived at within a given time, is an objective measure of an underlying unitary mechanism." An alternative approach is more clinical, i.e., addressing the particular strategies utilized by the person, and sensitive to variables such as sex, handedness, history, background, premorbid talents, medical history, psychiatric history, nature of the lesion and how it was incurred, and awareness of the emotional changes ensuing directly from brain damage, from the fright of the accident, and the stress of being injured and impaired.

A Somewhat Flexible Examination Is Recommended

I do not as a basic procedure use either one of the most popular unified batteries. Yet, procedures have been selected from both of them (Halstead–Reitan and Luria Nebraska; refer to Begali, 1987, p. 110; Hynd and Willis, 1988, pp. 146–159; Incagnoli, Goldstein, and Golden, 1986, for a critique of these procedures, including the application to children).

I would summarize the procedure as a relatively standardized but eclectic battery, with additions and deletions according to the age, clinical characteristics, occupation, etc., of the patient (see Chapter 14).

Balancing the Virtues and Faults of a Standardized Examination

The reader is entitled to a discussion concerning why procedures used by many neuropsychologists are not followed.

Advantages

1. *Research findings* extend the examiner's experience and understanding of the procedure's value and limitations.
2. *There is extended individual experience*, particularly with feedback from interviewing, records, clinical experience, etc.
3. *Local norms are developed* because of larger numbers.

Limitations

1. They are not designed for an outpatient population with primarily diffuse brain damage.
2. They do not assess adaptive functioning, personality, and emotional reactions.
3. The standard batteries ignore the personality, mood disorders, and sense of self of the brain-damaged victim.
4. There is a lack of national norms.
5. The latest version or revision of standard procedures are not used.
6. They are limited in the range of their exploration.
7. They use out-of-date theories or inappropriate theories.
8. Individuals with particular demographic characteristics may require special documentation.

The statement concerning the standard batteries will create some concern. The Halstead–Reitan procedure was developed in the 1940s. The Luria Nebraska procedure is based on Luria's (1980) theories concerning "Higher Cortical Functions in Man" and as amply documented subcortical connections are most significant, and subcortical damage is common. In any event secondary effects (see Chapter 4 on Trauma) *lead to diffuse damage and impact complex mental functions that are not well documented by these procedures. Moreover, there is an interaction of all systems, on the neuraxis, and off-axis structures, such as the cerebellum, glands, and autonomic nervous system, which also affect adaptation. There is even concern about electromagnetic influence on the brain.*

Experience Is Gained by a Relatively Standard Battery

Relatively standard procedures are used for each age range, e.g., preschool, school age, and age 18 and beyond (see Chapter 21). For example, one would usually interview the patient and/or parents or other collaterals, administer an IQ test, the Rorschach Inkblot Test, and various other neuropsychological and clinical procedures, and perform a sensorimotor examination. Even such a procedure as a preferred IQ test may require substitutions, depending on how many times it was previously administered (practice effect), demands for verbalizations or manipulation, etc. Thus, a final choice is modified according to the age, and demographic characteristics of the patient, and problems requiring documentation. This is determined by record review, or after meeting with the patient and collaterals.

New or different procedures are substituted as they become available, if they have better norms, or assess functions found to be of neuropsychological significance better than their predecessors.

Examine for a Wide Range of Functions

The examiner should be open to a wide range of possible dysfunctions in terms of current knowledge of TBI. The range of deficits and patient characteristics to be examined is potentially so large that many procedures must be available that are not routinely used. It is clear that among TBI's effects are dysfunctions whose primary neurological locus is subcortical or brainstem, or which are integrated with these areas even if there is a significant cerebral cortical component. Thus, the examiner should attempt to assess as broad a range of deficits as possible, not merely the "entire cerebral cortex" or cerebral hemispheres as emphasized by Reitan (1988).

Since the record of dysfunction or actual patient complaints are likely to be unrepresentative (see Chapter 16 on Expressive Deficits), a broad-range examination can bring forth considerable new information. Children and severely impaired individuals will have particular difficulties in stating their problems.

Select Procedures that Test Complex Functions

Tests tapping complex functions are most useful. These not only reflect naturalistic demands, but avoid the error of by-passing impairment because the task is too simple. Relatively pure or simple tasks overestimate a person's ability by not sampling reality situations in which complexity, efficiency, style, and personality play a role. Lyon, Moats, and Flynn (1988) put it well: "Truncated, structured, single ability measures...do not sample adequately the cognitive characteristics most relevant to academic performance and adaptation in general." To which I add the value of using measures permitting observation of motivation and style.

Practical intelligence is dependent on integration of many abilities and functions. Choosing measures of complex functions offers assurance that a patient's success samples ability, rather than simple or narrow functions and/or processing speed.

Application of this principle leads to problems in deciphering deficits. For example, if the person receives a relatively low score in Digit Symbol, where is the difficulty? A wide-range examination might include testing for visual memory (e.g., Bender Gestalt Recall), psychomotor speed (tapping speed), coordination (pencil movements from drawings; stringing beads), reading symbols (spelling or reading recognition tests), etc. The clinician then scans features of the examination related to the test in question, to look for related elements and patterns. In this example, visual memory may be unimpaired, but psychomotor speed or coordination could slow down performance.

Select Procedures that Have a High Ceiling and Low Floor

Use relatively complex tasks exploring a given area (verbal, spatial, etc.) with a high ceiling. Tasks with a low ceiling, e.g., (simple arithmetic) give the illusion of success, when the presence of more difficult items would permit assessment of capacity in ranges that may be more appropriate to the individual.

The Stanford Binet Intelligence Scale, 4th Ed., violates this principle. This scale has other procedural deficits that have caused me (and others) to abandon it. It gives no score for inability to get credit for a subtest (e.g., a scaled score of 1 on tests such as the Wechsler and Kaufman procedures, see Chapter 21). It recommends that when a child does so poorly as not to receive credit for a given subtest, it should be ignored (Thorndike, Hagen, and Sattler, 1986, p. 145). This procedure causes an artificial enhancement in measured level due to the deletion of information about functioning in which there has been conspicuous failure. In matters of litigation, the neuropsychologist who indicates that he did not report functioning in which there was so grievous a deficit would have his objectivity questioned.

The S-B IV offers other examples of unsound neuropsychological practice. For many subtests at many ages, a relatively low or high score for a given age is normed toward the center of an ideal distribution, preventing the examiner from learning the relative rank for that performance.

Moreover, an "adaptive-testing format" (Thorndike et al., 1986, p. 5), i.e., one in which not all examinees of the same chronological age will be given the same tasks, makes it difficult to actually compare children of the same age, which is the true meaning of the IQ. It is one thing to say that a smart child may not be given very easy items on a given subtest. It is another to say that his performance will be predicted in advance to be so good that one will not even bother to measure ability, in the name of saving time. This leads to the next principle.

Administer and Report the Entire Test

I have often observed that individual subtests of larger scales (e.g., the Wechsler Scales) are often deliberately eliminated, ostensibly to save time. This is a poor procedure for several reasons. Since the deleted subtests are each useful in their way for eliciting information, the examination becomes incomplete. Moreover, there are numerous studies showing that substantial differences exist between abbreviated scales and the completely administered scale. Thus, this procedure is essentially an error. Moreover, since the examiner of a brain-damaged person should assume that his or her report enters a permanent record, and, sooner or later, will be used for its information, and as a baseline for estimating change, significant information is not available for the subsequent examiner who is likely to need it to make a comparison (see also reporting results, below).

Many screening procedures estimate ability on the basis of simple tasks (e.g., similarities and analogies, administered to adults) sometimes taken from children's level items of tests such as earlier editions of the Stanford–Binet. With no norms, they do not indicate whether there has been a deviation from a higher baseline. An adult may pass them, but deficits from a baseline will not be revealed.

Procedures Should Be Appropriate to the Characteristics of the Patient

Choose tasks likely to have adaptive significance for educability or the patient's usual employment. The available battery should be appropriate for a range of victims of TBI: those who are immigrants or poorly acculturated, well or poorly educated, or involved in unskilled or highly skilled occupations. The functions to be documented may vary widely. The craftsman requires measures of nonverbal and spatial ability, psychomotor agility, and strength. The college professor's verbal and problem-solving abilities must be challenged. A person who is unskilled and marginally educated requires some measures of educational achievement, since even a slight loss can be impairing in shopping, following instructions, driving, etc. The findings are then compared with a baseline (inferred or prior examinations).

In my opinion, even immigrants can be assessed with a Verbal Scale if they have been in the United States around 3 years, and particularly if the Vocabulary subtest is not administered.

One may illustrate the principle of selecting procedures according to the needs of a particular examination. If there is a question of whether a patient is dysarthric, one may consider the Gray Oral Reading Test (Wiederholt & Bryant, 1986). It has a measure of verbal fluency (as well as reading comprehension). The Reading Comprehension subtest of the Woodcock Reading Mastery Tests – Rev (Woodcock, 1987), on the other hand, requires less overt verbal expression, in its one word response. It does require a higher level of verbal expression, not merely comprehension. Thus, it is useful in estimating aphasic problems, and reading comprehension, but does not document suspected dysarthria.

Some Functions Require Standardized Tests

These are of particular value in assessing intellectual level and educational achievement. Their reliability is known, and their correlates (other tests, other cognitive functions, etc.) contribute to knowledge of what they assess. They have the great advantage of offering results based on national norms, with standard scores and/or percentiles that can be compared with previous findings for a baseline, or other current findings with the same or similar procedures, for pattern analysis.

I have given up psychometric tests for personality assessment since they do not offer the range of personality styles, personalized material, and level of affective expression, hidden content, etc., that projective and graphomotor tests do (in particular the Rorschach and House–Tree–Persons Drawings).

Nonstandardized Procedures Can Be Integrated with Standardized Ones

Clinical observations, i.e., approach to the task, relatedness, affect, motivation, efficiency, etc., contribute to diagnosis and general assessment. More precise measurements serve as a guideline to judge the significance of a response. For example, if an adult is of above average intelligence, but is using trial-and-error behavior, is careless in eye–hand tasks, etc., one may hypothesize about regression from a more controlled level of functioning.

As an example of a useful, though nonstandardized procedure, I assess gross motor coordination by asking patients to string 10 beads on a knotted shoelace, using materials from an old edition of the Stanford–Binet Intelligence Scale (see Chapter 21). It is possible to observe how the child or adult approaches the task [holding the string and beads off the table, or resting it more efficiently on the table, whether they begin with the long end of the string (which is knotted at one end), or the short end; whether the patient remembers the instructions to stop after 10 beads, etc.]. After a few trials, the examiner can estimate effectiveness of a patient's relative performance. One observes demeanor, judgment and thinking, vocabulary usage, etc. and compares these to an assumed unimpaired person with similar characteristics (see observation outline in Appendix).

Use the Most Recent Edition of a Test

Many psychologists continue using a procedure after it has been superseded, since they are familiar with patterns and weaknesses. Bornstein (1987) points out the problems involved of utilizing a new edition of a test, or giving one up and becoming familiar with a new one. Nevertheless, when a psychometrically sound new edition of a test is available, it should be administered with the older edition for a few trials, until familiarity is achieved. One ought not to ignore progress in test construction and its application to a rapidly developing neuroscience.

Using out-of-date norms leads to inaccurate results. For eample, important deviations in mean score downward for the same subjects were detected for these comparisons: Wechsler Adult Intelligence Scale and subsequent WAIS-Revised; Wechsler Intelligence Scale for Children, WISC-Rev; 1937 Stanford–Binet and its 1960 revision (Wechsler, 1981, pp. 47–48; Lippold and Claiborn, 1983). The same person achieved a higher relative rank when older norms were utilized. The earlier test was easier.

This may be related to a significant but poorly explained phenomenon (Flynn, 1984). "Every Stanford–Binet and Wechsler standardization sample from 1932 to 1978 established norms of a higher standard than its predecessor . . . Representative samples of Americans did better and better on IQ tests over a period of 46 years" (mean IQ raise of 13.8 IQ points). Looking at this problem from another viewpoint, a patient's ability, represented by relative rank in the most currently standardized version of a test, would be higher if measured by a test with older standards. If it is assumed that apparent overall level of intelligence is higher at the time of the later standardization, the person then is compared with a seemingly less able group, raising the IQ, which is only a relative rank.

Integrating Flynn's research with the first observation, when an out-of-date norm is utilized, an artificial increment is given to the score, making it less likely that a deficit will be detected.

If possible, procedures should have nationally standardized norms. Percentile ranks are useful to compare different subtests and tests from different sources. However, different standardization groups introduce an unknown degree of error.

To utilize as a criterion of brain damage a certain number of errors increases the likelihood of over- or underestimating the presence of brain damage. The average number of errors achieved by some experimental criterion group may be exceeded by a score of an impaired, but before-injury above average person, who had sufficient reserves to reach the criterion, but still be less effective due to TBI.

An Appropriate Baseline Should Be Specified

An example of ignoring this principle is the Benton Visual Retention Test (Benton, 1974), still being distributed. It approaches the question of detecting brain damage as a deviation between number of responses (reproduction after 10 seconds of exposure to a drawing) correct or in error, based on achievement of groups of different levels of estimated premorbid IQ. Neither the scale utilized nor the means of estimating premorbid IQ is offered. This is a quasiprecise evaluation.

What If Suitable Norms Are Not Available?

If matched norms by age, occupation, or education are not available, well-standardized tests can still be useful. An example would be using for an adult patient the norms of high school seniors for tests of academic functions. (I use the Wide Range Achievement Test Revised and Woodcock–Johnson Tests of Achievement, which have national norms over a wide range of ages for children and adults; see Chapter 21).

If an examiner wishes to use a procedure because it is deemed useful, though proper norms are unavailable, then it requires subjective evaluation. One takes into account educational and vocational achievement, age, place of origin, etc. The examiner should make it clear, to himself and to the reader, the line of reasoning by which conclusions are drawn. For example, I utilize a quantitative approach to Rorschach assessment. This permits general statements, but not specific predictions of overt behavior from scores on quantitatively scored components.

What About Immigrants?

When the examiner assesses people who have poor or no command of the English language, or have not been exposed to the culture of their community for a long period, utilizing a good translator permits a reasonably complete and valid assessment. Occasionally a family member plays this role. They are given guidance. For example, if they are aiding with a self-report procedure (questionnaire or interview), they are told: "I am interested in so-and-so's response. Even if you have an idea as to what an answer should be, or you know the patient well enough to believe that a particular answer is correct, do not suggest anything."

Most portions of an intelligence scale can usually be administered. The examiner's clinical judgment is necessary to estimate any loss due to cultural reasons. A decision would be made in advance as to which subtests or items are substantially unreasonable. For intelligence tests, a Vocabulary subtest will not be administered. In balance, I believe that there is only a slight trend for immigrants to be penalized when highly culture-oriented subtests and items are deleted. The estimate of ability is not precise, but using preinjury information as a baseline, the experienced practitioner can estimate whether the person is showing intelligence and other adaptive skills to approach the tasks, or whether there is dysfunctioning.

Use Procedures that Permit Observation of Both Efficiency and Style

For example, I often choose the older Wechsler Intelligence Scale for Children—Revised over the more recently standardized Kaufman Assessment Battery for Children. The former gives a finer opportunity to observe performance through its choice of materials, both manipulative (Object Assembly, Block Design) and verbal expression (Similarities, Information, Comprehension, Vocabulary). However, a new factor analytic approach converts the Achievement Scale into Verbal Intelligence and Reading Standard scores, and contributes to a Global Intelligence Standard Score extending its utility (Kamphaus and Reynolds, 1987, Chapter V).

Avoid a Practice Effect

It may be necessary to substitute a different test for one previously administered. Children, for example, may be administered repeatedly the Wechsler Intelligence Scale for Children—Revised. A practice effect may create an exaggerated measure of mental level. My practice is to substitute a different examination, e.g., the Kaufman Assessment Battery for Children. However, this creates the problem that changes in percentile level are not as comparable. Moreover, in forensic work, where direct comparison with the same procedure to indicate any change of level is convincing to an attorney or jury, direct comparison with the same procedure is necessary. Therefore, when a person has had repeated exposure to a test, one may wish to extend the examination of cognitive level by using an additional intelligence test (recognizing that proper assessment requires additional time).

Be Aware of Drug Effects

There are numerous side effects on cognition, mood, speed of processing, alertness, etc., caused by chemical substances prescribed and other substances. A summary (Clinicians Research Digest, 1989) includes symptoms such as paranoia, anxiety, fear, anger, insomnia, nightmares, agitation, depression, confusion, and aggression (as well as hallucinations, catatonia, confusion, etc.). This is a good reason to inquire about medication and recreational drugs, in addition to implications about prior history and effect of a trauma.

Age Norms Are Preferred to Educational Norms

The question arises as to how to compare different measurements. Errors are introduced when such procedures are normed on different populations, but the problem is not enhanced when a common metric and type of norm is applied. In terms of availability, percentile by appropriate age group is the best. Thus, while individual scores should also be included in a report (e.g., age-scaled WAIS-R scores), where available, percentiles should be included. For children, educational norms may also be available, but these serve a different purpose, i.e., determining progress, rather than comparing ability. Since the traumatized person may have missed one or more years of school, comparing performance to age mates, but ignoring chronological age, can give a false impression of success.

21
Some Assessment Procedures

This chapter describes a wide-range examination for the assessment of TBI victims of various ages. The procedures, and the report format described in Chapter 22, are selected to assess the range of potential dysfunctions described in the Taxonomy. There will be a general description of different phases of the examination, with further explication for adults and children where appropriate.

A fixed battery for individuals of a given age is not prescribed; rather an approach to a comprehensive examination that utilizes varied procedures is suggested. The purpose is to obtain a rounded picture of a person who is known, or suspected, to have incurred traumatic brain injury. Individuals who do not speak the language are accompanied by a translator, a completely practical procedure for the purpose of assessing possible impairment.

The examination of an adult requires about 8 or more hours of testing, and 7 hours for a child or adolescent (including a 1-hour interview with the parent). It is generally accomplished in 1 day. The patient is instructed to bring a sandwich to avoid delays of leaving the office to go out for lunch. Another 8 or more hours is needed to prepare a detailed report, depending on the length of educational and/or medical records.

Review of Records

Records serve a variety of purposes, including establishing a baseline, information concerning the kind of injury, prior treatment (medical and psychological, etc.), medical and functional after-effects, current level of adaptation, and symptoms that require detailed exploration.

Baseline Information

A baseline may be defined as an estimated level of performance before an injury. The information elicited is used to compare pre- and postinjury functioning, and to trace the effect of the injury on the person, including evidence for improvement, permanency, or impairment. The sources include medical, school, employment, and military records. Inferences about impairment are made, and integrated with, or disputed by the evidence of the examination.

Preinjury areas to be explored include prior health, personality qualities, level of intellectual and emotional maturity achieved, psychiatric history, academic and vocational performance, social qualities, and capacity for independent functioning.

Postinjury areas include impairment, prognosis, injury, regression, symptoms, developmental level and progress, intellectual level, specific cognitive deficiencies, recovery, etc.

Special Considerations

Medical records should be reviewed to determine whether any preexisting condition existed. I find it useful to write a chronological summary, listing details of unconsciousness, nurses observations, physicians' notes, examination reports, ambulatory treatment, etc. Then the material is analyzed as "neuropsychological implications," i.e., have the objective findings, subjective complaints, and other indications of the patient's experience provided evidence for brain damage and emotional distress. Even where the evidence for brain damage is conclusive, it is necessary for the neuropsychological examination to document the nature of impairment. Where the results are ambiguous, it may provide more conclusive evidence that brain damage and impairment exist. It may simply indicate that no evidence exists, or that further exploration with other procedures (various imaging techniques) would be useful.

School records are explored for young adults. For details of the review of these records, see below under children's examination.

Adult achievement is explored in terms of vocational achievement (salary, responsibilities, development) and leisure time activities (art and crafts, for example). A veteran's military occupational specialty (MOS) and assignments often give evidence of the ability to learn complex psychomotor and cognitive functions. Preinjury earnings, skilled functioning, the ability to assume responsibility and supervisory functions, and the ability to work efficiently and without supervision are compared with the current level of performance.

Suggestions for Specific Examination

Significant information from the records is used to select procedures not ordinarily administered, and to focus relevant information. If a person was an engineer or skilled craftsman, nonverbal cognitive procedures will be selected. An individual in a profession or highly verbal trade would be given a reading comprehension test. A person with athletic skills or leisure activities would have coordination explored in greater than usual detail.

Interview with Collaterals

A spouse, friends, children, etc., are useful sources of information, and should be interviewed wherever possible. Useful information can be obtained in an extensive telephone interview, if it is difficult for them to come in.

The examiner explores what is known about the patient's development and preinjury behavior, including the possibility of a preexisting condition, and what effect the injury had on behavior, what changes have occurred since the accident, e.g., personality, academic functioning, social relationships, anxiety, restriction of interests, nightmares, signs of impaired functioning and stress, etc. Can the patient be trusted to be left alone, or travel alone, or is his or her judgment so defective that this imposes a risk? Does the person participate as before in family social gatherings, or activities with children, spouse, etc., or has withdrawal occurred because of preference, or emotional disturbance such as anger, irritability, shame, etc.?

Clinical Observation

The examiner's clinical impression is very significant for many areas of functioning. An outline for direct observation is offered in Appendix 1, which is useful for both children and adults. The examiner observes appearance (dress, visible scars, height and weight as reported, handedness), independence (punctuality and whether accompanied), social quality, alertness and concentration, problem-solving style, reaction to the event (the accident, and resulting impairment), emotional behavior (anxiety, depression, anger, voice, reactivity, etc.), morale, communications, physiological reactions (including ability to proceed for long periods, excessive use of the toilet or need for water), and movement or coordination problems.

Ruff et al. (1989) deal with the criticism of neuropsychological assessment that cognitive functioning can be influenced by the patient's cooperation, motivation, mood fluctuations, and preexisting limitations. These can be a consequence of the neuropathology, and should be evaluated and integrated into the clinical picture. The examiner should be alert to mood, variable efficiency, paradoxical levels of expressive output, inappropriate affect, whether the patient is socially related or withdrawn, reactions to the examiner's interventions, and how the patient handles difficulties in performing the tasks. Direct observation is made concerning alertness and attention, concentration, communication (comprehensibility, comprehension of the examiner, and clarity of speech). The level of emotional expression (spontaneous, bland, or uncontrolled) is compared with other evidence for reactivity level and quality (reports of temper outbursts or irritability, withdrawal, etc.), intense inner life as revealed by the Rorschach, etc. This may be used for evidence whether there is reduced emotional expressivity, corresponding to a cerebral personality syndrome (see Chapter 13).

The examiner's experience contributes to assessment of problem-solving style, which corresponds to the Taxonomic area of Efficiency. With experience, the examiner can judge, for example, whether the way of approaching problems emphasizes the immature form (trial and error) or more mature development (preplanning responses), and at what level of difficulty mental control is abandoned for random responses. The level of performance is compared to the baseline, the patient's age, occupation, etc., to determine whether a significant level of inefficiency exists to indicate impairment. Any performance can contribute to this, I find particular Wechsler subtests to be revealing (Object Assembly; Block Design).

Interviewing can lead to incorrect estimates of intellectual status. It is easy to be misled about the level of a patient's mental level. Why? It takes very little mental ability to answer questions about daily life, familiar activities, and community interests, such as watching TV. Simply asking an individual how he or she spends his time, or what activities have been performed recently, can bring forth a deceptively adequate answer. Perhaps a 10-year-old child could respond adequately to questions that are asked by professional people in their evaluations of current status.

The examiner should be alert to deficits of the "higher" cognitive functions. Verbal and comprehension deficits can be missed unless a thorough examination is performed. A patient may be seriously amnestic for new information, but be able to discourse on previously learned materials relating to his or her profession. This gives the illusion of retained general ability.

Use of the Brain Damage/Emotional Stress Checklist

I believe that very valuable information can be obtained from the patient's Personal Statement, which comprises the Brain Damage/Stress checklist and the Interview (Appendix 1). However, the effect of expressive deficits on self-report measures of TBI patients is noted by Burke, Smith, and Imhoff (1989). These include cognitive deficits and comprehension, fatigue, memory, an attempt to make oneself look good, and a marked tendency to deny or be unaware of personal problems. The potential for a test to create stress is observed by Stuss et al. (1989) for test selection. However, I believe that looking for procedures that are "relatively independent of moderator variables such as age and education" leads to the exploration of rather narrow facets of behavior. These have their place, but, with exceptions, for TBI victims, time is better spent in assessing more complex functions.

The Checklist symptoms are organized by areas of the neuropsychological Taxonomy. The list of symptoms evolved from the clinical literature on TBI, supplemented by reports from my patients and their collaterals (see Appendix 1). This self-description is used to select procedures to document the patient's condition. The value of a focused checklist is that it helps to overcome expressive deficits, i.e., the inability of the patient to tell the examiner about impairment.

The checklist is administered first in the battery. The patient is instructed to check every condition that has occurred since the accident, or was made worse, and to ignore other possibilities. They can underline problems of great importance, or write their comments on the printed form. These serve for further exploration in the interview, which follows.

If the patient is illiterate, the examiner reads the questions and explains them. If the patient does not speak English, a translator reads it, and is instructed not to prejudice the response.

Interviewing

Content of the Interview

The interview (see Intake Procedures in Appendix 1) covers place of origin and language spoken, health and accident history, educational history, preinjury vocational history, including skilled positions and responsibilities, how the accident took place, questions of consciousness and amnesia (anterograde and posterograde), areas of the body injured, anxiety, memory, difficulties in adapting (problems of employment, independence), family and social relationships, mood changes, what the patient experiences as the worst effect of the injury, the effect on goals of pain, loss of ability, or self-confidence, fearfulness, pain, cosmetic effects, etc., and the effect on the ability to enjoy life.

Be Aware of Expressive Deficits (see Chapter 16)

Obtaining a complete and objective report of posttraumatic personal difficulties from the patient can be extremely difficult, even when there is concern with injury and impairment. One should assess whether there is truly a full report from the patient concerning their current condition. Expressive deficits (see Chapter 16) include formal communications problems, poor motivation to communicate for reasons of self-esteem, and distortions in communication due to litigation. Westermeher and Wahmenholm (1989) point out the difficulties of assessing victimized patients directly due to their dysphoria, and the additional problem of relating their symptoms to a given injury.

Self-awareness shortly after injury may be relatively low. It has been established that shortly after an accident, poorly oriented individuals will offer unreliable information on questionnaires (Priddy, Mattes, & Lam, 1988), due to a memory deficit. In the early stages the patient may lack self-understanding or be motivated by denial (Lam, McMahon, Priddy, & Gehred-Schultz, 1988). They may also be too poorly oriented, or have amnestic symptoms, so that they cannot give a reliable self-report (Priddy et al., 1988).

Deception

The examiner also has to be aware of exaggeration of symptoms, and concealment of recovery or of a prior condition. Deception includes (1) concealing preexisting conditions, (2) concealing the extent of recovery, and (3) deliberately inventing or exaggerating symptoms. This is discussed further under "malingering."

Inquire About Prior Injury

One should routinely inquire whether there has been an earlier accident or neurological illness. Victims of TBI may not report injuries or see the connection between present problems and previous injuries. Therefore, professionals who render service to individuals should routinely inquire whether an accident or neurological illness has occurred before the period under exploration. Jacobson and Richardson (1987) note that assault is ignored in psychotherapy. Inquiry will often elicit a significant prior condition, which has been ignored in the records.

I have often had a patient state after an interview that this was the first time they could associate some personality or cognitive change with an accident. Ask about problems that arose after each accident. Was there recovery? Were the effects of the second accident different than the first, or did they render a previous difficulty worse?

Inquiry Concerning Preexisting Medical or Emotional Conditions

Prior conditions include abnormal development, previous accidents, illnesses, alcoholism, use of drugs, medical illnesses, learning disabilities, etc. Bornstein (1987) observes that the patient's physical status and education can have a considerable effect on the relative difficulty of a test, apart from any psychometric considerations of level psychological measurement.

Inquire About the Details of the Accident

There can be considerable information to be learned about how the person was injured (e.g., direction of impact), memory (anterograde and retrograde amnesia), loss of consciousness, etc. The neuropsychologist should always ask a patient whether they lost consciousness, or were dizzy or dazed, and whether there have been earlier injuries or illnesses. This information is often inaccurate in formal medical records, since observations were made after recovery.

Sensorimotor Examination

The sensorimotor examination is useful for detecting deficits of adaptive importance, and alerting the neuropsychologist to brainstem deficits, which are not tested directly by the classical battery. A useful sensorimotor examination is described in Appendix 2.

Many accident victims are unaware that vague discomforts are effects of the accident or injury. This will be particularly true if there has not been a careful neurological examination. A person may state that he bumps into things, without realizing that this symptom arose after an accident. Examination of peripheral visual fields often reveals that the field of vision is generally restricted, or restricted in one area, causing the individual not to see to one side. Sometimes the individual is cautioned about driving.

The examiner will organize information, within the context of medical reports, other observations, etc., as to whether dysfunctions are related to peripheral damage to the sense organs and tracts, at higher levels before decussation of the tracts, brainstem deficits (e.g., deficits of internal and external ocular muscles), cerebellar (kinesthesis), or perhaps cortical (problems of muscular strength and directing action). Tests of strength, particularly when one hand is unexpectedly stronger than the other or there is a loss of strength, are sensitive to peripheral or central damage.

Sensory deficits contribute to localizing the damage (see Chapter 2 on Neuroanatomy). The preferred hand should be stated in the report, and used as a rough guide to the dominant hemisphere. There is a discussion in Filskov and Catanese (1986) about handedness, lateralization, preferred strategy of task completion, and sex of the examiner, as issues that affect performance. Lateralization of spatial and verbal abilities is greater in males, from which it would be inferred that they are more vulnerable to focal brain damage. Where sex norms are available, they should be utilized, and the examiner should be aware of trends of sex differences (e.g., in Finger Tapping and Grip Strength, where even the apparatus shape may effect the results). Cut-off scores may create false negatives for females, where the sex distributions differ, e.g., the Halstead Impairment Index. It has been established that higher scores are obtained by the preferred hand on psychomotor tasks.

Cognitive Functioning in Structured Situations

It is useful to compare functioning in structured and unstructured situations. These are defined in Chapter 9 on Intellectual Functioning. I use full-scale IQ as a representative of functioning in structured situations, differentiating between measures of general intelligence and measures of academic achievement, although these are highly correlated. Scores on achievement test are loaded with prior ability to learn, retrieval from long-term memory, and problem solving.

General intelligence is sometimes ignored in screening examinations for brain damage for reasons of time. This is unfortunate for two reasons:

1. The significance of a particular score may derive from its deviation from a measure of cognitive level. For example, a person may have high retained general intelligence, but reduced memory, concentration, or ability to detect errors. This deviation creates the suspicion that some narrowly defined, but significant function has been impaired as a result of injury.
2. Impairment is best detected by utilizing complex tasks with a high ceiling. Most screening tasks utilize relative simple functions that would miss deficits

in an intelligent person who is dysfunctional but still performing above the ceiling of the test.

Wechsler Adult Intelligence Scale—Revised

For interpretation of cognitive level, age-scaled scores, not standard scores should be utilized. Calculate Factor means using age-scaled scores (Silverstein, 1982; Atkinson & St. Cyr, 1984).

Verbal Factor: Information and Vocabulary (former verbal learning, old learning), Comprehension and Similarities (contemporary verbal processing);
Perceptual Organization: Picture Completion, Block Design, Object Assembly;
Freedom from Distractibility/Numerical (FD/N): Arithmetic, Digit Span, Digit Symbol;
Sequential processing: I assume that this is measured by Picture Arrangement.

The Verbal and Perceptual Organizational Factors are purer measures of verbal and nonverbal or holistic reasoning than the Verbal and Performance IQs. The FD/N Factor seems to be a measure of short-term memory. Individuals who are well motivated to succeed perform relatively well, sometimes better than on the other factors. Clinical experience suggests that a two point difference is the beginning of reliable information concerning cognitive differences between Factors.

Administer the entire test. Abbreviated tests eliminate significant information, distort the actual performance level, and prevent comparison over time with more complete examinations. [The previous edition (WAIS) is not recommended. There are substantial differences in scores due to changes in standardization of WAIS-R (Smith, 1983) and other psychometric problems (see Chapter 20).]

A preinjury IQ baseline can be calculated, using age and education (Matarazzo and Herman, 1984). For interpreting differences between Verbal and Performance IQs, tables assessing reliability of a given difference are offered by various sources (Naglieri, 1982; Knight, 1983; Matarazzo and Herman, 1985; Bornstein et al., 1987). The significance of a level of intrasubtest scatter is offered by Matarazzo, Daniel, Prifitera and Herman (1988) in terms of Scaled Scores, rather than Age Scaled Scores. One's estimate of the significance of Verbal–Performance IQs can be conditioned by trends such as the following: (1) After brain damage, mean Performance IQ is reduced relative to Verbal IQ (Farr et al., 1986); (2) With higher levels of education, a higher proportion of high Verbal IQs is found; with lower levels of education, a higher proportion of higher Performance IQ's is found. These trends will help in determining deviations from an estimated baseline, although considerable variability exists.

Wide Range Achievement Test—Revised: Level 2 (Age 12–74)

The subtests include printed arithmetic, oral spelling, and reading individual words. It is a well-standardized test that reflects prior educational level. Individuals with visuoperceptual dysfunctioning tend to do relatively poorly on the visually presented arithmetic problems, compared to the orally administered arithmetic of WAIS-R. The reading test is also a measure of visual channel input. It should be supplemented by a test of reading comprehension (see Chapter 20 for a discussion of the Woodcock–Johnson and Gray Oral Reading Tests). Percentile ranks are compared to percentile ranks for the intelligence test as a measure of baseline functioning, i.e., long-term memory representing prior level of achievement.

Woodcock–Johnson Tests of Cognitive Ability and Tests of Achievement

The Revised Edition (1989) comprises 33 subtests, scaled both by age (2–90!) and by grade (up to college graduate). I have not used all of the materials, but they are divided into primary and supplementary tests for the two major groupings. Different kinds of problems, achievement, short-term and long-term memory, etc. are assessed. The range of materials is so broad, and the norms so superior to what has been available for many other functions, that it may be expected that some of them will become significant parts of the neuropsychological armamentarium. The reader is encouraged to explore these tests to find areas of interest that they measure. It is expensive, and the scoring procedures are complex. Computer-assisted scoring is available.

I recommend the Standard Battery of the Tests of Achievement (one hour plus). It includes reading comprehension, arithmetic, writing, and retrieval of information from pictures. This subtest, and the Picture Vocabulary Subtest of the Tests of Cognitive Ability, have norms that are far superior to the widely used Boston Naming Test.

The Tests of Cognitive Ability do not seem to tap verbal understanding as thoroughly as the Wechsler Scales (which seem unique in this regard). How the general measure of Broad Cognitive Ability (analogous to the IQ) will compare in effectiveness to the Wechsler IQ for measuring general adaptive ability remains to be seen. As with the Achievement Battery, the Standard and Supplemental Batteries have many subtests that measure functions of neuropsychological importance.

For tests of reading comprehension, the following are recommended. There is a description of their features in Chapter 20. It is recommended that this skill be assessed when baselines indicate that reading accomplishment or vocational usage is important.

Gray Oral Reading Test – Revised (Wiederholt & Bryant, 1986): Standardized scores for verbal comprehension and precision of articulation.

Woodcock Reading Mastery Tests – Revised: Visual-auditory associations measure the ability to associate symbols with oral stimuli (as would be used in learning to read); various verbal processes; reading comprehension. The Passage Comprehension subtest supplements the WRAT-R.

For varied procedures concerning assessment of aphasic deficits and verbal ability, see Gordon (1985).

Cognitive Functioning in Unstructured Situations

It is extremely useful to see how a person reacts in a free situation, as a measure of the ability to perform in unfamiliar and unsupervised conditions. Functioning in an unstructured situation predicts employment capability, ability to care for oneself, etc.

Rorschach

The Rorschach procedure has earned its place in personality assessment, offering a range of both cognitive and emotional data not obtainable through any other procedure. References include Piotrowski (1957) for interpretation, Klopfer, Ainsworth, Klopfer, and Holt (1954) for scoring, Exner (1986) for form accuracy scoring and information concerning cognitive functioning, and Goldfried, Stricker, and Weiner (1971) for a review of studies on brain damage.

Ordinarily, Rorschach performance is relatively less effective than an analogous level of ability represented by structured tests. This is due to the availability of familiar cues, retrieval of long-term memory, etc. Occasionally cognitive functioning is far superior on the Rorschach than on IQ-type tasks, and one may wonder why. A rich record, from the viewpoint of imagination, complexity etc., can be obtained when the intelligence test results seem low or impaired. The level and style of cognitive performance reveal not only current level, but can offer evidence concerning the preinjury baseline level. One looks for signs of maturity of personality development and use of mature cognitive processes. Signs of a well-developed preinjury functioning emphasize the significance of neuropsychological findings of regression, emotional emptiness, or cognitive inefficiency.

I feel that the Rorschach plus a questionnaire, and a symptom checklist provide more vivid and complete information than psychometric assessment alone. It differs from more psychometric tools (e.g., MMPI) that do not reveal a style or vivid self-image. Above all *it offers samples of personal expression that are unexcelled by any other procedure*, e.g., feelings about the self in relationship with others, self-awareness, guilt, and impulsivity.

Administration

The patient is told that "It is a test of imagination. Please tell me what they remind you of. I will hand them to you in a certain position, but you can turn them around if you want to." The plate is presented for 45 seconds, then they are permitted to reject it. On plates I–III the patient is encouraged to see more than one response. To measure the cognitive difficulty of the task, mean initial reaction time for the 10 plates is measured, as indicated by the time for the first noun, or other scorable response. To assess emotional dullness, and/or depression, if there are no color responses, and color vision has not been tested, the patient is asked to name the colors on one of the plates.

Inquiry is active. I recommend Piotrowski's suggestions (1957, pp. 55–57) for obtaining associations to the percept. It has been established that valuable evidence concerning the sense of identity can be obtained by a planned and active inquiry (Parker and Piotrowski, 1965). During or after the inquiry, the patient is asked: "Do you have any sense of action in this response . . . Tell me more . . . How do they feel?" If there is doubt whether the examiner suggested a determinant (formal characteristic of the response, e.g., color, shading, movement), the patient is asked: "Did you think of this before, or did I suggest it to you?" Specifically, though discretely, the examiner should inquire for movement, color, shading, darkness, and how the human figures feel.

Active inquiry often yields intrusive anxiety content. Examples of examiner query are offered: "Eyes." (Whose?) "The devil, looking at you." "Tyrannosaurus rex walking toward you." (E. Toward whom?) "Towards me." "Two girls washing." (How do they feel?) "If they feel like me, they feel badly." "Dentures." (Tell me about them.) "They are in bad condition." Active inquiry can elicit statements of direct threat by the inkblot, a response not apparently previously described.

Neuropsychological Features of the Rorschach

I use the Rorschach inkblot test for all patients in assessment of TBI. Some quantitative findings illustrating how it can differentiate between patients subjected to serious stress alone, and those who have incurred traumatic brain injury, are offered in Appendix 3, Table A1.

The task is to isolate an area or utilize the whole inkblot, and then associate a name, activity, or mood from one's experience by interpreting the stimulus and labeling it through retrieval of information stored in long-term memory as images and verbal concepts. As a multidimensional evaluation procedure, responding well requires many cognitive skills: complex visual analysis, verbal associations and expression, ability to perceive accurately, to organize ideas, to associate external stimulation with feelings and experiences in long-term memory, to express overtly what it has associated and retrieved, and to recognize and reject errors. The data are organized as follows:

Ability to create complex ideas: The number of accurate responses integrating an entire inkblot.
Productivity: The number of responses that meet minimal standards of accuracy and sharp articulation ("Good" R, i.e., are accurate and lack any vagueness whatsoever).
Conformity with group norm: The number of populars, and lack of idiosyncratic responses that are peculiar and inaccurate.
Creativity/range of ideas: The range of content and number of accurate original responses.
Judgment and reality testing: Deficits of monitoring are detected, i.e., inability to recognize and avoid perceptual errors, as revealed by peculiar thinking, and reduced extended form accuracy and judgment (ext F+%, see Appendix 3). This is measured by extended form accuracy. Reduced F+% is an indicator that

errors are not detected, or, if they are, are not rejected.

Overall expressiveness: Whether the protocol reveals personal experiences, in particular attitudes toward the self or stress-related content, or there is blandness, suppression, etc.

Objectivity: Whether intrusive anxiety impairs cognitive processes. The influence of feelings on cognitive processes are explored, i.e., preoccupations, intrusive anxiety, etc.

Developmental level: The current level of functioning, as revealed by good form, integration of form with color, shading, use of good human movement.

Overt pathology: Whether there are signs of psychosis or gross loss of ability to recognize reality (revealed by very low extended form accuracy, see Appendix 3). The clinician comes to a judgment about whether measures of dysphoria are outside the normal range, even taking into account TBI. Examples include psychopathology, e.g., psychosis, levels of dysphoria (anger, anxiety, depression, withdrawal).

The neuropsychological implications of these findings are then summarized.

Additional Cognitive Evaluation (Efficiency)

The Mental Efficiency system (see Chapter 11) is sampled by the following procedures. I routinely administer those marked with an asterisk.

House-Tree-Man-Woman Drawings* (Naglieri scoring-PsychCorp): This test assesses cognitive level and nonverbal reasoning. Norms are available for ages 5–17 for Man, Woman, Self, and Total score. This is useful for assessing relative cognitive level, but the procedure does not take into account the frequently bizarre and asymmetrical drawings produced by TBI patients.

Bender Gestalt and Recall*: A test for nonverbal reasoning, specific deficits found in brain damage, speed, and visual memory after distractions. Lacks' (1984) scoring is helpful in identifying perceptual errors, but has the familiar deficit of offering a cut-off score (5) independent of baseline measures of intelligence, age, occupation, etc.

Boston Naming Test (Lea & Febiger): Useful for detecting word-naming difficulties, i.e., retrieval of verbal information from long-term storage. The norms are very inadequate, and, curiously, reveal that the procedure is insensitive to differences of education (12 years or less versus more than 12 years). The description of results by aphasia level are contradictory, with increasing levels of severity. I feel that this test may be supplanted by the following:

Memory Subtests of Woodcock-Johnson Tests of Cognitive Ability: Short-term memory (Memory for Sentences); retrieval after interference (Memory for Names), and retrieval from long-term memory (Picture Vocabulary).

Trail Making Test*: A measure of remembering instructions, alternating ideas, speed, and generally functioning in a complex environment. I use only Form B (alternating numbers and letters scattered on a page), with regression equations standardizing the timed scores for age and education (Alekoumbides, Charter, Adkins, & Seacat, 1987).

Wechsler Memory Scale—Rev (PsychCorp): This requires 70–75 minutes, but offers comparison of memory with auditory and visual stimuli, mental control, and delayed recall. A full issue of *The Clinical Neuropsychologist* (Vol. 2, March 1988) describes its development and some applications. The preliminary reports do not encourage assessment of right/left cerebral hemisphere damage as measured by visual and auditory memory indices (Loring, Lee, Martin, & Meador, 1989).

Stroop Word and Color Test (Golden): Assesses speed of recognition of printed color names, reading colors directly, and suppression of reading colors printed as inappropriate color names. There is an opportunity to observe articulation. The norms are primitive, and the test may be supplanted by the following listed test. However, a correction for age offers some continuing utility for children.

*Stroop Neuropsychological Screening Test** (Trenerry et al., published by Psychological Assessment Resources, 1989): Deletes color naming from the above Stroop procedure, but probably has more reliable norms. My impression is that only major deficits of visuoperceptual monitoring and processing are detected.

Wisconsin Card Sorting Test (Psychological Assessment Resources): This test (20–25 minutes) requires the subject to match cards against models, using the principles of color, form, and equal number. It requires problem-solving ability, monitoring, and flexibility of decision making. Of particular interest is the tendency to perseverate errors that have been continued, although a different perceptual category has been announced as correct, or the current one stated to be incorrect. It is claimed to be sensitive to frontal lobe dysfunction. Although this test is widely used, the baseline norms are inadequate, and I have observed that severely injured people can succeed.

Embedded Figures (Valciukas and Singer, 1982): Used for individuals whose background included visuospatial skills (mechanics, engineers, etc.). Norms are dichotomized by age and education.

Peabody Picture Vocabulary Test—Revised (American Guidance Service): Receptive Vocabulary, a measure of retrieval from long-term memory. Norms are available from 2–6 to 40.

Diagnosis and Personality Evaluation

The neuropsychologist is concerned with the patient's diagnosis, stress-related emotional disturbance, mood, impulse control, morale (sense of optimism and ability to solve problems of living), sense of identity, potential to have a pleasant and meaningful life, possible withdrawal, and world-view (Weltanschauung). Examination findings are integrated and compared with any other information within or outside of the examination.

The evidence for the physiological and experiential basis for various posttraumatic stress reactions was reviewed in Chapter 15 on Stress. Since no patient has yet, in my practice, associated the stress reaction to prior experience, I conclude that persistent posttraumatic stress results from physiological reactions causing "intrusive" anxiety (discussed above), the imprinting of frightening experiences in memory and nightmares, and the reaction to being impaired and perhaps scarred. However, level of impairment is reduced by prompt rehabilitation, social support, and an assertive, positive attitude.

The diagnosis and personality are assessed through the personal statements (interview, checklist), statements made by collaterals, records, clinical impression, and projective testing (Rorschach and House-Tree-Persons Drawings, and occasionally the Thematic Apperceptive Test). Here the traditional clinical psychological approaches make a significant contribution. In particular, projective tests contribute information unavailable because of expressive deficits. This section is a continuation of the application of the Rorschach to TBI (see Unstructured Situations, above).

The Rorschach reveals inner experience in the absence of clinically observed or psychometric indices of anxiety. A 5-year-old girl scarred on the face by a projecting portion of a car offered the following responses calmly and quietly: "It looks like a monster, eyes, scratches on his face, walking around scaring everybody; Dracula killing a person; Dinosaur's body inside"; "Two people carrying a bag." (Is it easy or hard?) "Its hard." (?) "They don't look good." (Mood?) "They're in pain."

Assessing Posttraumatic Stress

Emotional distress is more varied than the formal posttraumatic stress disorder, i.e., one may diagnose anxiety reaction, depressive reaction, regression to a former psychosis, etc. The tendency toward release of obsessive compulsive symptoms was reviewed in Chapter 15. After stress, individuals can react in opposite directions, i.e., suppression or expression; thus diagnosis requires access to a wide range of materials. Chronic distress can lead to relatively bland Rorschachs, i.e., affective dullness. On the other hand, there can be gross unhappiness that is revealed only by projective exploration, in the presence of a bland affect caused by cerebrally caused depression, expressive deficits (unwillingness to reveal feelings).

A classification of stress-related Rorschach responses is offered in Appendix 3.

Mood

The assessment may begin with the level of anxiety (e.g., whether intrusive, normal range, or suppressed). Examples of anxiety level and defenses against it are offered in Appendix 3 (Rorschach Stress-Related Content, The Experience of Anxiety). Additionally, the presence of depression, tension (Reactive: "Dysphoric Mood"), and problems of self (self-esteem and self-concept, "Identity") is noted (see Case 20, p. 215).

A tragic example of the contrast between inner distress and overt constriction of affect is offered by the suicide of a 45-year-old man, a college graduate, struck by a bus, who could not maintain his small business. He stated that he was unconscious for a few minutes, though the medical record indicated no loss of consciousness, but abrasions to his forehead. He was being treated for

depression, and diagnosed with posttraumatic stress disorder and organic delu-
sional syndrome. On examination his affect was dull and unresponsive. He suffered
an estimated loss of 21 points of Full Scale IQ. The Rorschach indicated only 3
good W and 13 R, of which only 10 were "good," ExF+ was 85%, with relatively
little stress-related ideation. Cognitive difficulties were suggested by comments
such as "The shape is not perfect; I only see blots of ink; interesting colors but no
specific image." He perceived "dancers, rotating, opposing each other," which was
interpreted as a feeling of loss of control, with constricted feeling level.

Level of Emotional Reaction

This is diagnostically significant for both cerebral emotional disorder and PTSD.
Clinical observations are reviewed (dull, appropriate, hyperaroused), and then
compared to the Rorschach protocol (use of chromatic and achromatic color,
stress-related content, etc.). It is assumed that the Rorschach reflects inner experience (dull, constricted intense, pleasant, manic, dysphoric, etc.). Deviation
between expressed and experienced affect contributes diagnostic information
relative to cerebral disturbance of affect, i.e., whether released, blunted (exaggerated moods without modification by control), deeply experienced although
lacking overt expression (perhaps due to cerebral personality syndrome), the
presence of stress-related anxiety that is not overtly expressed, depression which
conceals expression of distress, etc.

Dynamic Influences on Cognitive Functioning

See Unstructured Situations, above.

Attitudes Towards the World

This is detected through content, Weltanschauung, i.e., feelings of dangerous-
ness, bleakness, wondering about the meaning of life, the idea that one's world
has been destroyed.

Feelings About the Self

The feeling of being a victim, mutilated, unattractive, helpless, and other indicators of being devalued, are revealed in "Identity."

Assessment of Children

The neuropsychological examination contributes to neurological assessment of
children (Hynd and Willis, 1988, p. 141):

1. Charting the extent of recovery or deterioration after injury, stroke, etc.;
2. Making a differential diagnosis between such a functional disorder as a conversion reaction and an organic disorder;

3. Contributing to decisions concerning medication of attentional deficit disorder;
4. Correlating dysfunctioning with such suspected disorders as a tumor;
5. Contributing to the differential diagnosis of deficits of higher cognitive function, severe learning disabilities, etc.

Prior to two years, examination of developmental milestones is significant (Larsen, 1986). A neuropsychological examination may be performed for children from approximately age 2 years and older. By that age, children may be expected to have some grasp of language, to follow directions, to express themselves, etc. Many procedures suitable for adults (e.g., the sensorimotor examination) have to be modified since the child is not expected to have achieved certain functions, and there are problems of cooperation and opportunity to learn (e.g., coin recognition).

With children up to the age of middle teens, I routinely recommend reexamination in 3 years. It may take that interval for impaired cognitive development to express itself academically, or in assessment procedure performance. Hynd and Willis (1988, p. 154) observe that functions associated with the frontal lobes develop in a step-wise, multistage fashion (from 6 to 12 or older). Thus, observation or assessment before maturity (which may occur even later) would preclude observations of undeveloped behavior attributable to an earlier accident.

Procedure

Available records are reviewed before the child is examined. Since children frequently get restless after a period of time, I begin with only a brief overview of the parents' concerns before beginning the examination. Then the child is examined either completely, or for several hours. At that time, an extended interview with the parent is performed (see Appendix 1).

Parents

The parents are asked to bring in or send personal documents, i.e., before and after examples of writing, art, etc. They are interviewed, using the form detailed in Appendix 1: Intake Procedures. The procedure is introduced to them as having two goals, i.e., to inquire what their child's personality was like before the accident, and then what changes have taken place that concern them. The developmental and health history is utilized to explore any preexisting condition.

School Records

In general, I will not examine a child unless the school records are available. These are often difficult to obtain and difficult to utilize. The duplication may be poor, and/or exclude portions of a page. Test scores often use abbreviations unfamiliar to an outsider. Dates may not be included, or may not be duplicated. Psychological examinations are sometimes considered to be so secret that they are not made available without a court order or threat of suit. Thus, records should be requested as soon as possible to permit further inquiry.

The examiner scrutinizes academic performance, teachers' comments, local grades, nationally standardized test scores, psychological examinations, social service reports, etc. Utilization of age-scaled percentiles is preferred (see Chapter 20).

Sometimes several years must elapse before loss of ability can be detected. It may be necessary to group several years of scores together to obtain a reasonably reliable estimate of level to determine whether there is a difference between pre-and-postinjury functioning. Percentiles can be averaged, the proportions of grades at each level can be calculated, and changes noted for succeeding years. Teachers' comments provide evidence for personality functioning for areas such as concentration, social integration, and academic progress.

Sensorimotor Examination

Many children (and adults) have never had a medical examination, in particular a neurological examination, after one, or sometimes even two head injuries. The schools, in turn, often ignore a history of brain injury, following business as usual. The neuropsychologist makes a definite contribution to assessing a child's functional problems through a careful sensorimotor examination, since deficits of audition and vision may be detected (see Appendix 2, Sensorimotor Examination).

A parent is always present. First, for reasons of discretion. Second, it is useful to have some confirmation for marginal findings, e.g., questions of oculomotor movements or fine motor coordination. Parents often volunteer information about problems through their associations to the examiner's questions and procedures, e.g., deficits of coordination or balance. Orientation to this approach may be obtained from Begali (1987, pp. 63–72), Bigler (1987), Mutti, Sterling, and Spalding (1978), and various articles in Tupper (1987).

Cognitive Functioning in Structured Situations

I use an intelligence test, e.g., the various Wechsler Scales; Kaufman Assessment Battery for Children, and may supplement these with selected items from The Stanford–Binet, 4th Ed. Achievement is measured with the Wide Range Assessment Battery—Revised, or the Woodcock-Johnson Tests of Achievement Rev. (see above). For additional assessment of verbal comprehension and reading, the Gray Oral Reading Test—Revised and the Woodcock Reading Mastery Tests—Revised are recommended (see above).

Norms for The Kaufman Assessment Battery for Children start at 2–6 and the Woodcock–Johnson Tests of Cognitive Ability and of Achievement (revised 1989) start at 2–0. Standards for Rorschach interpretation begin at age 2 (Ames, Learned, Metraux, & Walker, 1952). The Stanford–Binet, 4th Ed., starts at age 2. I have stopped using this test as a complete battery for reasons discussed in Chapter 20. Some of the SB-IV materials are useful, e.g., the estimate of short-term memory. These have been supplemented in my office by Woodcock-Johnson memory tests (see above).

Cognitive Functioning in Unstructured Situations

I utilize the Rorschach routinely for individuals from age 2 up. Ames et al. discuss specific norms and characteristics of individuals of different ages: 1952, children; 1971, adolescents; 1954, old age. Clinical use of the Rorschach with children, including application to neurological dysfunctions, is found in Halpern (1953) and Francis-Williams (1968).

Additional Cognitive Evaluation

This serves to supplement evaluation of cognitive efficiency (e.g., concentration and planning), and to obtain more informational processing, detection and suppression of errors, and nonverbal and verbal abilities. Tests routinely used include Bender Gestalt and Recall, scored according to the Watkins system (1976, with norms from 5–14), and a system too new to be tried by the writer (Brannigan and Brunner, 1989, with norms from 4-6 to 8-5); Trail Making Test, Part B (Childrens Form); and Stroop Color and Word Test. Additional procedures are offered by Begali (1987, pp. 99–102), by function, by Barkley (1988), for attention, and by Boyd (1988) for memory.

The *Woodcock Reading Mastery Tests—Revised* has norms from age 5 to older adult, and by grades. Visual–auditory associations measure the ability to associate symbols with oral stimuli (as would be used in learning to read; reading comprehension).

Personality

The procedures are similar to the adult examination, but the question to be asked concerns lack of development, as well as regression, which may be observed in adult patients. In general, the children of all ages offer Rorschach stress-related content, so that the test is of great use in personality assessment.

22
The Integrated Neuropsychological Report

The Pre-Injury Baseline

A wide-range neuropsychological examination entails eliciting and communicating a great deal of information. Some of the considerations in drawing conclusions are considered here (estimation of baseline and impairment), and a model for organizing the report is presented.

Baseline Estimation

Estimating preinjury ability is not terra incognita. It is possible to estimate the level of ability and kind of skills that individuals have on the basis of their "track record."

A variety of informational sources contribute to a baseline: school percentiles, work requirements and performance, personal productions such as art, writing, etc., and also inferences concerning performance from the nature of employment. Even the neuropsychologist without vocational counseling experience, by inquiring into the work history of examinees, can reach some sophistication concerning dimensions important in vocational performance for a wide range of occupations.

What Are the Demands of an Occupation?

When we hear that someone is a plumber, electrician, school teacher, lawyer, or physician, we have a good idea as to their level of ability and kinds of skills that they probably have. There are some tables indicating averages and range of IQ for different occupations. The professional person is expected to have a high IQ, to read well, and to have a good vocabulary. Some types of professions require good calculation, writing, or speaking ability. The technician has good manual and visuospatial skills, such as reading diagrams. Basic mathematics is needed to measure distances for carpentry or plumbing, to make up bills, etc. The artist has a good imagination, and can draw well.

For example, a construction contractor would be expected to have high perceptual spatial ability and nonverbal intelligence. This was used as an estimated baseline. Test results manifested a low WAIS-R perceptual organizational factor score, and offered a poor House-Drawing, offering evidence of impairment.

Preinjury IQ Estimates

I propose the following rule for estimating preinjury IQ (see also Matarazzo & Herman, 1985): doctoral level, 125; masters, 120; college graduate, 114; high school graduate, 100; 8 years of school completed, 89.

Components of the Baseline

A. Health
B. Emotional and personality development
C. School reports: Grades, style, educational level achieved, IQ testing
             Nationally standardized achievement tests
             Behavior descriptions by teachers
D. Higher and technical education: college, professional or technical school, whether academic or trade
E. Employment: job title, duties, skills, responsibilities, personality, whether promoted
F. Adaptive qualities: lived independently, took care of family, house, social qualities and friends, interests, enjoyed life.

Questions Addressed in Estimating the Baseline

Adult: "How was the person functioning when the accident occurred?" "Are there any differences?"

Children: "What was the child's achievement and development at the time of the injury? What kind of a person would the child have developed into if the accident had not occurred?" "How long is it reasonable to wait before it is assumed that impairment does or does not exist?"

Case 40: Clinical Example Establishing the Adult Baseline

A woman suffered a minor automobile accident with severe jarring to her body causing multiple somatic injuries. She was dazed, and subsequently had considerable anxiety, muscular problems, headaches, pain, weakness, and difficulties with mobility. Several years later, a neurologist detected some problems of concentration and loss of memory, but did no objective testing, nor did he refer this woman for a comprehensive neuropsychological examination. Rather, he attributed her deficiencies to histrionics and hysteria. There was no evidence for a preexisting emotional or cognitive condition.

TABLE 22.1. IQ.

Scale	Current IQ	Percentile	Range	Estimated premorbid IQ	Deviation
Verbal	76	5	Borderline	105	−29
Performance	81	10	Low average	105	−24
Full Scale	78	7	Borderline	106	−28

Achievement: Wide-Range Achievement Test—Revised

	Standard score National %	
Reading (word recognition)	64	1
Spelling	65	1
Arithmetic	66	1

She has an AA degree, and holds a responsible position at a securities firm that requires skill, judgment, and ability to handle calculations rapidly. She believes that her ability to pursue a career in the securities industry is impaired.

The current IQ was determined from a Full Scale WAIS-R. The estimated premorbid IQ was found in Matarazzo and Herman, (1984), entering the information in Table 22.1 according to her age and education (14 years in this instance).

For two different approaches to current functioning (IQ and achievement level), her performance is grossly below that expected of a woman of her education and vocational background. There is a generalized reduction of mental ability, represented by a borderline IQ, 7th percentile, with an estimated loss of 28 points of Full Scale IQ. When her ability to perform familiar school-type tasks is assessed, she had third and fourth grade equivalents. Such gross deficits point to an inability to retrieve information from long-term memory.

Her ability is so extremely low as to be inconsistent with any high school achievement at all, much less an AA degree and employment in a securities firm requiring calculations accuracy. Moreover, in such an organization, capacity to work under pressure is well known. Observation revealed that she could not work under pressure and gave up prematurely. Additional deficits were detected in verbal ability, nonverbal problem-solving and holistic thinking, rote and long-term memory, and practical social information that would be expected to contribute to good judgment. In addition, she had many sensory and motor problems not reviewed here.

Estimating Impairment

Impairment may be regarded as equaling baseline minus injury. The degree of impairment is the deviation from the former level of functioning, or from a reasonable expected level of development, in the case of children. Only when the individual is challenged by difficult problems is it possible to detect inadequate performance compared to preinjury level. If TBI occurs, but the reserves between preinjury mental ability (including components of efficiency such as concentration, attention, and memory) and current demands on performance are sufficiently great, then the person may be able to perform without seeming to be impaired.

Impairment assessment is performed through comparing current performance with a known or estimated baseline. It is important to be aware that *emotional distress is directly and indirectly impairing, even without evidence for brain damage* (see Chapter 15 on Stress).

Some Evidence for Impairment

1. Change in performance of specific tasks, e.g., grades and employment.
2. Change in relative rank, e.g., percentiles in class or nationally.
3. Inability to learn new material, conceptualize, generalize, retrieve information from long-term storage, etc.
4. Reduced mental efficiency, including flexibility.
5. Inability to perform particular tasks that are known or inferred to be significant for occupation or leisure time activity.

Formulas Conceptualizing Impairment

Degree of impairment = Baseline − Current functioning (expressed in terms of inability to perform particular functions).

Impairment is manifested: Baseline − Impairment exceeds the reserves of former level of functioning (cannot meet current demands).

Reporting Results

Integrate Information

I recommend a report that is *organized according to categories of information, not test by test.* Information takes into consideration support and interference between functions and systems. To illustrate, effectiveness of mental ability involves both the IQ (understood as an estimate of general ability) and the patient's efficiency. Whether a given level of effectiveness is impairing depends on the demands in a particular situation. Thus, *the baseline, reserves, and demands on a person are a part of the thinking involved in a thorough assessment.*

Do Not Exaggerate the Thoroughness of the Examination Conducted

A common error made by many examiners is this conclusion: "I haven't found brain damage, so it doesn't exist!" The examiner should be open to the possibility that genuine dysfunctions exist that are not explored by the administered examination, and thus conclusions should be modest, and further referrals made!

Reporting Measurement Should Be Percentiles and Standard Scores

To facilitate comparison between individuals, and different measurements of one person's abilities, a particular standard is usually applied, i.e., the percentile rank of some appropriate, structured sample. This is often converted into standard scores (S.S.), which are defined in terms of deviations around the average, and converted into a percentile rank, using the fractions of a standard deviation (the middle 68% of the distribution as the measure, see any statistics text). For example, the widely used Wechsler series of tests represents the average score for a particular age group as IQ 100, and arbitrarily converts the distribution of scores into standard deviations of 15 points. Therefore, the 68th percentile is called IQ 115 (+ 1 SD), and the 16th percentile is 85 (− 1 SD).

Comparing Different Measurements

Errors are introduced when such procedures are normed on different populations. Some difficulties are avoided when a common metric and type of norm is applied. Percentile rank for the appropriate age group is the best. Yet, individual scores should also be included in a report (e.g., all age-scaled WAIS-R, scaled scores for WISC-R, etc.). Where available percentiles should be included. Next equivalents are most useful for patients of all ages.

Educational Norms

It is necessary to be careful in using grade equivalents. Some tests, e.g., for academic achievement, may offer several scores including grade equivalents, or educational norms. These serve a different purpose, i.e., determining progress, rather than comparing ability. There are many possible errors when impairment is judged from grade or educational norms. Comparing performance to others in the same grade, but ignoring chronological age, can give a false impression of success: the traumatized child may have missed one or more years of school; a child may have been advanced in grade, started school early or late, or have been out of school for reasons of injury or illness.

Reporting both grade equivalents and age percentiles sometimes leads to ambiguous results, i.e., one wonders why a particular percentile represents a particular grade assignment. Thus, although determining what the relative rank is compared to children in that grade may be important for educational counseling, it can be highly misleading in terms of development.

What Should Be Reported?

All results can be used if each score makes a point. However, due to differences of the meaning of standard scores and SDs between tests, it is recommended that in every case a percentile be reported.

Organization of the Report

I use the following organization, which the reader may follow and then modify according to the details and requirements of individual practices. Recommended procedures for each section are detailed in Chapter 21 and also in the Appendix.

After each major section there is a brief paragraph, entitled "Neuropsychological Implications," serving as a summary with inferences drawn.

CONFIDENTIAL NEUROPSYCHOLOGICAL REPORT

Name:	Referral source:
Date of Examination:	Age at injury:
Date of injury:	Elapsed time since injury:
Present age:	Injury:

Reason for Referral:

Procedures:

Annex (copies of drawings, Bender Gestalt and Recall, personal documents, etc.):

Review of Medical Records:

Personal Statement (see Appendix 1):

Interview:

Responses to Brain Injury Symptom Checklist:

Clinical Impression (see Appendix):

Sensorimotor Functions (preferred hand):

Intellectual Functioning in Structured Situations: This section is divided into two subsections: I.Q. test(s) and achievement test(s). The estimated preinjury IQ and current IQ are compared, with reasons offered why the results are reasonable or unreasonable in terms of the clinical history. The significance of the factor scores, differences between them, and the meaning of particular subscales are discussed. Finally samples of responses are offered by subscale, where appropriate to retained or impaired abilities.

Model for Communicating IQ Findings

Wechsler Adult Intelligence Scale – Revised (WAIS-R)

			Premorbid IQ	
Scale	Current IQ	Percentile	Estimate	Deviation
Verbal				
Performance				
Full Scale				
Factors (related subtests)			Average	Percentile
Verbal (V)				
Perceptual Organizational (PO)				
Freedom from Distractibility (FD)				

Wechsler Adult Intelligence Scale — Revised (WAIS-R) (cont.)

Subtests		
Verbal	Performance	
Age Score Percentile	Age Score Percentile	
Information (V)		
Digit Span (FD)	Picture Completion (PO)	
Vocabulary (V)	Picture Arrangement	
Arithmetic (FD)	Block Design (PO)	
Comprehension (V)	Object Assembly (PO)	
Similarities (V)	Digit Symbol (FD)	

Intellectual Functioning in Unstructured Situations (Rorschach)

The details are discussed in Chapter 21.

1. Ability to create complex ideas.
2. Productivity.
3. Conformity with group norms.
4. Creativity/range of ideas.
5. Judgment and reality testing.
6. Overall expressiveness of Rorschach protocol.
7. Anxiety intrudes into intellectual functioning.
8. Developmental level.
9. Overt pathology.

   Other cognitive functions: Here, the results of supplementary neuropsychological procedures and their implications are detailed.

Personality

Formulation

This represents a summary, and a focus for organizing a great deal of information.

Background. What information is relevant to the victim's present situation, e.g., education, preexisting medical or psychological conditions, job history?

Baseline. This is related to estimated preinjury level, based on demographic characteristics, job and school records, and personal documents.

Injury. A summary of the trauma is included (histological and historical).

Impairment Evaluation. This corresponds to the Taxonomy of Dysfunctions.

   I. Consciousness and Orientation:
  II. Sensorimotor Systems:
 III. Physiological Functions:
  IV. Ability and Cognition:

V. Concentration, Planning, and Control:
VI. Learning: Short-Term Memory/Retrieval from Long-Term Memory:
VII. Communications:
VIII. Organic Personality Reactions:
IX. Personality Functioning:
Personality Integration:
Stress Reaction:
   Intrusive Anxiety:
   Identity:
   Morale:
   Sense of Impairment:
World View:
Reactive:
   Mood:
   Defensive/Restitutive:
Social:
Report of Pain:

Diagnosis. Is this an identifiable condition? Although the American Psychiatric Association's Diagnostic and Statistical Manual, 3rd Ed. Rev. (DSM-3R), has been popular with the insurance companies, I have seen increasing reference to the ICD-9-CM codes (U.S. Government). Diffuse brain damage and other specific neurological injuries are not coped with by DSM-3R. Therefore, its terminology is used only for strictly behavioral disorders, e.g., posttraumatic stress disorder, depression, anxiety reaction, etc. ICD includes skull fractures, intracranial injury, concussion with differing loss of consciousness, and other damage that is not directly observed by the neuropsychologist, but can be inferred.

Attribution. Can the dysfunctions documented be attributed to a particular injury?

Prognosis for Adaptability, Employment, Development. Will the individual be able to resume his former activities, or can a child develop normally? Are the deficits permanent? How does the injury affect the ability to function in the areas of work, education, independence, family, and social situations?

Implications for Quality of Life. Will the person be able to enjoy his or her life, or will deficits, scarring, loss of mobility, anxiety, social rejection, or other conditions prevent personal fulfillment and meeting personal goals?

Recommendation. Samples of treatment referrals include: psychotherapy, stress reduction to alleviate pain, anxiety, and muscular tension; further neurological or other medical study, sensory examination of vision and hearing; cognitive rehabilitation; biofeedback; various forms of stress reduction; remedial education; family therapy, etc. Since proper assessment of TBI requires varied sources of information, ambiguous results, or need for additional documentation, should lead to referral for modern exploratory techniques, including different kinds of neuroimaging.

Some Considerations in Counseling Testees

Procedure for Advising the Patient

At the end of a comprehensive examination, the neuropsychologist may have some idea concerning ultimate findings, but in balance, most of the analysis remains to be performed. Without scoring the tests, one is likely to have an incorrect idea as to the actual level achieved, intersubtest and subtest scatter, etc. Therefore, it is usually imprudent to convey information to the patient or family before the report is complete.

I follow this procedure. I state that: "Yes, it appears that the patient has suffered some level of impairment. However, a definitive statement requires integrating all of the information with the records, scoring, thinking about it, etc." If the patient or parent asks for a report he or she is told: "I will send the report to any professional person that you name. If you give me a release now, it will go out when it is ready. Later on, I will still send it out, but you will have to write to me to give me authorization. I prefer to let the explanation be given to you by somebody in whom you have confidence and with whom you will have contact. I cannot mail it to you because it will be complicated and technical and you might misunderstand it with some bad effect. After you have had a counseling session with some other professional, if you still want to talk to me about the results of this examination, then I will be glad to make a two hour appointment with you."

The Sensorimotor Examination Leads to Effective Counseling

An exception to the principle of conveying little or no information at the time of the examination is sometimes made during the sensorimotor examination. Many accident victims are unaware that vague discomforts are effects of an accident. This will be particularly true if there has not been a careful neurological examination. A person may state that he bumps into things, without realizing that this symptom arose after an accident. Examination of peripheral visual fields often reveals that the field of vision is generally restricted, or restricted in one area, causing the individual not to see to one side. They may not be aware of the implications of altered consciousness or seizures, and must be cautioned about driving.

Forensic Considerations

The forensic examination for neuropsychologically impaired patients differs in some significant regards (though not ethically) from the usual professional procedure. The issues, levels of proof, techniques of presentation, and above all standards of care are different than the usual clinical practice. For further information, refer to Dennis (1989), Matarazzo (1987), and Barth et al. (1986).

Since there may be millions of dollars at stake (I have performed one examination of a child who received a settlement valued at $21,500,000 over a lifetime) the reception of your report is highly adversarial. Therefore, be prepared from the moment the client enters your office to have to explain and properly document in a court of law any action, conclusion, or inference that you draw. Do not mutilate or lose any materials. Assume that any notes or test results will be examined by the other side, perhaps by a competent neuropsychologist or knowledgeable attorney, and may have to be presented in court.

At the outset it should be stated that the forensic psychological examination of civil and criminal issues such as competency to stand trial, child custody, determining the credibility of a child who has allegedly been the victim of rape or molestation, etc., is a separate specialty from examination of the TBI victim. If the psychologist accepts a referral for an examination, and is not familiar with the requirements of his particular jurisdiction, it is important to talk to the attorney to determine the standards of proof in his jurisdiction, the key issues of the particular case, and what level of documentation is needed.

I usually give many details of test findings in the report (specific scores, examples of performance, and interpretation) since in the jurisdictions within which I practice most attorneys prefer to avoid the costs and uncertainties of taking a case to trial. Therefore, in the process of "discovery" they exchange information with the opposition, and lay their cards on the table. To the extent that they can properly document dysfunctioning (or its absence, in the case of defendants) they usually wish to do so in pretrial negotiations.

Issues

The primary concern in examining a personal injury victim is impairment, implications for prognosis, and whether the deficits are reasonably related to the injury. Damages in law are estimated from factors such as lost earnings and reduced quality of life. The examiner is required to come to a conclusion "with reasonable neuropsychological certainty" as to whether a given trauma may have caused the damages (impairment) that have been alleged and whether such impairment is permanent, and to describe its effects on the person's life, development of a child, etc. The issues discussed in this book are all relevant to the forensic neuropsychological examination (to which my practice is almost exclusively directed).

Establishing a baseline is vital to establishing dysfunctioning and maladaptiveness. This should be performed carefully, since there is a stereotype among some attorneys and judges that this is impossible.

Standards

There are substantial differences between ordinary clinical practice and forensic neuropsychological examinations. In forensic cases, from the moment the patient walks in the door, the writer assumes that anything said or written may be scrutinized, and, by inference, only the highest standards can apply. Matarazzo (1987) observes that in the courtroom an adversary relationship may exist between the psychologist and patient that does not occur in ordinary clinical practice. Indeed, other psychologists may be called in to examine the (subpoenaed) records to attempt to discredit the conclusions. The writer can attest that the examination of one's examination in a courtroom can be jarring. With a skillful attorney on the attack it is not at all comparable to a presentation of findings at a case conference!

An extremely high level of accuracy and comprehensiveness is required. I concur with Matarazzo (1987), who observes that the courts require a higher level of validity of procedures than the usual collegial relationship in a hospital or clinic. One's records may be authorized by the patient to be given to the other side for scrutiny, or subpoenaed for trial. The psychologist may also be called by one side or the other. In my experience there is no examination of one's professional competence to perform a particular service, and what one has actually done, that is as hostile, scrutinizing, gruelling, and public. Many attorneys, retained by the opposing side (defendant or plaintiff-victim), have done their homework, examined the report and supporting records in advance, and have consulted a neuropsychologist to determine what weak points to probe. Having one's procedures, assumptions, and conclusions examined in open court by a hostile attorney with large amounts of money at stake focuses the mind considerably.

The scientific component is high. The forensic neuropsychological examination requires thoroughness, and provides an opportunity to integrate a wide range of information, e.g., available records should be summarized, with their neuropsychological implications, scientific background, development since previous examinations, employment and family considerations, technical background, personality and neuroscience theory, etc. For the psychologist who enjoys an intellectual challenge it is ideal.

An examination performed without integrating information about trauma, neurotoxins, vocational considerations, personality theory, etc. is incomplete. The neuropsychological examiner draws on special principles and procedures of neuropsychology, neuroscience, medicine, physiology, chemistry, physics, neurology, clinical psychology, career counseling, child development and educational psychology, general science, technology, vocational counseling, education, sociology, etc. A good library is essential. Data base searches provide access to modern sources of information about brain functioning and pathology, toxins, etc. Biosis Connection can provide references to the most recent 12 weeks of world literature. Medline and other data bases provide sources for the older literature. UMI, Inc. can provide reprints of most technical sources.

The forensic examination requires specific knowledge to overcome old stereotypes: mild head injury does not produce impairment, no loss of consciousness means nothing happened, malingering and secondary gains are commonplace, apparent recovery indicates that no subclinical deficits exist, posttraumatic stress is mostly in the head, etc. These issues are discussed elsewhere in this volume.

Malingering

Because of the frequency with which TBI is associated with litigation, the examiner will have to consider the possibility of malingering. Yet, although "secondary gains" to obtain compensation (Denny, Robinowitz, & Penk, 1987) are well known, its extent is grossly exaggerated, causing prejudice against the majority of impaired accident victims.

Malingering has been defined as the falsification or exaggeration of a disorder or symptom for personal gain. The motivation and pattern of an insanity defendant are likely to differ from the personal injury claimant (Lees-Haley, 1989). Conversion symptoms (the hysteric) are motivated to avoid personal responsibility, and may be characterized by bland indifference (Solomon and Masdeu, 1989). Indifference may be a component of an organic emotional disorder, so the examiner should guard against the mistake of diagnosing hysteria incorrectly.

The frequency of malingering in cases of personal injury is controversial (Grant & Alves, 1987, for review). Lishman (1987, pp. 150–151, 170) states that "impending litigation can strongly motivate the aggravation and prolongation of disability . . . The injured person is invited to complain . . . repeatedly . . . to a number of specialists." Significant forensic issues include whether someone is at fault, and whether compensation is feasible. Gross neurotic complaints are associated with male sex, road accidents, low social status, and large employment organizations. More severe injuries are inversely associated with neurotic disability. Actually, in these cases the patient is suffering from some cerebral personality disorder, and/or an expressive deficit. Long-lasting postconcussional symptoms are attributed to psychogenic mechanisms since they are not related to the extent or severity of injuries. However, the literature cited by Lishman is old (not later than 1961).

Similarly, "compensation neurosis" is considered to be colored by persistence of pain in the head, neck, and lower back. Long delay of settlement is considered to prolong disability. Multiple symptoms, including those resembling hysteria, are considered characteristic (unexplained symptoms mimicking neurological disease, e.g., seizures, amnesia, motor and sensory loss, narrowly confined pain). Objective assessment of the injury and psychiatric status, with rapid settlement, is recommended (Adams & Victor, 1989, p. 114, pp. 1193, 1196).

I would resolve this question by distinguishing between diagnosable neurological damage, and the posttraumatic stress reaction, through a wide-range examination of personality and other functions.

Control over Records

Unfortunately, when one claims a personal injury, at a certain point confidentiality is lost. One may have one's mental health, personal habits, impairment, etc., revealed or even maligned in open court. Although few people usually attend these sessions, nobody can be excluded either. Therefore, when a patient comes for an examination, he or she is warned that all statements ultimately will be exposed to the adversary, through their opportunity for examinations, obtaining medical and other records, etc. They are alerted that their only job for the day is to tell the truth, to state whatever their complaints are, but to add nothing nor to exaggerate.

I will not respond to an authorization to release records that are over 6 months old. Sometimes patients change lawyers, and, therefore, what they have authorized is no longer valid (i.e., for some reason the opposing party delayed requesting the authorized information). Moreover, the adversary may play games with improper subpoenas for records that they are not entitled to. Therefore the psychological examiner must become familiar with the rules of discovery in his jurisdiction, and, in general, when a request for records is received, check with the retaining attorney. If the examination has been performed outside of the forensic jurisdiction, i.e., on self-referral or conventional professional referrals, then the examiner should consult with a knowledgeable attorney. *Warning*: Improper release of records, even with an official looking document, could make you liable for violating the patient's confidentiality.

Conclusion

A practical and comprehensive examination can be performed, using as a guiding concept a wide-range Taxonomy of potential deficits of the TBI victim. The clinical skills of the examiner, and the willingness to utilize technical and social information of many kinds, are essential to a comprehensive exploration. Considerable information is integrated to assess the ability of the person to function in his usual milieu.

23
Therapeutic Considerations

The brain-damaged impaired person has special characteristics, and, therefore, special therapeutic needs, which must be given priority before more conventional psychodynamic considerations are treated. It should be remembered that a patient may not connect an accident with various symptoms, and therefore a general familiarity with traumatic brain injury should be part of the psychotherapist's armamentarium, and lead to further inquiry and referral for examination.

If a patient has had an impairing accident, before or during psychotherapy, one should assume that there will be a variety of emotional disturbances. These should be actively explored. Most characteristic are problems of anger, violence, and irritability, reduced motivation and apathy, depression (with various symptoms), inability to understand one's own reactions and those of others, lability, and apathy. Also, pathological laughing, euphoria, crying, rage, fear, temper, and irritability can occur. Some emotional disturbances can be a sign of partial seizures (so called, but possibly inaccurately so, "temporal lobe epilepsy").

The range of deficits (described in the Taxonomy) have psychotherapeutic implications that require a fundamentally different approach than treatment of other types of patients. Consultation with a TBI or other brain-damaged victim will use all of your previous knowledge, but one also enters a different professional world in terms of approach and technical background.

Some Characteristics of the TBI Victim

Brain Damage Is Impairing

The TBI patient's very organ of adaptational control is defective.

Many Aspects of Brain Damage Mimic Unrelated Personality Disorders

The etiology of affective problems such as temper, impulsivity, and depression is in part not related to familiar and well-studied psychodynamic reasons.

The TBI Victim May Not Be Able to Express His Distress or Inefficiency

Expressive deficits prevent communication and insight. For purposes of litigation or secondary gain, they may exaggerate deficit. Perhaps they will exaggerate improvement to gain the esteem of family or therapist. Also, the extreme expressive deficit is avoiding or denying discussion of impairment.

Inflexibility and Loss of Foresight

Repeating the same response time after time (perseveration), i.e., lack of flexibility in responding to errors or change of circumstances, is characteristic of many patients with TBI. This will certainly slow therapeutic progress, and render the patient vulnerable to the anger of members of the community (e.g., employer, family, etc.) when complaints are not responded to. Foresight and monitoring of ongoing activity are defective, therefore problems are created or not remedied that would be avoided or corrected in non-brain-damaged people.

The Degree of Emotional Stress Is Typically Great

The persistence and etiology of anxiety are due in part to a posttraumatic stress reaction, and release of physiological functions, whose treatment and symptoms vary from other sources of anxiety. Inability to deal with change and complexity is characteristic, and emotional distress is increased by reduced resistance to stress and tolerance of frustration. Inability to express one's deficits, and concurrent depression, may make the patient a suicidal risk.

The Prognosis Is Poor in Many Cases

Various studies have shown (see Chapter 18 on Recovery) that with severe brain injury, even so fundamental an adaptive task as returning to work may occur at less than the 50% rate. Indeed, with severely brain injured individuals, even with intensive rehabilitation efforts, improvement in cognitive and social functioning may be modest, nonexistent, and unpredictable as to who will benefit or whether recovery is essentially spontaneous without requiring treatment (Blair & Lanyon, 1987).

Intake Considerations

In daily therapeutic practice, one should always inquire as to the possibility of an accident. The patient may not understand that significant functional deficits are related to an accident that happened at some time in the past, until the professional person, with sympathetic awareness of the effects of brain damage, inquires into its existence, and then helps the patient to understand what has been perplexing for so long.

The psychotherapist or counselor is working with a patient who has special problems of self-understanding, and who will require far more than the usual amount of assistance to express deficits and distress. Appraisal of the accuracy of self-awareness is significant in rehabilitation (Lam et al., 1988). Minimal levels of communication can conceal comprehension, which in turn should not be confused with repression.

Insight contributes to a better outcome. The therapist might review at this point the varieties of Expressive Deficits (Chapter 16) since these will play a role in preventing information concerning the condition, loss of motivation, etc., from being communicated. Deficits of insight also prevent benefits from feedback within the therapeutic process and from the community.

When it is likely, or known, that a patient has had cerebral trauma, treatment should involve the advantage of a comprehensive neuropsychological study. This will help to prevent misinterpretation of disturbed emotional expression and personality problems. It will also alert the therapist to reduced efficiency, deficits of concentration and alertness, etc., which hamper assumption of normal responsibilities. In particular, premature return to work should be avoided.

Treatment planning will have to take into consideration whether particular cognitive deficits, common in TBI, are present: slow thinking, confusion, word seeking difficulties, problems of memory and repetition, etc. Therapy usually requires certain characteristics for self-understanding, which have been reviewed before (see Chapter 16 on Expressive Deficits): awareness, experiencing distress, remembering, sufficient intelligence and judgment, and motivation to communicate distress. All of these can be low in cases of TBI.

Inability to read is impairing in a variety of ways. Exploration can lead to further assessment of the patient's status, e.g., a problem of perception, ocular control, memory, and continued concentration. Reading deficits may be attributable to sensory loss, memory problems, etc., and illustrate that many TBI victims have never had any examination or only superficial ones, despite the likelihood of brain injury, or the presence of other injuries that invite further examination and consultation.

The characteristic self-concept of many brain-damaged victims may be out of the range of the ordinary psychotherapy patient. It is vaguer, regressed, and to the extent that it is understood, there can be profound feelings of valuelessness, vulnerability, and passivity in handling important problems. The person may feel depersonalized due to loss of sensory awareness, or to the gross change in self-concept after trauma.

Therefore, in beginning work with a brain-injured patient, comprehensive assessment is useful. Only too frequently, the neurological report (and sometimes these have never been performed) completely overlooks or makes inaccurate statements concerning these functions. Assessment of the level of patient understanding and insight is a component in treatment planning, since brain-damaged clients with self-awareness tend to have better treatment outcome (Lam et al., 1988).

Adaptive Survey

Since the TBI victim may not be able completely reveal current problems, it is useful to have a concrete approach to assessing daily activities of the brain-damaged victim. Use of a list can pinpoint problem areas that might be overlooked by the victim or professional. Valuable information can be elicited from collaterals (spouse, friends, children) concerning level of activity and pattern of successes and failures. Deviations from former levels of functioning invite either rehabilitative efforts or assistance from community resources. The following list of conventional adult activities is based on Morse and Morse (1988). Further adaptive surveys are referred to in Chapter 18 on Recovery.

1. *Self-care*, e.g., bathing, dressing, hygiene, eating.
2. *Household responsibilities*, e.g., cooking, cleaning, maintenance of the home.
3. *Child and family care.*
4. *Financial management* (budget, shopping, banking).
5. *Shopping* (food, clothing, household).
6. *Use of time* (planning, scheduling, awareness).
7. *Mobility* (use of public transportation, driving, knowing directions, oriented as to location).
8. *Use of community resources* (library, religious activities, clubs, movies, theaters).
9. *Enjoyment of life* (hobbies, sports, games, reading).
10. *Bodily movement* (domestic responsibilities, sports, driving).
11. *Work at the previously accustomed level.*
12. *Social life* (willingness to meet with family, friends, strangers).

Therapeutic Errors with Accident Victims

I have observed a number of errors by psychotherapists that represented considerable lack of understanding of their patients and the nature of their condition.

Resuming Psychoanalytically Oriented Treatment

Treatment should take into account genuine changes in effectiveness, the particular experience of posttraumatic stress, and problems in reaching insight. The patient can no longer participate in a treatment modality in which responsibility for his life, and for presenting issues, is his. The therapist must now take responsibility for raising issues, and some initiative in making interpretations, and often utilize a distinctly educational and directive approach.

Use of Developmental Theories of Personality and Treatment

The attempt to seek meaning in the emotional symptoms will ordinarily prove frustrating to the patient. They are preoccupied with their condition, and may have intrusive thoughts and/or nightmares about an accident. Even if there is a special significance to the patient's imaginational life, dreams, fantasies, etc., these should still take second place to aiding the patient's adaptive efforts, and controlling anxiety. Inability to describe problems accurately can be due to aphasia, and not denial or hysteria.

It can be a serious error to assume that there is an unconscious emotional cause for the symptoms, or a symbolic meaning to the accident. The reality is the extreme response of the stressed and brain-damaged person. When the therapist spends too much time interpreting in a dynamic way the circumstances of the patient's life, they experience this as demeaning. It "relegates to the periphery the importance of the emotional reactions to the trauma itself . . . [and may reinforce] the common irrational belief that they were somehow responsible for the tragedy" (Spiegel, 1988).

Mobilizing and Expressing Affect

This risks repeating the experience of loss of control over fear and other dysphoric feelings. The therapist must consider the possibility of poorly controlled anger, serious depression, and other affects and images that may be supported by a subclinical epileptic focus.

Not Recognizing Signs of Brain Damage

Sleepiness or other signs of disturbed consciousness may not be recognized as forms of epilepsy. The patient should be examined by a neurologist and in the interim advised not to drive, use power tools, etc.

Short-term memory, e.g., for a conversation, may be adequate, but long-term memory and/or retrieval can prevent new learning. This can affect the cognitive and social areas. In addition, different inputs, e.g., visual and auditory, may be differently retained. Thus, the patient may learn better in certain ways than others.

There are different forms of amnesia, including that for faces, only some of which may be psychogenic, while others are an apparent physiological loss of function, or inability to retrieve. Therefore, be loath to blame the patient for resistance and repression.

Inability to communicate is common, and conspicuous. It leads to withdrawal within the patient's life and evasion in discussing problems pertaining to therapy. Cues include word-naming deficits, circumlocutions, simplifications, and use of approximations in terms of general expression or single words.

Emotional distress is a common after-effect of brain damage, and one should not confuse it with psychogenic depression or anger. The dullness of a patient's speech can properly lead to the suspicion that there is a more general brain damage, i.e., the organic personality that is indicative of diffuse brain damage, perhaps centered in the right cerebral hemisphere.

Pain requires particular attention to reveal its meaning. Headaches may well be a result of soft-tissue damage after trauma. But in addition, the interaction of pain with depression, anger, inability to express other feelings, enhanced by tension, etc., common psychodynamics accompanying pain, must also be considered.

Overestimating the Prognosis

There may be relatively narrow deficits, within the context of generally maintained mental ability. These will create perplexity, and should they fall within the area of vocation, hobbies, or other frequent activities, the patient should be made aware of them and taught how to compensate. The likelihood of return to work may be less than 50% with certain injuries.

Some Treatment Considerations

Behaviors Interfering with Treatment Programs

After TBI certain patient characteristics can hamper therapeutic work: increased irritability, anxiety and frustration, reduced self-esteem and self-confidence, hyperactivity, impulsivity, egocentricity, emotional lability, inappropriate social judgment, mood swings, hypersexuality, loss of insight, denial of limitations, literal interpretation of situations, confusion, confabulation, perseveration, stimulus boundedness, lack of initiation of activity, impaired visual processing skills, easy fatiguability, slow mental processing, poor tolerance for extraneous visual and auditory stimuli, problems of motor control, and amnesia (Adamovich et al., 1985, p. 34).

Physiological Considerations

Biologically caused reactions affect adaptation, and should be considered by the therapist in planning interventions: symptoms mimicking anxiety, sexual problems, startle, hypo- and hyperarousal (this has been named the "conditioned Emotional Response," Kolb, 1986), with increases in blood pressure, heart rate, and muscle tension. Although this response is conditioned to circumstances reminiscent of the trauma, social frustrations arousing fear, anger, or helplessness lead to their recurrence. Pain can lead to problems with prescribed medication, as well as alcohol, drugs, and regressive life styles. Drugs and alcohol increase the likelihood of dissociation, and are probably poorly handled at best by TBI victims. Loss of energy and changes in sexuality can be directly related to brain injury.

After long periods of stress, the TBI victim may be suffering from a form of opiate withdrawal, i.e., irritability, overreaction, hyperarousal, and rapid heartbeat. Sleep disorders are common, allied to overarousal, and every effort to control them should be instituted (relaxation, medication) since fatigue is a serious stressor and increases vulnerability to every other weak point in the personality and adjustment.

The patient's health may be impaired as a consequence of the immediate injury, damage to the endocrine system or neuroimmune functions, inability to take care of one's health due to handicaps or lack of funds, etc. Children may show developmental problems, requiring endocrinological intervention.

Some conditions caused by brain damage are slow to be expressed. Be alert to changes of health and physiological activity. Children may not grow and mature (see Chapter 8 on the Hypothalamic–Pituitary Axis and Chapter 19 on Children's Brain Damage).

Psychopharmacological

Drugs serve a variety of purposes (see Appendix 4).

Reducing physiological hyperarousal facilitates retrieval of memories, which can then be placed into historical perspective, rather than considered to be contemporary experiences (van der Kolk, 1988). Drug treatment for restlessness, irritability, and explosiveness is described in Kolb (1986). In addition, the somatic effects of arousal and anxiety are distracting and disconcerting, and it may be useful to relieve the patient of this discomfort.

Treating endogenous depression can have an energizing effect, and also reduce the possibility of suicide brought on by frustration and dark feelings. Endogenous depression is susceptible to psychopharmacology. The nonmedical therapist is advised to collaborate with a physician sympathetic and knowledgeable about the problems of the TBI patient.

Reestablishing Control over Their Lives

Treatment planning must take into account expressive deficits, in particular, offering a misleading appearance of indifference or apathy. Also, traumatized individuals may be unwilling to face their helplessness, first, at the time of an injury, and then, subsequently, helplessness as a daily experience. The initial stress and subsequent impairment lead to the experience of goals and personal values as being unattainable. Their future is extremely grim and unhappy. There may be reasons to believe that former goals are unattainable. It is a special challenge for the therapist or counselor to help the TBI victim to get back on his feet, or at least to establish a life with more independence, pleasure, and meaning.

The brain-damaged person has a poor morale, i.e., does not expect his situation to improve, and, therefore, may be unable or unwilling to deal with future planning and events.

Inappropriate behavior is common, and is a serious sign, particularly if counseling or attention to this matter by family matters does not lead to modification. This would be a classic example of inability to establish ego controls, particularly as it signifies inability to learn from experience.

Reassurance and Counseling Concerning the Nature of the Disorder

TBI victims are confused by what happened. They are extremely perplexed by their condition. Brain-damaged victims are poorly prepared to comprehend their situation, i.e., why they cannot function or have maladaptive emotional responses. *It is reassuring, often, to be told that this is due to an injury, not to an emotional disorder, i.e., they are not crazy.* The permanency of many aspects of impairment is disturbing, but may be better accepted than the idea that symptoms are unaccounted for, and by inference that the patient is strange or crazy.

One impaired professional man described his depression as "strange." I explained to him that it was normal for him to feel depressed because of the ruination of his life-style (inability to work, loss of friends, loss of his girlfriend), and because depression was a usual consequence of brain damage. He felt relieved and thanked me for the explanation. I continued and pointed out that his temper outbursts and mood swings were a consequence of the brain damage. He accepted this well because he had thought of himself as peculiar and disturbed because of his emotional life. He did not previously understand it as an unhappy direct consequence of an injury.

The patient should be advised that brain damage is cumulative, and that each subsequent injury reduces the ability to function. Deficits of vision, coordination, etc., should be explored to determine vulnerability.

The Question of Confronting Denial

Denial ranges from literal physiological unawareness of lack of stimulation ("neglect," "phantom limbs," see Chapter 7) to refusal to understand that impairment is both serious and permanent. Psychodynamically based denial is a significant therapeutic issue. Although it preserves hope, it also interferes with motivation for change. It may be directed at serious problems such as seizures, headaches, sensorimotor problems, etc. I cannot recommend a vigorous attack on denial since one runs the risk of a "catastrophic reaction," frustration-generated seizure, etc. Probably, taking a positive approach, and attempting to have the patient reconstitute his life is a reasonably efficacious modality, with a more reasonable self-assessment evolving from attempts to achieve what is possible.

Some Practical Considerations

- Planning and use of time need special attention.
- If they cannot remember, have them learn to use notebooks or other reminders.
- Problems of foresight, monitoring, attention, and concentration are grossly impairing, and should be remedied, e.g., through cognitive rehabilitation.

Working Through Resistance Carefully

The patient who has expended so much effort to ward off remembering the trauma is likely to work through anxiety only when a strong bond has been established. Therefore, it is recommended that the approach to trauma-related material should be gradual (van der Kolk, 1988).

The psychotherapeutic session may be an opportunity to express unresolved issues. Difficulties in maintaining one's responsibilities and personal relationships in a usual or competent manner are hard to acknowledge. Feelings such as shame, guilt, grief, rage, tender memories, fear, and loathing may be admixed so that patients are confused by their own feelings (Westermeyer & Wahmenholm, 1989). As cognitive problems recede, emotional factors may become more important in overall adjustment (Novack et al., 1984).

Placing the Accident in Perspective

The concept of survivor guilt is well known. The accident victim, in most circumstances, is not the cause of his own distress and impairment. It is true that some self-blame may occur, as the young woman who was seriously injured when she was in a car with a man of whom her mother disapproved. Such a problem is within the familiar context of the psychotherapeutic relationship. The accident victim may have to develop a different self-image, and learn to accept himself as an impaired person. This approach is surely a trial of the therapist's kindness, devotion, and skill.

Social Withdrawal Is Common

Most therapists would consider helping a patient to overcome withdrawal to be an essential of their work, and perhaps even a sign of success. Nevertheless, in the case of TBI, this has to be thought through. Your patient may have reduced or no income, be less able to comprehend or to communicate, be embarrassed by scarring, gait disorder, inability to travel, or to undertake former activities due to anxiety. Overcoming withdrawal remains a significant therapeutic problem, but it requires special empathy and ingenuity with the TBI victim.

Involving Collaterals

As documented earlier, the families of brain-damaged victims are part of the therapeutic system, and they are the sufferers in many ways as well as the primary patient. They will need considerable support since emotional dissatisfaction grows over time, sometimes even reflecting a worsening rather than recovering condition. The family has to cope with the inability to assume responsibilities, to participate in many former activities, the willingness to visit others, and withdrawal, loss of income, and reduced self-esteem.

Above all, they have to be brought to understand that the patient's personality difficulties and even misbehavior, while real enough, need not be the result of deliberate provocativeness or self-indulgence. Rather, they are the expression of a very serious injury. In particular, when there has been a diagnosis of mild head injury or concussion, it should not be taken at face value, i.e., there can be long-term impairment.

Lack of foresight or comprehension makes the patient vulnerable to danger. It may be that the family should be alerted to this as a problem, and their intervention may be needed. They may create dangers around the house, be unaware that difficulties with vision or coordination make them poor drivers, etc.

The therapist may have to help collaterals of the patient understand the patient, i.e., family, friends, and employer. These people may also be unsympathetic. They are uncomfortable when a formerly competent and independent person is now incompetent, unpleasant to deal with, and dependent. The family may have to be informed as to the degree of impairment and the likelihood of permanency.

Their best interest is represented by a combination of tolerance, support, and lack of inappropriate pressure. Many brain-damaged victims are urged to return to work before the recovery process is complete, adding to frustration and unnecessary failure. On the other hand, here, as elsewhere in therapy, truth is required. Many accident TBI victims are so badly impaired that their employability is ruined, their capacity to be independent is slight or nonexistent, and their ability to create pleasure for the members of the family is minimal.

The family may not be aware of certain symptoms, e.g., seizures, because the patient is too embarrassed to reveal them. They should also be informed of the need for their cooperation with rehabilitation, since the likelihood of return to work may be poor.

Hypnosis Is Recommended

Hypnosis is recommended with PTSD victims for handling dissociation. Modifying and coping with memories under hypnotherapy have proven to be useful (Kolb, 1986; Spiegel, 1988).

Dealing with Return to Work

Employment often requires rather specific areas of application, as well as the other components of efficiency. Reduced comprehension leads to reduced standards of performance, of which the patient may not be aware. Jobs that are in a noisy or uncontrolled environment create special problems of attention and concentration, i.e., problems of filtering out stimuli, sensory loss, and hypersensitivity.

Therefore, ability to work should be thoroughly explored. Deficits may cause the patient to be unable to resume prior employment, though able to work elsewhere where lesser demands are made on impaired areas.

You Are the Advocate

It is quite common that the brain-damaged person has no one in their personal life to help with very significant matters. The counselor will often be placed in the position of offering practical advice and counsel, far beyond the professional preferences of many therapists. This could include applying for Social Security Disability, public assistance, getting an attorney, or contacting the attorney, or even helping to obtain one who will take better care of the disabled person's legal needs.

Group Therapy

Kolb (1986) describes this procedure as useful in treatment of posttraumatic stress disorders, which in some form are characteristic of TBI victims. Of course, the group experience can be stressful, and I would warn the group leader to be sensitive to signs of overloading, inability to achieve insight, etc., or other demands beyond the ability to cope of the TBI patient (Parker, 1972a,b).

Further Reading

For further discussion see Allen and Lewis (1986).

Conclusion

The victim of TBI requires psychotherapy, counseling, and rehabilitation that differ from other patients. Since their brain, the organ of adaptation, is injured, the therapist in a real sense has to be a kindly and dedicated ego until the patient can reestablish his life. This work is difficult in many ways, but can be accomplished only by therapists who are willing to enter into a professional environment and conceptual framework different than that in which most of us were trained.

Indeed, when one comes to grips with a patient whose capacity to reestablish a life is poor, then at least we may then be dedicated to reducing the avoidable causes of brain damage, a truly gross and hidden epidemic.

References

Acklin, M. W., & Bernat, E. (1987). Depression, alexithymia, and pain proness disorder. Rorschach study. *Journal of Personality Assessment*, **51**(3),462–479.

Adamovich, B. B., Henderson, J. A., & Auerbach, S. (1985). *Cognitive Rehabilitation of Closed Head Injured Patients*. San Diego, CA: College Hill Press.

Adams, J. H., Mitchell, D. E., Graham, D. I., & Doyle, D. (1977). Diffuse brain damage of immediate impact type: Its relationship to 'primary brain-stem damage' in head injury. *Brain*, **100**, 489–502.

Adams, J. H., Graham, D. I., & Gennarelli, T. A. (1985). Contemporary neuropathological considerations regarding brain damage in head injury. In Becker, D. B., & Povlishock, J. T. (Eds.), *Central Nervous System Trauma Status Report*, pp. 65–77. National Institute of Neurological and Communicative Disorders and Stroke, National Institutes of Health.

Adams, R. D., & Victor, M. (1985). *Principles of Neurology*, 3rd ed. New York: McGraw-Hill.

Adams, R. D., & Victor, M. (1989). *Principles of Neurology*, 4th ed. New York: McGraw-Hill.

Addonzio, G., & Shamoian, C. A. (1986). Depression and dementia. In Jeste, D. V. (Ed.), *Neuropsychiatric Dementias*, pp. 73–109. Washington, DC: American Psychiatric Press.

Ader, R., & Cohen, N. (1984). Behavior and the immune system. In Gentry, W. D. (Ed.), *Handbook of Behavioral Medicine*. New York: Guilford.

Adler, R. (1989). Experts urge control of aerospace toxics. *The APA Monitor*, **20**(5), 1,14,15.

Alarie, Y., Cain, W., et al. (1987). Trigeminal chemoreception. Olfaction and Taste. *Annals of the N.Y. Academy of Science*, **150**, 127–129.

Alekoumbides, A., Charter, R. A., Adkins, T. G., & Seacat, G. F. (1987). The diagnosis of brain damage by the WAIS, SMS, and Reitan Battery utilizing standardized scores corrected for age and education. *International Journal of Clinical Neuropsychology*, **9**, 11–27.

Alexander, L., & Ax, A. F. (1951). Rorschach studies in combat flying personnel. In Hoch, P. H., and Zubin, J. *Relation of Psychological Tests to Psychiatry*, pp. 219–243. New York: Grune & Stratton.

Alexander, M. P., Naeser, M. A., & Palumbo, C. L. (1987). Correlations of subcortical CT lesion sites and aphasia profiles. *Brain*, **110**, 961–991.

Allen, J. G., & Lewis, L. (Eds.) (1986). *Neuropsychology in a Psychodynamic Setting: Bulletin of the Menninger Clinic*, **50**.

Allen, J. G., Lewis, L., Peebles, M. J., & Pruyser, P. W. (1986). Neuropsychological assessment in a psychoanalytic setting: The mind-body problem in clinical practice. *Bulletin of the Menninger Clinic*, **50**, 5–21.

Alves, W. M. (1989). Obstacles to identifying and treating the consequences of mild and moderate brain injury. In Hoff, J. T., Anderson, T. E., & Cole, T. M. (Eds.), *Mild to Moderate Head Injury*, pp. 187–202. Boston: Blackwell Scientific Publications.

Alves, W. M., & Jane, J. A. (1985). Mild brain injury: Damage and outcome. In Becker, D. P., & Povlishock, J. T. (Eds.), *Central Nervous System Trauma Status Report—1985*, pp. 255–270. National Institute of Neurological and Communicative Disorders and Stroke, National Institutes of Health.

American Psychiatric Association. (1985). *Diagnostic and Statistical Manual of Mental Disorders*, 3rd ed. rev. Washington, DC: Author.

Ames, L. B., Learned, J., Metraux, R. W., & Walker, R. N. (1952). *Child Rorschach Responses*. New York: Hoeber-Harper.

Ames, L. B., Learned, J., Metraux, R. W., & Walker, R. N. (1954). *Rorschach Responses in Old Age*. New York: Hoeber-Harper.

Ames, L. B., Metraux, R. W., & Walker, R. N. (1971). *Adolescent Rorschach Responses*. New York: Brunner/Mazel.

Andermann, F., Remillard, G. M., Zifkin, B. G., Trottier, A. G., & Drouin, P. (1988). Epilepsy and driving. *Canadian Journal of Neurological Science*, **15**, 371–377.

Anderson, A. (1982). Neurotoxic follies. *Psychology Today*, **7**(22), 30–42.

Andreassi, J. L. (1980). *Psychophysiology: Human Behavior and Physiological Response*. New York: Oxford University Press.

Antelman, S. M., & Caggiula, A. R. (1980). Stress-induced behavior: Chemotherapy without drugs. In Davidson, J. M., & Davidson, R. J. (Eds.), *The Psychobiology of Consciousness*, pp. 65–104. New York: Plenum.

Aram, D. M., & Ekelman, B. L. (1988). Scholastic aptitude and achievement among children with unilateral brain lesions. *Neuropsychologia*, **26**, 903–916.

Arato, M., Banki, C., Nemeroff, C. B., & Bisette, G. (1986). Hypothalamic-pituitary-adrenal axis and suicide. In Mann, J. J., & Stanley, M. (Eds.), *Psychobiology of Suicidal Behavior. Annals of the N.Y. Academy of Science*, **487**, 243–270.

Asnis, G. M., & Lemus, C. S. (1987). Cortisol secretion in psychiatric disorders. In Nemeroff, C. B., & Loosen, P. T. (Eds.), *Handbook of Clinical Psychoneuroendocrinology*. pp. 369–383. New York: Guilford.

Atkinson, L., & St. Cyr, J. J. (1984). Factor analysis of the WAIS-R: Psychiatric and standardization samples. *Journal of Consulting and Clinical Psychology*, **52**, 714–716.

Atteberry-Bennett, J., Barth, J. T., Loyd, B. H., & Lawrence, E. C. (1986). The relationship between behavioral aned cognitive deficits, demographics, and depression in patients with minor head injuries. *International Journal of Clinical Neuropsychology*, **8**, 114–117.

Baddeley, A., Harris, J., Sunderland, A., Watts, K. P., & Wilson, B. A. (1987). Closed head injury and memory. In Levin, H. S., Grafman, J., & Eisenberg, H. M. (Eds.), *Neurobehavioral Recovery from Head Injury*, pp. 295–317. New York: Oxford University Press.

Bajandas, F. J., & Kline, L. B. (1987). *Neuro-Opthamology Review Manual*, 2nd ed. Thorofare, NJ: Slack, Inc.

Bakay, L., Glasauer, F. E., & Alker, G. J. (1980). *Head Injury*. Boston: Little, Brown.

Bakay, R. A. E., & Wood, J. H. (1985). Pathophysiology of cerebrospinal fluid in trauma. In Becker, D. P., & Povlishock, J. T. (Eds.), *Central Nervous System Status Report— 1985*, pp. 89–122. National Institute of Neurological and Communicative Disorders and Stroke, National Institutes of Health.

Banki, C. B., Arato, M., & Kilts, C. D. (1986). Aminergic studies and cerebrospial fluid cations in suicide. In Mann, J. J., & Stanley, M. (Eds.), *Psychobiology of Suicidal Behavior. Annals of the N.Y. Academy of Science*, **487**, 221–230.

Barkley, R. A. (1988). Attention. In Tramontana, M. G., & Hooper, S. R. (Eds.), *Assessment Issues in Child Neuropsychology*, pp. 145–176. New York: Plenum.

Barnes, D. M. (1986). Steroids may influence changes in mood. *Science.* **232**, 1344–1345.

Barr, M. L., & Kiernan, J. A. (1983). *The Human Nervous System*, 4th ed. New York: Harper & Row.

Barr, M. L., & Kiernan, J. A. (1988). *The Human Nervous System*, 5th ed. New York: Harper & Row.

Barth, J. T., & Macciocchi. (1986). Dementia: Implications for clinical practice and research. In Filskov, S. B., & Boll, T. J. (Eds.), *Handbook of Neuropsychology*, pp. 398–425. New York: Wiley.

Barth, J. T., Gideon, D. A., Sciara, A. D., Hulsey, P. H., & Anchor, K. N. (1986). Forensic aspects of mild head trauma. *The Journal of Head Trauma Rehabilitation*, **12**, 63–70.

Barton, W. A. (1985). *Recovering for Psychological Injuries*. Washington, DC: Association of Trial Lawyers of America.

Beatty, J., Barth, D. S., Richer, F., & Johnson, R. A. (1986). Neuromagnetometry. In Coles, M. G. H., Donchin, E., & Porges, S. W. (Eds.), *Psychophysiology: Systems, Processes, and Applications*, pp. 26–40. New York: Guilford.

Becker, D. B., & Povlishock, J. T. (1985). *Central Nervous System Trauma Status Report*. National Institute of Neurological and Communicative Disorders and Stroke, National Institutes of Health.

Beckman, D. L. (1985). Pulmonary responses to experimental brain injury. In Becker, D. B., Povlishock, J. T. (Eds.), *Central Nervous System Trauma Status Report— 1985*, pp. 417–424. National Institute of Neurological and Communicative Disorders and Stroke, National Institutes of Health.

Begali, V. (1987). *Head Injury in Children and Adolescents*. Charlottesville, VA: Charlottesville Public Schools.

Benedek, E. P. (1985). Children and psychic trauma. A brief review of contemporary thinking. In Eth, S., & Pynoos, R. S. (Eds.), *Post-traumatic Stress Disorder in Children*, pp. 1–16. Washington, DC: American Psychiatric Press.

Bennett, T. L., & Krein, L. K. (1989). The neuropsychology of epilepsy: Psychological and social impact. In Reynolds, C. R., & Fletcher-Janaen, E., *Handbook of Clinical Child Neuropsychology*, pp. 419–441. New York: Plenum.

Benson, D. F. (1985). Aphasia. In Heilman, K. M., & Valenstein, E. (Eds.), *Clinical Neuropsychology*, 2nd ed., pp. 17–47. New York: Oxford University Press.

Benson, D. F., & Cummings, J. L. (1986). A scheme to differentiate the dementias. In Jeste, D. V. (Ed.), *Neuropsychiatric Dementias*, pp. 1–26. Washington, DC: American Psychiatric Press.

Benson, D. F., & Geschwind, N. (1985). Aphasia and related disorders: A clinical approach. In Marsulam, M., *Principles of Behavioral Neurology*, pp. 193–238. Philadelphia: F.A. Davis.

Benton, A. (1974). *Revised Visual Retention Test*. San Antonio, TX: The Psychological Corporation.

Benton, A. (1985a). Body schema disturbances: Finger agnosia and right-left disorientation. In Heilman, K. M., & Valenstein, E. (Eds.), *Clinical Neuropsychology*, 2nd ed., pp. 115–129. New York: Oxford University Press.

Benton, A. (1985b). Visuoperceptual, visuospatial, and visuoconstructive disorders. In Heilman, K. M., & Valenstein, E. (Eds.), *Clinical Neuropsychology*, 2nd ed., pp. 151–185. New York: Oxford University Press.

Benyakar, M., Tadir, M. Groswasser, Z., & Stern, M.J. (1988). Dreams in head-injured patients. *Brain Injury*, 2, 351–356.

Berg, R. (1986). Neuropsychological effects of closed-head injury in children. In Obrzut, J. E., & Hynd, G. W. (Eds.), *Child Neuropsychology*, Vol. 2, pp. 113–135. New York: Academic Press.

Berndt, R. S., & Caramazza, A. (1981). Syntactic aspects of aphasia. In Sarno, M. T. (Ed.), *Acquired Aphasia*, pp. 157–179. New York: Academic Press.

Beutler, L. E., Engle, D., Oro-Beutler, M. E., Daldrup, R., & Meredith, K. (1986). Inability to express intense affect: A common link between depression and pain? *Journal of Consulting and Clinical Psychology*, 54, 752–759.

Biari, N., Cleeves, L., Findley, L., & Koller, W. (1989). Post-traumatic tremor. *Neurology*, 39, 103–106.

Bigler, E. D. (1988). The role of neuropsychological assessment in relation to other types of assessment with children. In Tramontana, M. G., & Hooper, S. R. (Eds.), *Assessment Issues in Child Neuropsychology*, pp. 67–91. New York: Plenum.

Bilder, R. M., & Goldberg, E. (1987). Motor perseverations in schizophrenia. *Archives of Clinical Neuropsychology*, 2, 1–19.

Biller, J., & Brazis, P. W. (1985). The localization of lesions affecting the cerebellum. In Brazis, P. W., Masdeu, J. C., and Biller, J. (Eds.), *Localization in Clinical Neurology*, pp. 225–238. Boston: Little, Brown.

Bisiach, E., Ballar, G., Perani, D., Papagno, C., & Berti, A. (1986). Unawareness of disease following lesions of the right hemisphere: Anosognosia for hemiplegia and anosognosia for hemianopia. *Neuropsychologia*, 24, 471–482.

Black, R. G. (1982). The clinical management of chronic pain. In Hendler, N. H., Long, D. M., & Wise, T. N. (Eds.), *Diagnosis and treatment of chronic pain*, pp. 211–224. Boston: John Wright.

Blackerby, W. (1987). Disruption of sexuality following a head injury. *Newsletter: National Head Injury Foundation*, 7(1), 2–8.

Blair, C. D., & Lanyon, R. I. (1987). Retraining social and adaptive living skills in severely head injured adults. *Archives of Clinical Neuropsychology*, 2, 33–43.

Blumstein, S. E. (1981). Phonological aspects of aphasia. In Sarno, M. T. (Ed.), *Acquired Aphasia*, pp. 129–155. New York: Academic Press.

Bolter, J. F. (1986). Epilepsy in children. In Obrzut, J. E., & Hynd, G. W. (Eds.), *Child Neuropsychology*, Vol. 2, pp. 59–81. Orlando: Academic Press.

Bond, M. (1984). The psychiatry of closed head injury. In Brooks, B. (Ed.), *Closed Head Injury: Psychological, Social, and Family Consequences*, pp. 148–178. New York: Oxford University Press.

Bond, M. R.. (1983a). Standardized methods of assessing and predicting outcome. In Rosenthal, M., Griffith, E. R., Bond, M. R., and Miller, J. R. (Eds.), *Rehabilitation of the Head Injured Adult*, pp. 97–113. Philadelphia: F. A. Davis.

Bond, M. R. (1983b). Effects on the family system. In Rosenthal, M., Griffith, E. R., Bond, M. R., & Miller, J.R. (Eds.), *Rehabilitation of the Head Injured Adult*, pp. 209–217. Philadelphia: F.A. Davis.

Bond, M. R. (1986). Neurobehavioral sequelae of closed head injury. In Grant, I., & Adams, K. M. (Eds.), *Neuropsychological Assessment of Neuropsychiatric Disorders*, pp. 347–373. New York: Oxford University Press.

Bondy, S. C., & Prasad, K. N. (1988). *Metal Neurotoxicity*. Boca Raton, FL: CRC Press.

Bornstein, R. A. (1984). Unilateral lesions and the Wechsler Adult Intelligence Scale-Revised. *Journal of Consulting and Clinical Psychology*. **52**, 604–608.

Bornstein, R. A. (1987). The WAIS-R in neuropsychological practice: Boon or bust? *The Clinical Neuropsychologist*, **1**, 185–190.

Bornstein, R. A. (1988). Entry into clinical neuropsychology: Graduate, undergraduate, and beyond. *The Clinical Neuropsychologist*, **3**, 213–220.

Bornstein, R. A., Suga, L., & Prifitera, A. (1987). Incidence of verbal-performance IQ discrepancies at various levels of education. *Journal of Clinical Psychology*, **43**, 387–389.

Bossert, S., Berger, M., Krieg, J.-C., Schreiber, W., Junker, M., & von Zerssen, D. (1988). Cortisol response to various stressful situations: Relationship to personality variables and coping styles. *Neuropsychobiology*, **20**, 36–42.

Bouvet, J-F., Delaleu, J-C., & Holley, A. (1987). Does the trigeminal nerve control the activity of the olfactory receptor cells? Olfaction and Taste. *Annals of the N.Y. Academy of Science*, **150**, 187–189.

Bowen, M. (1989). Frontal lobe function. *Brain Injury*, **3**, 109–128.

Boyd, T. A. (1988). Clinical assessment of memory in children. In Tramontana, M. G., & Hooper, S. R. (Eds.), *Assessment Issues in Child Neuropsychology*, pp. 177–204. New York: Plenum.

Brannigan, G. G., & Brunner, N. A. (1989). *The Modified Version of the Bender Gestalt Test for Preschool and Primary School Children*. Clinical Psychology Publishing Co.

Braun, C. M. J., et al. (1989). Processing of pragmatic and facial affective information by patients with closed-head injuries. *Brain Injury*, **3**, 5–17.

Brazis, P. W., Masdeu, J. C., & Biller, J. (1985). *Localization in Clinical Neurology*. Boston: Little, Brown.

Brodal, A. (1981). *Neurological Anatomy in Relation to Clinical Medicine*, 3rd ed. New York: Oxford University Press.

Brooks, N. (1984). Head injury and the family. In Brooks, N. (Ed.), *Closed Head Injury*, pp. 121–147. New York: Oxford University Press.

Brooks, N., Symington, C., Beattie, A., Campsie, L., Brydens, J., & McKinlay, W. (1989). Alcohol and other predictors of cognitive recovery after severe head injury. *Brain Injury*, **3**, 235–246.

Brown, G. M., Chik, C. L., & Ho, A. K. (1988a). The pineal gland. In Collu, R., Brown, G. M., & Van Loon, G. R. (Eds.), *Clinical Neuroendocrinology*, pp. 475–489. Boston: Blackwell Scientific Publications.

Brown, G. M., Steiner, M., & Grof, P. (1988b). Neuroendocrinology of affective disorder. In Collu, R., Brown, G. M., & Van Loon, G.R. (Eds.), *Clinical Neuroendocrinology*, pp. 461–474. Boston: Blackwell Scientific Publications.

Bruce, D. A. (1985). Cerebrovascular dynamics following brain insults. In James, H. E., Anas, N. G., & Perkin, R. M. (Eds.), *Brain insults in Infants and Children: Pathophysiology and Management*, pp. 83–88. New York: Grune & Stratton.

Bruno, R. S. (1984). The catastrophic reaction: Release of cortical inhibition following cortical lesion. *Newsletter: The New York Neuropsychology Group*, **3**(1), 1,5,6.2

Bryden, M. P., & Ley, R. G. (1983). Right hemispheric involvement in the perception and expression of emotion in normal humans. In Heilman, K. M., & Satz, P. (Eds.), *Neuropsychology of Human Emotion*, pp. 6–44. New York: Guilford.

Buchsbaum, M. (1986). Functional imaging of the brain in psychiatry. In Arieti, S. (Ed.), *American Handbook of Psychiatry*, Vol. 8, 2nd ed., pp. 236–248. New York: Basic Books.

Buckingham, H. W. (1981). Explanations for the concept of apraxia of speech. In Sarno, M. T. (Ed.), *Acquired Aphasia*, pp. 271–301. New York: Academic Press.

Burke, J. M., Smith, S. A., & Imhoff, C. L. (1989). The response style of postacute traumatic brain-injuried patients on the MMPI. *Brain Injury*, 3, 35–40.

Carpenter, M. B., & Sutin, J. (1983). *Human Neuroanatomy*, 8th ed. Baltimore: Williams & Wilkins.

Carpenter, M. B. (1985). *Core Text of Neuroanatomy*, 3rd ed. Baltimore: Williams & Wilkins.

Carr, A. (1984). Content interpretation re: Salley and Teiling's dissociated rage attacks in a Vietnam veteran: A Rorschach study. *Journal of Personality Assessment*, 48, 420–421.

Cartlidge, N. E. F., & Shaw, D. A. (1981). *Head Injury*. Philadelphia: W.B. Saunders.

Chadwick, O., & Rutter, M. (1983). Neuropsychological assessment. In Rutter, M. (Ed.), *Developmental Neuropsychiatry*, pp. 181–212. New York: Guilford.

Chang, L. W. (1987). Neuropathological changes associated with accidental or experimental exposure to organometallic compounds: CNS effects. In Tilson, H. A., & Sparber, S. B. (Eds.), *Neurotoxicants and Neurobiological Function: Effects of Organoheavy Metals*, pp. 83–116. New York: Wiley.

Chusid, J. G. (1985). *Correlative Neuroanatomy and Functional Neurology*, 19th ed. East Norwalk, CT. Appleton, Century Crofts.

Clasen, R. A., & Penn, R. D. (1987). Traumatic brain swelling and edema. In Cooper, P. R. (Ed.), *Head Injury*, 2nd ed., pp. 285–312. Baltimore: Williams & Wilkins.

Clifton, G. L., Robertson, C. S., & Grossman, R. G. (1985). Management of the cardiovascular and metabolic responses to severe head injury. In Becker, D. B., & Povlishock, J. T. (Eds.), *Central Nervous System Trauma Status Report – 1985*, pp. 139–159. National Institute of Neurological and Communicative Disorders and Stroke, National Institutes of Health.

Clinicians Research Digest. (8/1989). 7, 1, citing Meyer, J. D. (1989) *Professional Psychology: Research and Practice*, 20, 90–96.

Cocchi, D., & Muller, E. O. (1988). Control of anterior pituitary function. In Collu, R., Brown, G. M., & Van Loon, G. R. (Eds.), *Clinical Neuroendocrinology*, pp. 17–63. Boston: Blackwell Scientific Publications.

Code, C. (1987). *Language, Aphasia, and the Right Hemisphere*. New York: Wiley.

Cohen, S. B. (1986). Educational reintegration and programming for children with head injuries. *Journal of Head Trauma Rehabilitation*, 1(4), 220–229.

Cohen, R. M., Semple, W. E., Gross, M., Holcomb, H. H., Dowling, M. S., & Nordahl, T. E. (1988). Functional localization of sustained attention: Comparison to sensory stimulation in the absence of instruction. *Neuropsychiatry, Neuropsychology and Behavioral Neurology*, 1, 3–20.

Cooper, J. R., Bloom, F. E., & Roth, R. (1986). *The Biochemical Basis of Neuropharmacology*, (5th ed.), New York: Oxford University Press.

Cooper, P. (1985). Delayed brain injury: Secondary Insults. In Becker, D. B., & Povlishock, J. T. (Eds.), *Central Nervous System Trauma Status Report – 1985*, pp. 217–228. National Institute of Neurological and Communicative Disorders and Stroke, National Institutes of Health.

Cooper, P. R. (1987a). Skull fracture and traumatic cerebrospinal fluid fistulas. In Cooper, P. R. (Ed.), *Head Injury*, 2nd ed., pp. 89–107. Baltimore: Williams & Wilkins.

Cooper, P. R. (1987b). Post-traumatic intracranial mass lesions. In Cooper, P. R. (Ed.), *Head Injury*, 2nd ed., pp. 238–284. Baltimore: Williams & Wilkins.

Cooper, P. R. (Ed.). (1987c). Post-traumatic intracranial mass lesions. In Cooper, P. R. (Ed.), *Head Injury* (2nd ed.), pp. 238–284. Baltimore: Williams & Wilkins.

Cooper, P. R. (Ed.). (1987d). *Head Injury*, 2nd ed. Baltimore: Williams & Wilkins.

Corbett, J. A., & Trimble, M. R. (1983). Epilepsy and anticonvulsant medication. In Rutter, M. (Ed.), *Developmental Neuropsychiatry*, pp. 112–129. New York: Guilford.

Corkin, S., Cohen, N. J., Sullivan, E. V., Clegg, R. A., & Rosen, T. J. (1985). In Olton, D. S., Gamzu, E., & Corkin, S. (Eds.), *Memory Dysfunctions: An Integration of Animal and Human Research from Preclinical and Clinical Perspectives. Annals of the N. Y. Academy of Science*, **444**, 10–40.

Corkin, S. H., Hurt, R. W., Twitchell, T. E., Franklin, L. C., & Yin, R. K. (1987). Consequences of nonpenetrating and penetrating head injury: Retrograde amnesia, posttraumatic amnesia, and lasting effects on cognition. In Levin, H. S., Grafman, J., & Eisenberg, H. M. (Eds.), *Neurobehavioral Recovery from Head Injury*, pp. 318–329. New York: Oxford University Press.

Costanzo, R. M., Heywood, J. D., & Young, H. F. (1987). Neurosurgical applications of clinical olfactory assessment. In Roper, S. D., & Aterna, J. (Eds.), *Olfaction and Taste IX*, pp. 242–244. New York: The New York Academy of Sciences.

Cripe, L. I., & Dodrill, C. B. (1988). Neuropsychological test performances with chronic low level formaldehyde exposure. *The Clinical Neuropsychologist*, **2**, 41–48.

Crockett, D., Clark, C., & Klonoff, H. (1981). An overview of neuropsychology. In Filskov, S. B., & Boll, T. J. (Eds.), *Handbook of Neuropsychology*, pp. 1–37. New York: Wiley.

Crossen, J. R., & Wiens, A. N. (1988a). Wechsler Memory Scale-Revised: Deficits in performance associated with neurotoxic solvent exposure. *The Clinical Neuropsychologist*, **2**, 181–187.

Crossen, J. R., & Wiens, A. N. (1988b). Residual neuropsychological deficits following head-injury on the Wechsler Memory Scale-Revised. *The Clinical Neuropsychologist*, **2**, 393–399.

Cytowic, R. E., Stump, D. A., & Larned, D. C. (1988). Closed head trauma: Somatic, ophthalmic, and cognitive impairments in nonhospitalized patients. In Whitaker, H. A. (Ed.), *Neuropsychological Studies of Nonfocal Brain Damage*, pp. 226–264. New York: Springer-Verlag.

Dacey, G. R., & Dikmen, S. S. (1987). Mild head injury. In Cooper, P. R. (Ed.), *Head Injury*, 2nd ed., pp. 125–140. Baltimore: Williams & Wilkins.

Damasio, A. (1981). The nature of aphasia: Signs and syndromes. In Sarno, M. T. (Ed.), *Acquired Aphasia*, pp. 51–65. New York: Academic Press.

Damasio, A. R. (1985). Disorders of complex visual processing: Agnosias, achromatopsia, Balint's syndrome, and related difficulties of orientation and construction. In Marsulam, M. (Ed.), *Principles of Behavioral Neurology*, pp. 259–288. Philadelphia: F.A. Davis.

Damasio, A. R., & Van Hoesen, G. W. (1985). Emotional disturbances associated with focal lesions of the limbic frontal lobe. In Heilman, K., & Satz, P. (Eds.), *Neuropsychology of Human Emotion*, pp. 85–110. New York: Guilford.

Darby, J. K. (Ed.). (1985). *Speech and Language Evaluation in Neurology*. New York: Grune & Stratton.

Davidson, R. J. (1980). Consciousness and information processing. In Davidson, J. M., & Davidson, R. J. (Eds.), *The Psychobiology of Consciousness*, pp. 11–46. New York: Plenum.

Day, B. L., Rothwell, J. C., Thompson, P. D., De Noordhout, A. M., Nakashima, I., Shannon, K., & Marsden, C. D. (1989). Delay in the execution of voluntary movement by electrical or magnetic brain stimulation in intact man. *Brain*, **112**, 649–663.

Dean, J. H., Murray, M. J., & Ward, E. C. (1986). Toxic responses of the immune system. In Klaassen, C. D., Amdur, M. O., & Doull, J. (Eds.), pp. 256–286. *Casarett and Doull's Toxicology*. New York: Macmillan.

Dean, R. S. (1986). Neuropsychological aspects of psychiatric disorders. In Obrzut, J. E., & Hynd, G. W. (Eds.), *Child Neuropsychology*, Vol. 2, pp. 83–112. Orlando: Academic Press.

DeGroot, J., & Chusid, J. G. (1988). *Correlative Neuroanatomy*, 20th ed. East Norwalk, CT: Appleton & Lange.

De Renzi, E. (1986). Prosopagnosia in two patients with CT scan evidence of damage confined to the right hemisphere. *Neuropsychologia*, **24**, 385–389.

De Wied, D., & De Kloet, E. R. (1987). Pro-opiomelanocortin (POMC) as homeostatic control system. In Ganong, W., Dallman, M. F., & Roberts, J. L. (Eds.), *The Hypothalamic-Pituitary-Adrenal Axis Revisited*, pp. 328–337. New York: The New York Academy of Sciences.

Del Rey, A., Besedovsky, H., Sorkin, E., & Dinarello, C. (1987). Interleukin-1 and glucocorticoid hormones integrate an immunoregulatory feedback circuit. In Jankovic, B. D., Markovic, B. M., & Spector, N. H. (Eds.), *Neuroimmune Interactions: Proceedings of the Second International Workshop on Neuroimmunomodulation. Annals of the N.Y. Academy of Sciences*, **496**, 85–90.

Dennis, M. M. (1988). Language and the young damaged brain. In Boll, T., & Bryant, B. K. (Eds.), *Clinical Neuropsychology and Brain Function*, pp. 89–123. Washington, DC: American Psychological Association.

Denny, N., Robinowitz, R., & Penk, W. (1987). Conducting applied research on Vietnam combat-related post-traumatic stress disorder. *Journal of Clinical Psychology*, **43**(1), 56–66.

Depue, R. A., & Spoont, M. R. (1986). Conceptualizing a serotonin trait: A behavioral dimension of constraint. In Mann, J. J., & Stanley, M. (Eds.), *Psychobiology of Suicidal Behavior. Annals of the N.Y. Academy of Sciences*, **487**, 47–62.

Deschaux, P., & Rouhabhia, M. (1987). In Jankovic, B. D., Markovic, B. M., & Spector, N. H. (Eds.), *Neuroimmune interactions: Proceedings of the Second International Workshop on Neuroimmunomodulation. Annals of the N.Y. Academy of Sciences*, **496**, 49–55.

Di Rocco, D., & Velardi, F. (1986). Epidemiology and etiology of craniocerebral trauma in the first two years of life. In Raimondi, A. J., Choux, M., & Di Rocco, C. (Eds.), *Head Injuries in the Newborn and Infant*, pp. 125–140. New York: Springer-Verlag.

Dor-Shav, N. K. (1978). On the long-range effects of concentration camp internment on Nazi victims: 25 years later. *Journal of Consulting and Clinical Psychology*, **46**, 1–11.

Drake, M. E., Shuttleworth, E. C., & Kellum, J. B. (1988). Nonverbal memory disorder with right caudate hemorrhage. *Neuropsychiatry, Neuropsychology, and Behavioral Neurology*, **1**, 141–146.

Drummond, O. M. (1988). Delayed emergence of obsessive-compulsive neurosis following head injury. *British Journal of Psychiatry*, **153**, 939–842.

Ducharme, J. R. (1988). Puberty and its anomolies. In Collu, R., Brown, G. M., & Van Loon (Eds.), *Clinical Neuroendocrinology*, pp. 121–143. Boston: Blackwell Scientific Publications.

Dunn, A. J. (1987). Neurochemistry of stress. In Adelman, G. (Ed.), *Encyclopedia of Neuroscience, Vol II*, pp. 1146–1148. Boston: Birknauser.

Dyken, P. R., & McCleary, G. E. (1986). Dementia in infantile and childhood neurological disease. In Obrzut, J. E., & Hynd, G. W. (Eds.), *Child Neuropsychology*, Vol. 1, pp. 175–189. Orlando, FL: Academic Press.

Eames, P. (1988). Behavior disorders after severe head injury: Their nature and causes and strategies for management. *Journal of Head Trauma*, **3**(3), 1–6.

Ehrlich, J., & Barry, P. (1989). Rating communication behaviours in the head injured adult. *Brain Injury*, **3**, 193–198.

Eliott, F. A. (1976). Neurological factors in violent behavior. *The Bulletin of the American Academy of Psychiatry and the Law*, **4**, 297–315.

Elliott, G. R. (1986). Magnetic resonance and in vivo studies of the human brain. In *American Handbook of Psychiatry*, Vol. 8, 2nd ed., pp. 249–262. New York: Basic Books.

Ellis, A. W., & Young, A. W. (1988). *Human Cognitive Neuropsychology*. Hillsdale, NJ: Lawrence Erlbaum.

Ellis, D. W., & Christensen, A-L. (Eds.). (1989). *Neuropsychological Treatment after Brain Injury*. Boston: Kluver Academic Publishers.

Epstein, F. M., Ward, J. D., & Becker, D. P. (1987). Medical complications of head injury. In Cooper, P. R. (Ed.), *Head Injury*, pp. 390–421. Baltimore: Williams & Wilkins.

Eskenazi, B., Cain, W. S., Novelly, R. A., & Mattson, R. (1988). Odor perception in temporal lobe epilepsy patients with and without temporal lobectomy. *Neuropsychologia*, **24**, 553–562.

Eth, S., & Pynoos, R. S. (1985). *Post-traumatic Stress Disorder in Children*. Washington, DC: American Psychiatric Association.

Etkoff, N. L. (1986). The neuropsychology of emotional expression. In Goldstein, G., & Tarter, R. E. (Eds.), *Advances in Clinical Neuropsychology*, Vol. 3, pp. 127–177. New York: Plenum.

Everly, G. S., & Horton, A. M. (1988). Cognitive impairment and post-traumatic stress disorder. *Bulletin of the National Academy of Neuropsychologists*, **5**, 1.

Exner, J. E. (1986). *The Rorschach: A Comprehensive System*, Vol. I, 2nd ed. New York: Wiley.

Ewing-Cobbs, L., Fletcher, J. M., Landry, S. H., & Levin, H. S. (1985). Language disorders after pediatric head injury. In Darby, J. (Ed.), Examples include: visual (color, space, faces) auditory, and tactile (form recognition, fingers, body parts), (Ed.), *Speech and Language Evaluation in Neurology: Childhood Disorders*, pp. 97–111. New York: Grune & Stratton.

Fallon, J. H. (1988). Topographic organization of ascending dopaminergic projections. In Kalivas, P. W., & Nemeroff, C. B. (Eds.), *The Mesocorticolimbic Dopamine System, Annals of the New York Academy of Sciences*, Vol. 537, pp. 1–9. New York: The New York Academy of Sciences.

Farah, M. J., Wong, A. B., Monheit, M. A., & Morrow, L. A. (1989). Parietal lobe mechanisms of spatial attention: Modality-specific or supramodal? *Neuropsychologia*, **27**, 461–470.

Farber, S. D., & Zoltan, B. (1989). Visual-vestibular systems interaction: Therapeutic implications. *Journal of Head Trauma Rehabilitation*, **4**(2), 9–16.

Farr, S. P., Greene, R. L., & Fisher-White, S. P. (1986). Disease process, onset, and course and their relationship to neuropsychological performance. In Filskov, S. B., & Boll, T. J. (Eds.), *Handbook of Clinical Neuropsychology*, Vol. II, pp. 213–253. New York: Wiley.

Fay, G., & Janesbeski, J. (1986). Neuropsychological assessment of head-injured children. *The Journal of Head Trauma Rehabilitation*, **1**(4), 16–21.

Fenichel, G. M. (1985). *Neonatal Neurology*. New York: Churchill Livingston.

Fenichel, G. M. (1988). *Clinical Pediatric Neurology*. Philadelphia: Saunders.

Field, L. H., & Weiss, C. J. (1989). Dysphagia with head injury. *Brain Injury*, **3**, 19–26.

Filley, C. M., Cranberg, L. D., Alexander, M. P., & Hart, E. J. (1987). Neurobehavioral outcome after closed head injury in childhood and adolescence. *Archives of Neurology* **44**, 194–198.

Filskov, S. B., & Catanese, R. A. (1986). Effects of sex and handedness on neuropsychological testing. In Filskov, S. B., & Boll, T. J. (Eds.), *Handbook of Clinical Neuropsychology*, Vol. II, pp. 198–212. New York: Wiley.

Findling, J. W., & Tyrell, J. B. (1986). Anterior pituitary and somatomedins: I. Anterior pituitary. In Greenspan, F. G., & Forsham, P. H. (Eds.), *Basic and Clinical Endocrinology*, 2nd ed., pp. 43–94. Los Altos, CA: Lange Medical Publications.

Flood, J. F., Cherkin, A., & Morley, J. E. (1987). Antagonism of endogenous opioids modulates memory processing. *Brain Research*. **422**, 218–234.

Flor, H., & Turk, D. C. (1989). Psychophysiology of chronic pain: Do chronic pain patients exhibit symptom-specific psychophysiological responses? *Psychological Bulletin*, **105**, 215–259.

Flynn, J. R. (1984). The mean IQ gains of Americans: Massive gains 1932–1978. *Psychological Bulletin*, **95**, 29–51.

Francis-Williams, J. (1968). *Rorschach with Children*. Oxford: Pergamon Press.

Franck, J. E., et al. (1989). The limbic system. In Patton, H. D., Fuchs, A. F., Hille, B., Scher, A. M., & Steiner, R. (Eds.), *Textbook of Physiology*, Vol. I, pp. 693–717. Philadelphia: Saunders.

Frankowski, R. F., Annegers, J. F., & Whitman, S. F. (1985). The descriptive epidemiology of head trauma in the United States. In Becker, D. P., & Povlishock, J. T. (Eds.), *Central Nervous System Trauma Status Report 1985*, pp. 33–43. National Institute of Neurological and Communicative Disorders and Stroke, National Institutes of Health.

Frantz, A. G. (1988). Hyperprolactinemia. In Collu, R., Brown, G. M., & Van Loon, G. R. (Eds.), *Clinical Neuroendocrinology*, pp. 311–332. Boston: Blackwell Scientific Publications.

Frederick, C. J. (1985). Children traumatized by catastrophic situations. In Eth, S., & Pynoos, R. S. (Eds.), *Post-traumatic Stress Disorder in Children*, pp. 71–99. Washington, DC: American Psychiatric Association.

Fowler, P. C., Richards, H. D., Berent, S., & Boll, T. J. (1987). Epilepsy, neuropsychological deficits and EEG localization. In *Archives of Clinical Neuropsychology*, **2**, 81–92.

Fuchs, A. F., & Phillips, J. O. (1989). Association Cortex. In Patton, H. D., Fuchs, A. F., Hille, B., Scher, A. M., & Steiner, R. (Eds.), *Textbook of Physiology*, Vol. I, pp. 663–692. Philadelphia: Saunders.

Gaddis, W. H. (1981). An examination of the validity of neuropsychological knowledge in educational diagnosis and remediation. In Hynd, G. W., & Obrzut, J. E. (Eds.), *Neuropsychological Assessment and the School-Age Child*, pp. 27–84. New York: Grune & Stratton.

Gadisseux, P. (1985). Nutrition and CNS trauma. In Becker, D. P., & Povlishock, J. T. (Eds.), *Central Nervous System Trauma Status Report 1985*, pp. 207–216. National Institute of Neurological and Communicative Disorders and Stroke. National Institutes of Health.

Gale, A., & Edwards, J. E. (1986). Individual differences. In Coles, M. G. H., Donchin, E., & Porges, S. W. (Eds.), *Psychophysiology: Systems, Processes and Applications*, pp. 431–507. New York: Guilford.

Ganong, W. F. (1986). Neuroendocrinology. In Greenspan, F. G., & Forsham, P. H. (Eds.), *Basic and Clinical Endocrinology*, 2nd ed., pp. 31–42. Los Altos, CA: Lange Medical Publications.

Ganong, W. F., Dallman, M. F., & Roberts, J. L. (1987). *The Hypothalamic-Pituitary-Adrenal Axis Revisted*. New York: The New York Academy of Sciences.

Gelb, H., & Siegel, P. N. (1980). *Killing Pain without Prescription*. New York: Harper & Row.

Geneen, V., Legros, J-J., Franchimont, P., Defresne, M.-P., & Boniver, J. (1987). The thymus as a neuroendocrine organ. In Jankovic, B. D., Markovic, B. M., & Spector, N. H. (Eds.), *Neuroimmune interactions: Proceedings of the Second International Workshop on Neuroimmunomodulation. Annals of the N.Y. Academy of Sciences*, **496**, 56–66.

Gennarelli, T. M. (1987). Cerebral concussion and diffuse brain injuries. In Cooper, P. R. (Ed.), *Head Injuries*, 2nd ed., pp. 108–124. Baltimore: Williams & Wilkins.

Gilbert, A. N., Greenberg, M. S., & Beauchamp, G. K. (1989). *Neuropsychologia*, **27**, 509–511.

Gill, G. N. (1985). The hypothalamic-pituitary control system. In West, J. B. (Ed.), *Best and Taylor's Physiological Basis of Medical Practice*, 11th ed., pp. 856–871. Baltimore: Williams & Wilkins.

Gill, T., Calav, A., Greenberg, D., Kugelmass, S., & Lerer, B. (1990). Cognitive functioning in post-traumatic stress disorder. *Journal of Traumatic Stress*, **3**, 29–45.

Gold, P. W., Avgerinos, P. C., Kling, M. A., Loriaux, D. L., Calabrese, J. R., Chrousos, G. P., & Kalogeras, K. (1987). Physiological, diagnostic and pathophysiological implications of corticotropin-releasing hormone. In Nemeroff, C. B., & Loosen, P. T. (Eds.), *Handbook of Clinical Psychoneuroendocrinology*, pp. 85–105. New York: Guilford.

Goldberg, E., & Bilder, R. M. (1987). The frontal lobes and hierarchical organization of cognitive control. In Perecman, E. (Ed.), *The Frontal Lobes Revisited*, pp. 159–167. New York: IRBN Press.

Golden, C. (1986). Forensic neuropsychology: Introduction and overview. In Golden, G., & Strider, M. A. (Eds.), *Forensic Neuropsychology*, pp. 1–48. New York: Plenum.

Golden, C. J., Moses, J. A., Coffman, J. A., Miller, W. R., & Strider, F. D. (1983). *Clinical Neuropsychology*. New York: Grune & Stratton.

Goldfried, M. R., Stricker, G., & Weiner, I. B. (1971). *Rorschach Handbook of Clinical and Research Applications*. Englewood Cliffs, NJ: Prentice-Hall.

Goldstein, S., & Halbreich, U. (1987). Hormones and stress. In Nemeroff, C. B., & Loosem, P. T. (Eds.), *Handbook of Clinical Psychoneuroendocrinology*, pp. 460–469. New York: Guilford.

Golper, L. A. C. (1985). Nonverbal communication after hemispheric disease. In Darby, J. K. (Ed.), *Speech and Language Evaluation in Neurology: Adult Disorders*, pp. 297–322. New York: Grune & Stratton.

Goodglass, H., & Kaplan, E. (1983). *The Assessment of Aphasia and Related Disorders*, 2nd ed. Philadelphia: Lea & Febiger.

Goodwin, D. W. (1989). Alcoholism. In Kaplan, H. I., & Sadock, B. J. (Eds.), *Comprehensive Textbook of Psychiatry*, Vol. I, 5th ed., pp. 686–698. Baltimore: Williams & Wilkins.

Gordon, W. P. (1985). Neuropsychologic assessment of aphasia. In Darby, J. K. (Ed.), *Speech and Language Evaluation in Neurology: Adult Disorders*, pp. 161–196. New York: Grune & Stratton.

Gorman, J. R., & Locke, S. E. (1989). Neural, endocrine and immune interactions. In Kaplan, H. I., & Sadock, B. J. (Eds.), *Comprehensive Textbook of Psychiatry*, Vol. I, 5th ed., pp. 111–124. Baltimore: Williams & Wilkins.

Gosselin, R. W., Smith, R. P., & Hodge, H. D. (1984). *Clinical Toxicology of Commercial Products*, 5th ed. Baltimore: Williams & Wilkins.

Glover, H. (1988). Four syndromes of post-traumatic stress disorder: Stressors and conflicts of the traumatized with special focus on the Viet Nam combat veteran. *Journal of Traumatic Stress*, 1, 57–78.

Goyer, R. A. (1986). Toxic effects of metals. In Klaassen, C. D., Amdur, M. O., & Doull, J. (Eds.), *Casarett and Doull's Toxicology*, pp. 582–636. New York: Macmillan.

Grafman, J., et al. (1988). Intellectual function following penetrating head injury in Vietnam veterans. *Brain*, 3, 169–184.

Graham, D. I., Lawrence, A. E., Adams, I. H., Doyle, D., McClellan, D., & Gennarelli, T. A. (1989). Pathology of mild head injury. In Hoff, J. T., Anderson, T. E., & Cole, T. M. (Eds.), *Mild to Moderate Head Injury*, pp. 63–75. Boston: Blackwell Scientific Publications.

Graham, D. I., Adams, J. H., & Gennarelli, T. A. (1987). Pathology of brain damage in head injury. In Cooper, P. R. (Ed.), *Head Injury*, 2nd ed., pp. 72–88. Baltimore: Williams & Wilkins.

Grant, I., & Alves, W. (1987). Psychiatric and psychosocial disturbances in head injury. In Levin, H. S. Grafman, J., & Eisenberg, H. M. (Eds.), *Neurobehavioral Recovery from Head Injury*, pp. 233–261, Oxford University Press.

Gray, J. W., & Dean, R. S. (1986). Neuropsychological correlates of depression. *Archives of Clinical Neuropsychology*, 1, 298–299, abstract.

Green, A. H. (1985). Children traumatized by physical abuse. In Eth, S., & Pynoos, R. S. (Eds.), *Post-traumatic Stress Disorder in Children*, pp. 133–154. Washington, DC: American Psychiatric Association.

Greiffenstein, M. F., Verma, N. P., Nichols, C. D., & Delacruz, C. R. (1989). Neuropsychological validation of two dementia categories: A preliminary study. *Neuropsychiatry, Neuropsychology, and Behavioral Neurology*, 2, 21–30.

Grigsby, J. P. (1986). Depersonalization following minor closed head injury. *The International Journal of Clinical Neuropsychology*, 8, 65–68.

Guss, D. A. (1985). The head-injured patient: Prehospital care. *Trauma*, 2(1), 1–7.

Guthrie, R. (1986). Lead exposure in children: The need for professional and public education. In Wisniewski, H. M., & Snider, D. A. *Mental Retardation: Research, Education, and Technology Transfer. Annals of the New York Academy of Sciences*, Vol. 477. New York: New York Academy of Sciences.

Haas, D. C., & Ross, G. S. (1986). Transient global amnesia triggered by mild head trauma. *Brain*, 109, 251–257.

Hadden, J. W. (1987). Neuroendocrine modulation of the thymus-dependent immune system: Agonists and Mechanisms. In Jankovic, B. D., Markovic, B. M., & Spector, N. H. (Eds.), *Neuroimmune Interactions: Proceedings of the Second International Workshop on Neuroimmunomodulation. Annals of the N.Y. Academy of Sciences*, 496, 39–48.

Hadley, M. N., Sonntag, V. K. H., Rekate, H. L., & Murphy, A. (1989). The infant whiplash-shake injury syndrome: A clinical and pathological study. *Neurosurgery*, 24, 536–540.

Hales, R. E., & Yudofsky, S. C. (1987). *Textbook of Neuropsychiatry*. Washington, DC: American Psychiatric Press.

Hall, H. V., & McNinch, D. (1988). Linking crime-specific behavior to neuropsychological impairment. *International Journal of Clinical Neuropsychology*, 10, 113–122.

Halpern, F. (1953). *A Clinical Approach to Children's Rorschachs*. New York: Grune & Stratton.

Hans, S. L. (1980). Develomental consequences of prenatal exposure to methadone. In Hutchings, D. E. (Ed.), *Prenatal Abuse of Licit and Illicit Drugs. Annals of the N.Y. Academy of Sciences*, **562**, 195–207.

Hart, K., & Faust, D. (1988). Prediction of the effects of mild head injury: A message about the Kennard principle. *Journal of Clinical Psychology*, **44**, 780–782.

Hartig, B. (1984). Pain – Symptoms, causes and modes of treatment. Framingham, MA: National Head Injury Foundation.

Hartlage, L. C., & Hartlage, P. L. (1989). Neuropsychological aspects of epilepsy: Introduction and overview. In Reynolds, C. R., & Fletcher-Janaen, E. (Eds.), *Handbook of Clinical Child Neuropsychology*, pp. 409–417. New York: Plenum.

Hartlage, L. C., & Telzrow, C. F. (1986). *Neuropsychological Assessment and Intervention with Children and Adolescents*. Sarasota, FL: Professional Resource Exchange.

Hartman, D. E. (1987). Neuropsychological toxicology: Identification and assessment of neurotoxic syndromes. *Archives of Clinical Neuropsychology*, , 45–65.

Hartman, D. E. (1988). *Neuropsychological Toxicology*. New York: Pergamon.

Hartmann, E. (1988). Who has nightmares? Interview. *The Harvard Medical School Mental Health Letter*, **4**(4), 8.

Hass, W. K., & Hawkins, R. A. (1978). Bilateral reticular formation lesions causing coma: Their effects on regional cerebral blood flow, glucose utilization and oxidative metabolism, In Korein, J. (Ed.), *Brain Death: Interrelated Medical and Social Issues. Annals of the N.Y. Academy of Sciences*, **325**, 105–109.

Hastings, L., & Sun, T. (1987). Effects of cadmium on the rat olfactory system. In Roper, S. D., & Aterna, J. (Eds.), *Olfaction and Taste IX*, p. 355. New York: The New York Academy of Sciences.

Headlines. Coming to terms with sexuality and head injury. March/April 1988, 1–3.

Heaton, R. K. (1981). *Wisconsin Card Sorting Test Manual*. Odessa, FL: Psychological Assessment Resources.

Heilman, K. M., & Rothi, L. J. G. (1985). Apraxia. In Heilman, K. M., & Valenstein, E. (Eds.), *Clinical Neuropsychology*, 2nd ed., pp. 131–150. New York: Oxford University Press.

Heilman, K. M., Watson, R. T., & Bowers, D. (1983). Affective disorders associated with hemispheric disease. In Heilman, K. M., & Satz, P. (Eds.), *Neuropsychology of Human Emotions*, pp. 45–64. New York: Guilford.

Heilman, K. M., Watson, R. T., & Valenstein, E. (1985). Neglect and related disorders. In Heilman, K. M., & Valenstein, E. (Eds.), *Clinical Neuropsychology*, 2nd ed., pp. 234–293. New York: Oxford University Press.

Helzer, J. E., Robbins, L. N., & McEvoy, L. (1987). Post-traumatic stress disorder in the general population. *The New England Journal of Medicine*, pp. 1630–1634.

Hendler, N. (1981a). *Diagnosis and Nonsurgical Management of Chronic Pain*. New York: Raven.

Hendler, N. (1981b). Depression caused by chronic pain. *The Journal of Clinical Psychiatry*, **45**(3) (Reprint unpaged).

Herrenkohl, L. R. (1986). Prenatal stress disrupts reproductive behavior and physiology in offspring. In Komisaruk, B. R., Siegel, H. I., Cheng, M-F., & Feder, H. H. (Eds.), *Reproduction: A Behavioral and Neuroendocrine Perspective*, pp. 120–128. New York: New York Academy of Sciences.

Herskowitz, J., & Rosman, N. P. (1982). *Pediatrics, Neurology, and Psychiatry-Common Ground*. New York: Macmillan.

Heverly, L., Isaac, W., & Hynd, G. W. (1986). Neurodevelopmental and racial differences in tactile-visual (cross-modal) discrimination in normal black and white children. *Archives of Clinical Neuropsychology*, **1**, 139–145.

Hillyard, S. A., & Hansen, J. C. (1986). Attention: Electrophysiological Approaches. In Coles, M. G. H., Donchin, E., & Porges, S. W. (Eds.), *Psychophysiology: Systems, Processes, and Applications*, pp. 227–243. New York: Guilford.

Hinds, M. D. (1989). Bareheaded motorcyclists pressed anew to cover up. *New York Times*, 1/14/89, p. 50.

Hodges, J. R., & Ward, C. D. (1989). Observations during transient global amnesia: A behavioural and neuropsychological study of five cases. *Brain*, **112**, 595–620.

Holson, R. R., Ali, S. F., & Scallet, A. C. (1988). The effect of isolation rearing and stress on monoamines in forebrain nigrostriatal, mesolimbic, and mesocortical dopamine systems. In Kalivas, P. W., & Nemeroff, C. B. (Eds.), *The Mesocorticolimbic Dopamine System, Annals of the New York Academy of Sciences*, Vol. 537, 512–514. New York: The New York Academy of Sciences.

Horvath, T. B., Siever, L. J., Mohns, R. C., & Davis, K. (1989). Organic mental syndromes and disorders. In Kaplan, H. I., & Sadock, B. J. (Eds.), *Comprehensive Textbook of Psychiatry*, Vol. I, 5th ed., pp. 599–639. Baltimore: Williams & Wilkins.

House, J. S., Landis, K. R., & Umberson, D. (1988). Social relationships and health. *Science*, **241**, 540–545.

Hovind, H. (1986). Traumatic birth injuries. In Raimondi, A. J., Choux, M., & Di Rocco, C. (Eds.), *Head Injuries in the Newborn and Infant*, pp. 7–109. New York: Springer-Verlag.

Howard, J. H., Cunningham, D. A., & Rechnitzer, P. A. (1986). Personality (hardiness) as a moderator of job stress and coronary risk in type A individuals: A longitudinal study. *Journal of Behavioral Medicine*, **9**, 229–244.

Hutchings, D. E. (Ed.). (1989). *Prenatal Abuse of Licit and Illicit Drugs. Annals of the N.Y. Academy of Sciences*, **562**.

Hynd, G. W., Connor, R. T., & Nieves, N. (1990). Learning disabilities subtypes: Perspectives and methodological issues in clinical assessment. In Tramontana, M. G., & Hooper, S. R. (Eds.), *Assessment Issues in Child Neuropsychology*, pp. 281–312.

Hynd, G. W., & Willis, W. G. (1988). *Pediatric Neuropsychology*. New York: Grune & Stratton.

Incagnoli, T. G., Goldstein, G., & Golden, C. J. (1986). *Clinical Application of Neuropsychological Test Batteries*. New York: Plenum.

Inhoff, A. W., Diener, H. C., Rafa, R. D., & Ivry, R. (1989). The role of cerebellar structures in the execution of seria movements. *Brain*, **112**, 565–582.

Jacobson, A., & Richardson, B. (1987). Assault experiences of 100 psychiatric inpatients: Evidence of the need for routine inquiry. *American Journal of Psychiatry*, **144**, 908–913.

Jafek, B. W., Eller, P. M., Esses, B. A., & Moran, D. T. (1989). Post-traumatic anosmia: Ultrastructural correlates. *Archives of Neurology*, **46**, 300–304.

Jaffe, J. H. (1989). Drug dependence: Opioids, narcotics, nicotine (tobacco), and caffeine. In Kaplan, H. I., & Sadock, B. J. (Eds.), *Comprehensive Textbook of Psychiatry*, Vol. I, 5th ed., pp. 642–686. Baltimore: Williams & Wilkins.

Jaffe, K. M. (1986). Preface: Pediatric head injury. *Journal of Head Trauma Rehabilitation*, **1**(4), ix.

Jaffe, K. M., Hayes, R. M. (1986). Pediatric head injury: Rehabilitative medical management. *Journal of Head Trauma Rehabilitation*, **1**(4), 30–40.

Jankovic, B. D. (1987). Opening remarks. In Jankovic, B. D., Marcovic, B. M., & Spector,

N. H. (1987). *Neuro-immune Reactions*. Annals of the N.Y. Academy of Sciences, **496**, 1–2.

Janoff-Bulman, R. (1985). The aftermath of victimization: Rebuilding shattered assumptions. In Figley, C. R. (Ed.), *Trauma and Its Wake*, pp. 15–35. New York: Brunner/Mazel.

James, H. E. (1985). Evaluation of head injury in reference to therapy. In James, H. E., Anas, N. G., & Perkin, R. M. (Eds.), *Brain Insults in Infants and Children: Pathophysiology and Management*, pp. 237–244. New York: Grune & Stratton.

Jenkins, L. W., Lyeth, B. G., & Hayes. (1989). The role of agonist-receptor interactions in the pathophysiology of mild and moderate head injury. In Hoff, J. T., Anderson, T. E., & Cole, T. M. (Eds.), *Mild to Moderate Head Injury*, pp. 47–61. Boston: Blackwell Scientific Publications.

Jennings, J. R. (1986). Bodily changes during attending. In Coles, M. G. H., Donchin, E., & Porges, S. W. (Eds.), *Psychophysiology: Systems, Processes, and Applications*, pp. 269–289. New York: Guilford.

Jordan, F. M., Ozanne, A. E., & Murdoch, B. E. (1988). Long-term speech and language disorders subsequent to closed head injury in children. *Brain Injury*, **2**, 179–185.

Joseph, R. (1988). The right cerebral hemisphere: Emotion, music, visual-spatial skills, body-image, dreams and awareness. *Journal of Clinical Psychology*, **44**, 630–674.

Kales, A., & Kales, J. D. (1984). *Evaluation and Treatment of Insomnia*. New York: Oxford University Press.

Kaltenbach, K., & Finnegan, L. P. (1989). Children exposed to methadone in utero: Assessment of develomental and cognitive ability. In Hutchings, D. E. (Ed.), *Prenatal abuse of Licit and Illicit Drugs. Annals of the New York Academy of Sciences*, **562**, 360–362.

Kalivas, P. W., & Nemeroff, C. B. (Eds.). (1988). *The Mesocorticolimbic Dopamine System, Annals of the N.Y. Academy of Sciences*, Vol. 537. New York: The New York Academy of Sciences.

Kampaus, R. W., & Reynolds, C. (1987). *Clinical and Research Applications of the K-ABC*. Circle Pines, MN: American Guidance Service.

Kandel, E., & Freed, D. (1989). Frontal-lobe dysfunction and antisocial behavior: A review. *Journal of Clinical Psychology*, **45**, 404–413.

Kandel, E. R., & Schwartz, J. H. (1985). *Principles of Neural Science*, 2nd ed. New York: Elsevier.

Kaplan, E. (1988). A process approach to neuropsychogical assessment. In Boll, T., & Bryant, B. K. (Eds.), *Clinical Neuropsychology and Brain Function: Research, Measurement and Practice*. Washington, DC: American Psychological Association.

Karol, R. L. (1989). Duration of seeking help following traumatic brain injury: Thy persistence of symptom complaints. *The Clinical Neuropsychologist*, **3**, 244–249.

Katzman, R., & Pappius, H. M. (1973). *Brain Electrolytes and Fluid Metabolism*. Baltimore: Williams & Wilkins.

Kaufman, A. S. (1979). *Intelligent Testing with the WISC-R*. New York: Wiley.

Keefe, F. J., Wilkins, R. H., Cook, W. A., Crisson, J. E., & Muhlbaier, L. H. (1986). Depression, pain and pain behavior. *Journal of Consulting and Clinical Psychology*, **54**, 665–669.

Kelly, J. P. (1985). Reactions of neurons to injury. In Kandel, E. R., & Schwartz, J. H. (Eds.), *Principles of Neural Science*, 2nd ed., pp. 187–195. New York: Elsevier.

Kelly, R. E., & Smith, B. N. (1981). The post-traumatic syndrome. *Journal of the Royal Society of Medicine*, **74**, 275–277.

Kennedy, C. R., & Freeman, J. M. (1986). Posttraumatic seizures and posttraumatic epilepsy in children. *Journal of Head Trauma Rehabilitation*, **1**, 66–73.

Kewman, D. G., Yanus, B., & Kirsch, N. (1988). Assessment of distractibility in auditory comprehension after traumatic brain injury. *Brain Injury*, **2**, 131–138.

Kirshner, H. S., Casey, P. F., Kelly, M. P., & Webb, W. G. (1987). Anomia. *Neuropsychologia*, **25**, 701–705.

Kishore, P. R. S., & Hall, J. A. (1987). Radiographic evaluation. In Cooper, P. R. (Ed.), *Head Injury*, 2nd ed., pp. 51–71. Baltimore: Williams & Wilkins.

Klaassen, C. D., Amdur, M. O., & Doull, J. (Eds.). (1986). *Casarett and Doull's Toxicology*. New York: Macmillan.

Klauber, K. W., & Ward-McKinlay, C. (1986). Managing behavior in the patient with traumatic brain injury. *Topics in Acute Care and Trauma Rehabilitation*, **1**(1), 48–60.

Klopfer, B., Ainsworth, M. D., Klopfer, W., & Holt, R. R. (1954). *Developments in the Rorschach Technique: Vol. I*. Yonkers-on-Hudson, NY: World Book Co.

Knight, R. G. (1983). On interpreting the several standard errors of the WAIS-R: Some further tables. *Journal of Consulting and Clinical Psychology*, **51**, 671–673.

Kobassa, S. C. (1979). Stressful life events, personality and health: An enquiry into hardiness. *Journal of Personality and Social Psychology*, **37**, 1–11.

Kobassa, S. C., Maddi, S. R., & Zola, M. A. (1983). Type A. and hardiness. *Journal of Behavior Medicine*, **67**, 41–51.

Kodimer, C. (1988). Neuropsychological assessment and Social Security disability: Writing meaningful reports and documentation. *Journal of Head Trauma Rehabilitation*, **3**(1), 77–85.

Kolb, L. C. (1986). Treatment of chronic post-traumatic stress disorders. In Masserman, J. (Ed.), *Current Psychiatric Therapies*, pp. 119–127. New York: Grune & Stratton.

Kolb, L. C. (1987). A neuropsychological hypothesis explaining posttraumatic stress disorders. *American Journal of Psychiatry*, **144**, 989–995.

Kolb, L. C. (1988). A critical survey of hypotheses regarding post-traumatic stress disorders in light of recent research findings. *Journal of Traumatic Stress*, **1**, 291–304.

Kolb, L. C., Burris, B. C., & Griffiths, S. (1984). Propranolol and clinidine in treatment of the chronic posttraumatic stress disorders of war. In van der Kolk, B. A. (Ed.), *Post-Traumatic Stress Disorder: Psychological and Biological Sequelae*, pp. 59–79. Washington, DC: American Psychiatric Press.

Korein, J. (1978). *Brain Death: Interrelated Medical and Social Issues. Annals of the New York Academy of Sciences*, **325**.

Krane, R. J., Siroky, M. B., & Goldstein, I. (Eds.). (1983). *Male Sexual dysfunction*. Boston: Little, Brown.

Kraus, J. F., & Arzemanian. (1989). Epidemiologic features of mild and moderate brain injury. In Hoff, J. T., Anderson, T. E., & Cole, T. M. (Eds.), *Mild to Moderate Head Injury*, pp. 9–28. Boston: Blackwell Scientific Publications.

Kraus, J. F., Morgenstern, H., Fife, D., Conroy, C., & Nourijah, P. (1989). Blood alcohol tests, prevalence of involvement, and outcomes following brain injury. *American Journal of Public Health*, **79**, 294–299.

Kreitler, S., & Kreitler, H. (1988). Trauma and anxiety: The cognitive approach. *Journal of Traumatic Stress*, **1**, 35–56.

Kreutzer, J. S., & Zasler, N. D. (1989). Psychosexual consequences of traumatic brain injury: Methodology and preliminary findings. *Brain Injury*, **3**, 177–186.

Kreutzer, J. S., Wehman, P., Morton, M. V., & Stonnington, H. H. (1988). Supported employment and compensatory strategies for enhancing vocational outcome following traumatic brain injury. *Brain Injury*, **2**, 205–233.

Krystal, H. (1984). Psychoanalytic views on human emotional damages. In van der Kolk, B. A. (Ed.), *Post-traumatic stress disorder: Psychological and Biological Sequelae*, pp. 1–25. Washington, DC: American Psychiatric Press.

Krystal, J. H., Giller, E. L., & Cicchetti, D. V. (1986). Assessment of alexithymia in posttraumatic stress disorder and somatic illness: Introduction of a reliable measure. *Psychosomatic Medicine*. **48**, 84–89.

Kurtz, D. (1987). Trigeminal chemoreception. In Roper, S. D., & Aterna, J. (Eds.), *Olfaction and Taste IX*, pp. 127–129. New York: The New York Academy of Sciences.

Lam, C. S., McMahon, B. T., Priddy, D. A., & Gehred-Schultz, A. (1988). Deficit awareness and treatment performance among traumatic head injury adults. *Brain Injury*, **2**, 235–242.

Lamb, M. R., Robertson, L. C., & Knight, R. T. (1989). Attention and interference in the processing of global and local information: Effects of unilateral temporal-parietal junction lesions. *Neuropsychologia*, **27**, 471–484.

Langfitt, T. W., & Zimmerman, R. A. (1985). Imaging and in vivo biochemistry of the brain in head injury. In Becker, D. P., & Povlishock, J. T. (Eds.), *Central Nervous System Trauma Status Report–1985*, pp. 53–63. National Institute of Neurological and Communicative Disorders and Stroke. National Institutes of Health.

Laplane, D., et al. (1989). Obsessive compulsive and other behavioural changes with bilateral basal ganglia lesions. *Brain*, **112**, 699–725.

Larsen, M. (1986). Normal developmental milestones, the significance of delayed milestones, and neurodevelopmental evaluation of infants and young children. In Raimondi, A. J., Choux, M., & DiRocco, C. (Eds.), *Head injuries in the newborn and infant*, pp. 67–81. New York: Springer-Verlag.

Laufer, R. S., Brett, E., & Gallops, M. S. (1984). Posttraumatic stress disorder (PTSD) reconsidered: PTSD among Vietnam Veterans. In Van Der Kolk, B. A. (Ed.), *Post-Traumatic Stress Disorder: Psychological and Biological Sequelae*, pp. 59–79. Washington: American Psychiatric Association.

Lawson, G. W. (1988). Adverse reactions to drugs. In Lawson, G. W., & Cooperrider, C. A. (Eds.), *Clinical Psychopharmacology*, pp. 275–284. Rockville, MD: Aspen.

Lazarus, R. S., & Folkman, S. (1984). Coping and adaptation. In Gentry, W. D. (Ed.), *Handbook of Behavioral Medicine*, pp. 282–325. New York: Guilford.

Lecours, A. R., Mehler, J., et al. (1987). Illiteracy and brain damage-I. Aphasia testing in culturally contrasted populations (control subjects). *Neuropsychologia*, **25**, 231–245.

Lee, G. P., Arena, J. G., Meador, K. J., Smith, J. R., Loring, D. W., & Flanigin, H. F. (1988). Changes in autonomic responsiveness following bilateral amygdalotomy in humans. *Neuropsychiatry, Neuropsychology, and Behavioral Neurology*, **1**, 119–129.

Lees-Haley, P. R. (1989). MMPI-F and F-K Scales: Questionable indices of malingering. *American Journal of Forensic Psychology*, **7**, 81–83.

Leonard, G., Jones, L., & Milner, B. (1988). Residual impairment in handgrip strength after unilateral frontal-lobe lesions. *Neuropsychologia*, **26**, 555–564.

Levin, H. S. (1981). Aphasia in closed head injury. In Sarno, M. T. (Ed.), *Acquired Aphasia*, pp. 427–463. New York: Academic Press.

Levin, H. S. (1985), Outcome after head injury: Part II. Neurobehavioral Recovery. In Becker, D. P., & Povlishock, J. T. (Eds.), *Central Nervous System Status Report–1985*, pp. 281–299. National Institute of Neurological and Communicative Disorders and Stroke, National Institutes of Health.

Levin, H. S. (1987). Neurobehavioral sequelae of head injury. In Cooper, P. R. (Ed.), *Head Injury*, 2nd ed., pp. 442–463. Baltimore: Williams & Wilkins.

Levin, H. S., Benton, H. S., & Grossman, R. G. (1982). *Neurobehavioral Consequences of Closed Head Injury*. New York: Oxford University Press.

Levin, H. S., High, W. M., & Eisenberg, H. M. (1985). Impairment of olfactory recognition after closed head injury. *Brain*, **108**, 579–591.

Levin, H. S., Amparo, E. G., Eisenberg, H. M., Miner, M. E., High, W. M., Ewing-Cobbs, L., Fletcher, J. M., & Guinto, F. C. (1989). *Neurosurgery*, **24**, 223–227.

Levin, R. (1987). *Reducing Lead in Drinking Water*. Environmental Protection Agency, United States Environmental Protection Agency. (EPA Report-230-09-86-019).

Levine, P. (1986). Stress. In Coles, M. G. H., Donchin, E. & Porges, S. W. (Eds.), *Psychophysiology: Systems, Processes and Applications*, pp. 331–353. New York: Guilford.

Levy, D. W., Knill-Jones, & Plum, F. (1978). The vegetative state and its prognosis following nontraumatic coma. In Korein, J. (Ed.), *Brain Death: Interrelated Medical and Social Issues*, pp. 293–306. Annals of the N.Y. Academy of Science, **315**.

Lewis, D. O., Pincus, J. H., Feldman, M., Jackson, L., & Bard, B. (1986). Psychiatric, neurological, and psychoeducational characteristics of 15 death row inmates in the United States. *American Journal of Psychiatry*, **143**, 838–845.

Lewis, G. R., & Lawson, G. W. (1988). Heroin. In Lawson, G. W., & Cooperrider, C. A. (Eds.), *Clinical Psychopharmacology*, pp. 237–242. Rockville, MD: Aspen.

Lewis, R. J., Dlugokinski, E. L., Caputo, L. M., & Griffin, R. B. (1988). Children at risk for emotional disorders. *Clinical Psychology Review*, **8**, 417–448.

Lewis, R. S., & Harris, L. J. (1988). The relationship between cerebral lateralization and cognitive ability: Suggested criteria for empirical tests. *Brain and Cognition*, **8**, 275–280.

Lewis, W. H. (1936). *Gray's Anatomy*. Philadelphia: Lea & Febiger.

Lezak, M. (1983). *Principles of Neuropsychological Assessment*, 2nd ed. New York: Oxford University Press.

Libet, B. (1987). Consciousness: Consconscious, subjective, experience. In Adelman, G. (Ed.), *Encyclopedia of Neuroscience. I*, pp. 271–275. Boston: Birkhauser.

Lindberg, N., Basch-Kahre, E., & Lindberg, E. (1982). Psychotherapeutic examination of patients with suspected chronic solvent intoxication. *Psychotherapy and Psychosomatics*, **37**, 36–63.

Lippold, S., & Claiborn, J. M. (1983). Comparison of the Wechsler Adult Intelligence Scale and the Wechsler Intelligence Scale-Revised. *Journal of Consulting and Clinical Psychology*, **51**, p. 315.

Lishman, W. A. (1987). *Organic Psychiatry*. Boston: Blackwell Scientific Publications.

Livingston, R. B. (1985). Section IX. Neurophysiology. In West, J. B. (Ed.), *Best and Taylor's Physiological Basis of Medical Practice*, 11th ed., pp. 970–1295. Baltimore: Williams & Wilkins.

Loberg, Tor. (1986). Neuropsychological findings in the early and middle phases of alcoholism. In Grant, I., & Adams, K. M. (Eds.), *Neuropsychological Assessment of Neuropsychiatric Disorders*, pp. 415–440. New York: Oxford University Press.

Loring, D. W., Lee, G. P., Martin, R. C., & Meador, K. J. (1989). Verbal and visual memory index discrepancies from the Wechsler Memory Scale-Rev.: Cautions in interpretation. *Psychological Assessment*, **1**, 198–202.

Luerssen, T. G. (1985). Resuscitation of brain-injured children: Special considerations. *Trauma*, **2**(1), 20–25.

Luria, A. R. (1980). *Higher Cortical Functions in Man*, 2nd ed. New York: Basic Books.

Lyon, G. R., Moats, L., & Flynn, J. M. (1988). From assessment to treatment: Linkage to interventions with children. In Tramontana, M. G., & Hooper, S. R. (Eds.), *Assessment Issues in Child Neuropsychology*, pp. 113–142. New York: Plenum.

Lytton, W. W., & Brust, J. C. M. (1989). Direct dyslexia: Preserved oral reading of real words in Wernicke's aphasia. *Brain*, **112**, 583–594.

Mack, J. L. (1986). Clinical assessment of disorders of attention and memory. *Journal of Head Trauma Rehabilitation*, **1**(3), 22–33.

Maestroni, J. G. M., Conti, A., & Pierpaoli, W. (1987). The pineal gland and the circadian, opiatergic, immunoregulatory role of melatonin. In Jankovic, B. D., Markovic, B. M., & Spector, N. H. (Eds.), *Neuroimmune Interactions: Proceedings of the Second International Workshop on Neuroimmunomodulation. Annals of the N.Y. Academy of Sciences*, **496**, 67–77.

Mann, J. J., & Stanley, M. (1986). *Psychobiology of Suicidal Behavior. Annals of the N.Y. Academy of Sciences*, **487**.

Mark, V. H., & Ervin, F. R. (1970). *Violence and the Brain*. New York: Harper and Row.

Markowitsch, H. J. (1988). Diencephalic amnesia: A reorientation towards tracts? *Brain Research Bulletin*, **13**, 351–370.

Marmarou, A., & Tabaddor, K. (1987). Intracranial pressure: Physiology and pathophysiology. In Cooper, P. R. (Ed.), *Head Injury*, 2nd ed., pp. 159–176. Baltimore: Williams & Wilkins.

Marshall, E. (1983). EPA faults classic lead poisoning study. *Science*, **222**, 906–907.

Marshall, L. F., & Marshall, S. B. (1985a). Current clinical head injury research in the United States. In Becker, D. B., & Povlishock, J. T. (Eds.), *Central Nervous System Trauma Status Report—1985*, pp. 45–51. National Institute of Neurological and Communicative Disorders and Stroke, National Institutes of Health.

Marshall, L. F., & Marshall, S. B. (1985b). Epidemiological and descriptive studies. Part II: Current clinical head injury research in the United States. In Becker, D. P., & Povlishock, J. T. (Eds.), *Central Nervous System Trauma Status Report—1985*, pp. 45–51. National Institutes of Neurological and Communicative Disorders and Stroke, National Institute of Health.

Martin, J. H. (1985). Development as a guide to the regional anatomy of the brain. In Kandel, E. R., & Schwartz, J. H. (Eds.), *Principles of Neural Science*, 2nd ed., pp. 244–258. New York: Elsevier.

Masdeu, J. C. (1985a). The localization of lesions affecting the cerebral hemispheres. In Brazis, P. W., Masdeu, J. C., & Biller, J. (Eds.), *Localization in Clinical Neurology*, pp. 289–359. Boston: Little, Brown.

Masdeu, J. C. (1985b). The localization of lesions causing coma. In Brazis, P. W., Masdeu, J. C., & Biller, J. (Eds.), *Localization in Clinical Neurology*, pp. 381–405. Boston: Little, Brown.

Masdeu, J. C. (1985c). The localization of lesions in the oculomotor system. In Brazis, P. W., Masdeu, J. C., & Biller, J. (Eds.), *Localization in Clinical Neurology*, pp. 117–157. Boston: Little, Brown.

Matarazzo, J. D. (1987). Validity of psychological assessment: From the clinic to the courtroom. *The Clinical Neuropsychologist*, **4**, 307–314.

Matarazzo, J. D., & Herman, D. O. (1984). Relationship of education and IQ in the WAIS-R standardization sample. *Journal of Consulting and Clinical Psychology*, **52**, 631–634.

Matarazzo, J. D., & Herman, D. O. (1985). Clinical uses of the WAIS-R: Base rates of differences between VIQ and PIQ in the WAIS-R standardization sample. In Wolman, B. B. (Ed.), *Handbook of Intelligence: Theories, Measurements and Applications*, pp. 899–932. New York: Wiley.

Matarazzo, J. D., Bornstein, R. A., McDermott, P. A., & Noonon, J. V. (1986). Verbal IQ versus performance IQ differences scores in males and females from the WAIS-R standardization sample. *Journal of Clinical Psychology*, **42**, 965–974, as corrected by *JCP*, 1987, **43**, 293–297.

Matarazzo, J. D., Daniel, M. H., Prifitera, A., & Herman, D. O. (1988). Inter-subtest scatter in the WAIS-R standardization sample. *Journal of Clinical Psychology*, **44**, 941–950.

Mayes, C. D., Pelco, L. E., & Campbell, C. J. (1989). Relationships among pre- and post-injury intelligence, length of coma and age in individuals with severe closed head injuries. *Brain Injury*, **3**, 301–313.

McCaig, J., & Lawson, G. W. (1988). Marijuana. In Lawson, G. W., & Cooperrider, C. A. (Eds.), *Clinical Psychopharmacology*, pp. 243–250. Rockville, MD: Aspen.

McCarthy, R. A., & Warrington, E. K. (1987). Understanding: A function of short-term memory. *Brain*, **110**, 1565–1578.

McClellend, J. L. (1985). Distributed models of cognitive processes. In Olton, D. S., Gamzu, E., & Corkin, S. (Eds.), *Memory Dysfunctions: An Integration of Animal and Human Research from Preclinical and Clinical Perspectives*. *Annals of the N.Y. Academy of Science*, **444**, 1–9.

McComb, J. G. (1985). Impaired cerebrospinal fluid circulation: Alternative pathways. In James, H. E., Anas, N. G., & Perkin, R. M. (Eds.), *Brain Insults in Infants and Children: Pathophysiology and Management*. pp. 75–81. New York: Grune & Stratton.

McGaugh, J. L. (1983). Preserving the presence of the past: Hormonal influences on memory storage. *American Psychologist*, **38**, 161–174.

McGuire, T. A., & Rothenberg, M. B. (1986). Behavioral and psychosocial sequelae of pediatric head injury. *The Journal of Head Trauma Rehabilitation*. **1**(4), 1–6.

McKeny, R. (1983). Deficits in activities of daily living. In Rosenthal, M., Griffith, G., Bond, M., & Miller, J. D. (Eds.), *Rehabilitation of the Head Injured Adult*, pp. 143–153. Philadelphia: F.A. Davis.

McKeon, J., McGuffin, P., & Robinson, P. (1984). Obsessive-compulsive neurosis following head injury: A report of four cases. *British Journal of Psychiatry*, **144**, 190–192.

McMahon, E. A., & Satz, P. (1981). Clinical psychology: Some forensic applications. In Filskov, S. B., & Boll, T. J., (Eds.), *Handbook of Clinical Neuropsychology*, pp. 689–701. New York: Wiley.

McMordie, W.R., & Barker, S. L. (1989). The financial trauma of head injury. *Brain*, **2**, 357–364.

Mednick, S. A. (1980). Human nature, crime and society. *Annals of the New York Academy of Science*, **347**, 335–348.

Meltzer, H. Y., & Lowy, M. T. (1986). Neuroendocrine function in psychiatric disorders and behavior. *American Handbook of Psychiatry*, 2nd ed., Vol. 8, pp. 111–150. New York: Basic Books.

Menkes, J. H. (1985). *Textbook of Child Neurology*, 3rd ed. Philadelphia: Lea & Febiger.

Mercury Exposure (1980). *Science News*, **118**, 118.

Merriam, A. E. (1988). Emotional arousal-induced transient global amnesia. *Neuropsychiatry, Neuropsychology, and Behavioral Neurology*, **1**, 73–78.

Messing, R. B. (1987). Learning and memory dysfunction as selective neurotoxic effects. In Tilson, H. A., & Sparber, S. B. (Eds.), *Neurotoxicants and Neurobiological Function*, pp. 281–302. New York: Wiley.

Mesulem, M-Marsel. (1985). Attention, confusional states, and neglect. In Mesulam, M. (Ed.), *Principles of Behavioral Neurology*, pp. 125–168. Philadelphia: F.A. Davis.

Millan, M. J., & Emrich, H. M. (1981). Endophinergic systems and the response to stress. *Psychotherapy and Psychosomatics*, **36**, 43–56.

Miller, T. W. (1988). Advances in understanding the impact of stressful life events on health. *Hospital and Community Psychiatry*, pp. 615–622.

Miller, W. G. (1986). The neuropsychology of head injuries. In Wedding, D., Horton, A. M., & Webster, J. (Eds.), *The Neuropsychology Handbook*, pp. 347–375. New York: Springer.

Miner, M. E. (1985). Systematic effects of brain injury. *Trauma*, **2**(1), 75–83.

Mishkin, M., & Appenzeller, T. (1987). The anatomy of memory. *Scientific American*, **226**(6), 6/87, 80–89.

Moehle, K. A., & Fitzhugh-Bell, K. B. (1986). Lateralization of brain damage and emotional response in patients referred for neuropsychological testing. *Archives of Clinical Neuropsychology*. **1**, 264–265, abstract.

Moore, A. D. (1989). Stambrook, M., & Peters, L. C. (1989). Coping strategies and adjustment after closed-head injury: A cluster analytical approach. *Brain Injury*, **3**, 171–176.

Morse, P. A., & Morse, A. R. (1988). Functional living skills: Promoting the interaction between neuropsychology and occupational therapy. *Journal of Head Trauma Rehabilitation*, **3**, 33–44.

Muizellaar, J. P., & Obrist, W. D. (1985). Cerebral blood flow and brain metabolism with brain injury. In Becker, D. P., & Povlishock, J. T. (Eds.), *Central Nervous System Trauma Status Report—1985*, pp. 123–137. National Institute of Neurological and Communicative Disorders and Stroke, National Institutes of Health.

Murdoch, B. E., Chenery, H. J., & Kennedy, M. (1989). Aphemia associated with bilateral striato-capsular lesions subsequent to cerebral anoxia. *Brain Injury*, **3**, 41–49.

Mutti, M., Sterling, H. M., & Spalding, N. V. (1978). *Neurological Screening Test*, rev. ed. Novato, CA: Academic Therapy Publications.

Naglieri, J. A. (1982). Two types of tables for use with the WAIS-R. *Journal of Consulting and Clinical Psychology*, **50**, 319–321.

Naglieri, J. A. (1988). *Draw a Person: A Quantitative Scoring System*. San Antonio: The Psychological Corporation.

National Head Injury Foundation. (1987). Disruption of sexuality can have traumatic effect. *Newsletter*, **6**(1), 4–5.

National Institute for Occupational Safety and Health. (1977). *Occupational Diseases: A Guide to their Recognition*, rev. ed.

National Institutes of Health. (1984). *Head Injury: Hope Through Research*. NIH Publication No. 84-2478, August 1984.

Naugle, R. I. (1987). Catastrophic minor head trauma. *Archives of Clinical Neuropsychology*, **2**, 93–100.

Needleman, H. L., Gunnoe, C., Leviton, A., Reed, R., Peresie, H., Mahjer, C., & Barrett, P. (1979). Deficits in psychologic and classroom performance of children with elevated dentine lead levels. *The New England Journal of Medicine*, **300**, 689–694.

Neiss, R. (1988). Reconceptualizing arousal: Psychobiological states in motor performance. *Psychological Bulletin*, **103**, 345–366.

Neistadt, M. W. (1988). Sexuality and head injury. *Headlines* (New Medico Head Injury
System), March/April 1988, 4–6.

Nemeroff, C. B., & Loosen, P. T. (1987). *Handbook of Clinical Psychoendocrinology.*
New York: Guilford.

Nichelli, P., Bahmanian-Behbahani, G., Gentilini, M., & Vecchi, A. (1988). Preserved
memory abilities in thalamic amnesia. *Brain*, **111**, 1337–1353.

Nichols, P. L. (1987). Minimal brain dysfunction and soft signs: The collaborative perinatal project. In Tupper, D. E. (Ed.), *Soft Neurological Signs*, pp. 179–199. New York:
Grune & Stratton.

Nieuwenhuys, R. (1985). *Chemoarchitecture of the Brain.* New York: Springer-Verlag.

Nilsson, B., & Ponten, U. (1985). Metabolism and neurophysiological function following
head injury. In Becker, D. B., & Povlishock, J. T. (Eds.), *Central Nervous System
Trauma Status Report*, pp. 425–429. National Institute of Neurological and Communicative Disorders and Stroke, National Institutes of Health.

Nissen, M. J. (1986). Neuropsychology of attention and memory. *Journal of Head Trauma
Rehabilitation*, **1**(3), 13–21.

Norton, N. C. (1989). Three scales of alexythymia: Do they measure the same thing?
Journal of Personality Assessment, **53**, 621–637.

Norton, S. (1986). Toxic responses of the central nervous system. In Klaassen, C. D.,
Amdur, M. O., & Doull, J. (Eds.), *Casarett and Doull's Toxicology*, p. 386. New York:
Macmillan.

Norton, W. T. (1972). Formation, structure and biochemistry of myelin. In Siegel, G. J.,
et al. (Eds.), *Basic Neurochemistry*, pp. 74–99. Boston, Little Brown.

Novack, T. A., Daniel, M. S., & Long, C. J. (1984). Factors related to emotional adjustment following head injury. *International Journal of Clinical Neuropsychology*, **6**,
139–141.

Nuechterlein, K. H., & Asarnow, R. F. (1989). Perception and cognition. In Kaplan,
H. I., & Sadock, B. J. (Eds.), *Comprehensive Textbook of Psychiatry*, Vol. I, 5th ed.,
pp. 241–256. Baltimore: Williams & Wilkins.

Oddy, M. (1984). Head injury and social adjustment. In Brooks, N. (Ed.), *Closed Head
Injury: Psychological, Social and Family Consequences.* pp. 109–122. New York:
Oxford University Press.

Oddy, M., Humphrey, M., & Uttley, D. (1978). Subjective impairment and social recovery after closed head injury. *Journal of Neurology, Neurosurgery, and Psychiatry*, **41**,
611–616.

Ogden, J. A. (1988). Language and memory functions after long recovery period in left
hemispherectomized subjects. *Neuropsychologia.* **26**, 645–649.

Olton, D. S., Gamzu, E., & Corkin, S. (Eds.). (1985). *Memory Dysfunctions: An Integration of Animal and Human Research from Preclinical and Clinical Perspectives. Annals
of the New York Academy of Science*, **444**.

Ondrusek, G. (1988). Cocaine. In Lawson, G. W., & Cooperrider, C. A. (Eds.), *Clinical
Psychopharmacology*, pp. 201–235. Rockville, MD: Aspen.

Ornstein, R. E. (1977). *The Psychology of Consciousness*, 2nd ed. New York: Harcourt
Brace Jovanovich.

Pacyna, S. (1985). Management of intra-cranial pressure in the ICU. *Trauma*, **2**(1), 63–74.

Palkovitz, M. (1987). Anatomy of neural pathways affecting CRH secretion. In Ganong,

W. F., Dallman, M. F., & Roberts, J. L. (Eds.), *The Hypothalamic-Pituitary-Adrenal Axis Revisted*, pp. 139–148. New York: The New York Academy of Sciences.

Pansky, B., Allen, D. J., & Budd, G. C. (1988). *Review of Neuroscience*, 2nd ed. New York: Macmillan.

Panzeri, M., Semenza, C., & Butterworth, B. (1987). Compensatory processes in the evolution of severe jargon aphasia. *Neuropsychologia*, **25**, 919–933.

Parker, K. (1983). Factor Analysis of the WAIS-R at nine age levels between 16 and 74 years. *Journal of Consulting and Clinical Psychology*, **51**, 302–308.

Parker, R. S. (1972a). Can group therapy be harmful to the individual? *Journal of Clinical Issues in Psychology*, **3**, 22–24.

Parker, R. S. (1972b). The patient who cannot express pain. In Parker, R. S. (Ed.), *The Emotional Stress of War, Violence and Peace*, pp. 71–85. Pittsburgh: Stanwix House.

Parker, R. S. (1981). *Emotional Common Sense*, 2nd ed. New York: Harper & Row.

Parker, R. S. (1983). *Self-Image Psychodynamics*. Englewood-Cliffs, NJ: Prentice-Hall.

Parker, R. S. (1987). Recognizing employees who have suffered brain damage. *EAP Digest* (Employees Assistance Program), **7**, March/April, 55–60.

Parker, R. S. (1988). Brain damage victims: They may not be the best witnesses for themselves. *Trial*, **24**(2), 68–73.

Parker, R. S. & Piotrowski, Z. A. (1965). The acceptability and expression of attitudes associated to the Rorschach Human Movement Response (M). *Journal of Projective Techniques*, **29**, 82–92.

Parmellee, D. X., Kowatch, R. A., Sellman, J., & Davidow, D. (1989). Ten cases of head-injured, suicide-surviving adolescents: challenges for rehabilitation. *Brain Injury*, **3**, 301–313.

Pattison, E. M., & Kahan, J. (1986). Personal experience as a conceptual tool for modes of consciousness. In Wolman, B. B., & Ullman, M. (eds.), *Handbook of States of Consciousness*, pp. 199–245. New York: Van Nostrand Reinhold.

Peacock, W. J. (1986). The postnatal development of the brain and its coverings. In Raimondi, A. J., Choux, M., & Di Rocco, C., (Eds.), *Head Injuries in the Newborn and Infant*, pp. 53–66. New York: Springer-Verlag.

Peck, E., Ettigi, P., Narasimhachari, & Mishra, A. (1986). Neurochemical, neuroendocrine, and neuropsychological correlates of post head injury depression. *Archives of Clinical Neuropsychology*, **1**(1) 63–64.

Pelletier, G. (1988). Anatomy of the hypothalamic-pituitary axis. In Collu, R., Brown, G. M., & Van Loon, G. R. (Eds.). *Clinical Neuroendocrinology*, pp. 1–15. Boston: Blackwell Scientific Publications.

Penfield, W., & Roberts, L. (1959). *Speech and Brain Mechanisms*. Princeton NJ: Princeton University Press.

Penn, C., & Cleary, J. (1989). Compensatory strategies in the language of closed head injured patients. *Brain Injury*, **2**, 3–18.

Perkin, R. M. (1985). Pathophysiology of childhood shock syndromes. In James, H. E., Anas, N. G. and Perkin, R. M. (Eds.), *Brain Insults in Infants and Children*, pp. 191–198. New York: Grune & Stratton.

Pfeffer, C. (1985). Children's reactions to illness, hospitalization and surgery. In Kaplan, H. I., & Sadock, B. J. (Eds.), *Comprehensive Textbook of Psychiatry*, 4th ed., pp. 1836–1842. Baltimore: Williams & Wilkins.

Pierpaoli, W., Balakrishnan, J., Sache, E., Choay, J., & Maestroni, G. J. M. (1987). Neuroendocrine and bone marrow factors for control of marrow transplantation and tissue regeneration. In Jankovic, B. D., Markovic, B. M., & Spector, N. H. (Eds.),

Neuroimmune Interactions: Proceedings of the Second International Workshop on Neuroimmunomodulation. Annals of the NY Academy of Sciences, **496**, 27–38.

Pincus, J. H., & Tucker, G. J. (1985). *Behavioral Neurology*, 3rd ed. News York: Oxford U. Press.

Piotrowski, Z. (1937). The Rorschach inkblot method in organic disturbances of the central nervous system. *Journal of Nervous and Mental Disorders*, **86**(5), 525–537.

Piotrowski, Z. A. (1957). *Perceptanalysis*. Privately reproduced in 1965, Philadeophia: Ex Libris.

Pirozzoli, F. J., & Papanicolaou, A. C. (1986). Plasticity and recovery of function in the central nervous system. In Obrzut, J. F., & Hynd, G. W. (Eds.), *Child Neuropsychology*, Vol. 1, pp. 141–154. New York: Academic Press.

Plotsky, P. M. (1987). Regulation of hypophysiotropic factors mediating ACTH secretion. *The Annals of the N. Y. Academy of Sciences*, **512**, 218–236.

Pogach, L. M. & Vaitukaitis, J. L. (1983). Endocrine disorders associated with erectile dysfunction. In Krane, R. J., Soroky, M. B., & Goldstein, I. (Eds.), *Male Sexual Dysfunction*. (pp. 63–76). Boston: Little, Brown.

Posner, J. B. (1978). Coma and other states of consciousness: The differential diagnosis of brain death. In Korein, J. (Ed.), *Brain Death: Interrelated Medical and Social Issues. Annals of the N.Y. Academy of Sciences*, **315**, 215–227.

Posner, M. I. (1988). Structures and function of attention. In Boll, T., & Bryant, B. K. (Eds.), *Clinical Neuropsychology and Brain Function*, pp. 169–202. Washington, DC: American Psychological Association.

Povlishock, J. T. (1985). The morphologic responses to experimental head injuries of varying severity. In Becker, D. B., & Povlishock, J. T. (Eds.), *Central Nervous System Trauma Status Report*, pp. 443–452. National Institute of Neurological and Communicative Disorders and Stroke, National Institutes of Health.

Pribram, K. (1980). Mind, brain and consciousness: The organization of competence and conduct. In Davidson, J. M., & Davidson, R. J. *The Psychobiology of Consciousness*, 47–63. New York: Plenum Press.

Priddy, D. A., Mattes, D., & Lam, C. S. (1988). Reliability of self-report among nonoriented head-injured adults. *Brain Injury*, **2**, 249–253.

Pritchard, P. B. (1983). Personality and emotional complications of epilepsy. In Heilman, K. M., & Satz, P. (Eds.), *Neuropsychology of Human Emotion*, pp. 165–192. New York: Guilford.

Pynoos, R. S., & Eth, R. S. (1985). Children traumatized by witnessing acts of personal violence: Homicide, rape, or suicide behavior. In Eth, S., & Pynoos, R. (Eds.), *Post-Traumatic Stress Disorder in Children*, pp. 17–43.

Pynoos, R. S., Frederick, C., Nader, K., Arroyo, W., Steinberg, A., Eth, S., Nunez, F., & Fairbanks, L. (1987). Life threat and posttraumatic stress in school-age children. *Archives of General Psychiatry*, **44**, 1057–1063.

Puente, A. E. (1987). Social Security disability and clinical neuropsychological assessment. *The Clinical Neuropsychologist*, (1), 353–363.

Raines, G. N., & Broomhead, E. (1945). Rorschach studies on combat fatigue. *Diseases of the Nervous System*, **5**, 250–256.

Ramsey, D. J. (1986). Posterior pituitary gland. In Greenspan, F. G., & Forsham, P. H., (Eds.), *Basic and Clinical Endocrinology*, 2nd ed., pp. 132–142. Los Altos, CA: Lange Medical Publications.

Randolph, C., & Miller, M. H. (1988). EEG and cognitive performance following closed head injury. *Neuropsychobiology*, **20**, 43–50.

Ranson, S. W., & Clark, S. L. (1959). *The Anatomy of the Nervous System*. Philadelphia: Saunders.

Rao, L., Stefan, H., & Bauer, J. (1989). Epileptic but not psychogenic seizures are accompanied by simultaneous elevation of serum pituitary hormones and cortisol levels. *Neuroendocrinology*, **49**, 33–39.

Rao, N., & Costa, J. L. (1989). Recovery in non-vascular locked-in syndrome during treatment with Sinemet. *Brain Injury*, **3**, 207–211.

Reichmister, J. P. (1982). Differential diagnosis of neck and shoulder pain. In Hendler, N. H., Long, D. M., & Wise, T. N. (Eds.), *Diagnosis and Treatment of Chronic Pain*, pp. 153–160. Boston: John Wright.

Reiser, L. W., & Reiser, M. F. (1985). In Kaplan, H. I., & Sadock, B. J. (Eds.), *Comprehensive Textbook of Psychiatry*, 4th ed., pp. 1167–1178. Baltimore: Williams and Wilkins.

Reitan, R. M. (1988). Integration of neuropsychological theory, assessment, and clinical applications. *The Clinical Neuropsychologist*, **4**, 331–349.

Reitan, R. M., & Wolfson, D. (1985). *Neuroanatomy and Neuropathology*. Tuscon, AZ: Neuropsychology Press.

Reus, V. I. (1989). Psychoneuroendocrinology. In Kaplan, H. I., & Sadock, B. J. (Eds.), *Comprehensive Textbook of Psychiatry*, Vol. I, 5th ed., pp. 105–111. Baltimore: Williams and Wilkins.

Reus, V. I., & Collu, R. (1988). Endocrine effects of stress. In Collu, R., Brown, G. M., & Van Loon, G. R. (Eds.), *Clinical Neuroendocrinology*, pp. 435–459. Boston: Blackwell Scientific Publications.

Rey, M., Dellatolas, G., Bancaud, J., & Talairach, J. (1988). Hemispheric localization of motor and speech functions after early brain lesion: Study of 73 epileptic patients with intracarotid amytal test. *Neuropsychologia*, **26**, 167–172.

Riddoch, M. J., & Humphreys, G. W. (1987). A case of integrative visual agnosia. *Brain*, **110**, 1431–1462.

Rimel, R. W., Giordani, B., Barth, J. T., Boll, T. J., & Jane, M. A. (1981). Disability caused by minor head injury. *Neurosurgery*, **9**, 221–228.

Rimel, R. W., Giordani, B., Barth, J. T., & Jane, M. A. (1982). Moderate head injury: Completing the clinical spectrum of brain trauma. *Neurosurgery*, **11**, 344–351.

Riva, D., & Cazzaniga, L. (1986). Late effects of unilateral brain lesions sustained before and after age one. *Neuropsychologia*, **24**, 423–428. Abstract.

Robinson, R. G., & Benson, D. F. (1981). Depression in aphasic patients: Frequency, severity, and clinical-pathological correlations. *Brain and Language*, **14**, 182–291.

Rosner, M. J. (1985). Systemic response to experimental brain injury. In Becker, D. B., & Povlishock, J. T. (Eds.), *Central Nervous System Trauma Status Report*, pp. 405–415. National Institute of Neurological and Communicative Disorders and Stroke, National Institutes of Health.

Ross, E. D. (1985). Modulation of affect and nonverbal communication by the right hemisphere. In Mesulam, M. (Ed.), *Principles of Behavioral Neurology*, pp. 239–257. Philadelphia: F. A. Davis.

Ross, E. D., Anderson, B., & Morgan-Fisher, A. (1989). Crossed aprosodia in strongly dextral patients. *Archives of Neurology*, **46**, 205–209.

Roth, W. T., & Pfefferbaum, A. (1986). *American Handbook of Psychiatry*, Vol. 8, 2nd ed., pp. 189–212. New York: Basic Books.

Rouit, R. L., & Murali, R. (1987). Injuries of the cranial nerves. In Cooper, P. R. (Ed.), *Head Injury*, 2nd ed., pp. 141–158. Baltimre: Williams and Wilkins.

Roy, A., Virkkunen, M., Guthrie, S., & Linnoila, M. (1986). Indices of serotonin and glucose metabolism in violent offenders, arsonists, and alcoholics. In Mann, J.J., and

Stanley, M. (Eds.), *Psychobiology of Suicidal Behavior. Annals of the N.Y. Academy of Sciences*, **487**, 202–220.

Ruckdeschel-Hibbard, M., Gordon, W. A., & Diller, L. (1986). Affective disturbances associated with brain damage. In Filskov, S. B., and Boll, T. J. (Eds.), *Handbook of Clinical Neuropsychology*, Vol. II, pp. 335–337. New York: Wiley and Sons.

Ruff, R. M., Buchsbaum, M. S. Tropster, A. I., Marshall, L. F., Lottenberg, S., Somers, L. M., & Tobias, M. D. (1989). Computerized tomography, neuropsychology, and positron emission tomography in the evaluation of head injury. *Neuropsychiatry, Neuropsychology, and Behavioral Neurology*, **2**, 103–123.

Ruff, R. M., Buchsbaum, M. S., Tropster, A. I., Marshall, L. F., Lottenberg, S., Somers, L. M., & Tobias, M. D. (1989). Computerized tomography, neuropsychology, and positron emission tomography in the evaluation of head injury. *Neuropsychiatry, Neuropsychology, and Behavioral Neurology*, **2**, 103–123.

Ruff, R. M., Evans, R., & Marshall, L. F. (1986). Impaired verbal and figural fluency after head injury. *Archives of Clinical Neuropsychology*, **1**, 87–102.

Rutter, M. (Ed.). (1983a). *Developmental Neuropsychiatry*. New York: Guilford.

Rutter, M. (1983b). Cognitive deficits after lateralized brain injuries seem less specific in children than in adults (Chadwick & Rutter, 1983). Issues and prospects in developmental neuropsychiatry. In Rutter, M. (Ed.), *Developmental Neuropsychology*, pp. 577–598. New York: Wiley.

Rutter, M., Chadwick, O., & Shaffer, D. (1983). Head injury. In Rutter, M. (Ed.), *Developmental Neuropsychology*, pp. 83–111. New York: Wiley.

Sackheim, H. A., Putz, E., Vingiano, W., & McElhiney, M. (1988). Lateralization in the processing of emotionally laden information. I. Normal functioning. *Neuropsychiatry, Neuropsychology and Behavioral Neurology*, **1**, 97–110.

Salley, R. D., & Teiling, P. A. (1984). Dissociated rage attacks in a Viet Nam Veteran: A Rorschach study. *Journal of Personality Assessment*, **48**, 98–104.

Sapolsky, R. M., Krey, L. C., & McEwen, B. S. (1984). Glucocorticoid-sensitive hippocampal neurons are involved in terminating the adrenocortical stress response. *Proceedings of the National Academy of Sciences*, U.S.A. **81**, 6174–6177.

Sarno, J. (1981). Emotional aspects of aphasia. In Sarno, M. T. (Ed.), *Acquired Aphasia*, pp. 465–484. New York: Academic Press.

Sarno, M. T. (Ed.). (1981a) *Acquired Aphasia*. New York: Academic Press.

Sarno, M. T. (1981b). Recovery and rehabilitation in aphasia. In Sarno, M. T., *Aphasia*, pp. 485–529. New York: Academic Press.

Schilder, P. (1950). *The Image and Appearance of the Human Body*. New York: Wiley.

Schilder, P. (1964). *Contributions to Developmental Neuropsychiatry*. New York: International Universities Press.

Schneider, S. K., & Kaplan, S. M. (1989). Secondary mania resulting from a closed-head injury. *The Clinical Neuropsychologist*, **3**, 230–234.

Schwartz, G. E. (1986). Emotion and psychophysiological organization: A systems approach. In Coles, M. G. H., Donchin, E., & Porges, S. W. (Eds.), *Psychophysiology: Systems, Processes and Applications*, pp. 354–377. New York: Guilford.

Schwartz, J. H. (1985). Synthesis and distribution of neuronal protein. In Kandel, E. R., & Schwartz, J. H. (Eds.), *Principles of Neural Science*, 2nd ed., pp. 37–48. New York: Elsevier.

Schwartzkroin, P. A. & Fuchs, A. F. (1989). Physiological bases of learning, memory and, adaptation. In Patton, H. D., et al., (Eds.), *Textbook of Physiology*, Vol. I, pp. 718–735. Philadelphia: Saunders.

Seliger, G., Cosman, F., Abrams, G. M., & Lindsay, R. (1989). Case study: Hypercalcae-
mia causing declining cognitive function in a head injured patient. *Brain Injury*, **3**,
315–318.

Sergent, J. (1987). A new look at the human split brain. *Brain*, **110**, 1375–1392.

Shapiro, D. L. (1984). *Psychological Evaluation and Expert Testimony*. New York: Van
Nostrand Reinhold.

Shapiro, K. (1985). Head injury in children. In Becker, D. B., & Povlishock, J. T. (Eds.),
Central Nervous System Trauma Status Report—1985. pp. 243–253. National Institute of
Neurological and Communicative Disorders and Stroke, National Institutes of Health.

Shapiro, K. (1987). Special considerations for the pediatric age group. In Cooper, P. R.
(Ed.), *Head Injury*, pp. 367–389. Baltimore: Williams and Wilkins.

Signoret, J-L. (1985). Memory and amnesias. In Mesulam, M. (Ed.), *Principles of Behavioral Neurology*, pp. 169–192. Philadelphia: F.A. Davis.

Silverstein, A. B. (1982). Factor structure of the Wechsler Adult Intelligence Scale-
Revised. *Journal of Consulting and Clinical Psychology*, **50**, 661–664.

Singer, R., & Scott, N. E. (1987). Progression of neuropsychological deficits following
toluene diisocyanate exposure. *Archives of Clinical Neuropsychology*, **2**, 145–154.

Siroky, M. B., & Krane, M. B. (1983). Neurophysiology of erection. In Krane, R. J.,
Soroky, M. B., & Goldstein, I. (Eds.), *Male Sexual Dysfunction*, pp. 9–18. Boston:
Little, Brown.

Sloviter, R. S., Valiquette, G., Abrams, G. M., Ronk, E. C., Sollas, A. L., Paul, L. A.,
& Neubort, S. (1989). Selective loss of hippocampal granule cells in the mature rat brain
after adrenalectomy. *Science*, **243**, 535–538.

Smith, A., Walker, M. L., & Myers, G. (1988). Hemispherectomy and diaschisis: Rapid
improvement in cerebral functions after right hemispherectomy in a six year old child.
Archives of Clinical Neuropsychology, **3**, 1–8.

Smith, D. K. (1989). The K-ABC and preschool assessment. *Assessment Information
Exchange* (American Guidance Service), Spring 1989, p. 12.

Smith, R. S. (1983). A comparison study of the Wechsler Adult Intelligence Scale and the
Wechsler Adult Intelligence Scale-Revised in a college population. *Journal of Consulting and Clinical Psychology*, **51**, 414–419.

Social Security Administration. (1986). *Disability Evaluation under Social Security*. SSA
Publication No. 05-90089, Feb. 1986.

Solomon, S., & Masdeu, J. C. (1989). Neuropsychiatry and behavioral neurology. In
Kaplan, H. I., & Sadock, B. J. (Eds.), *Comprehensive Textbook of Psychiatry*, 5th ed.,
Vol. I. pp. 217–240. Baltimore: Williams and Wilkins.

Speed, W. G. (1982). Headaches. In Hendler, N. H., Long, D. M., & Wise, T. N. (Eds.).
Diagnosis and treatment of chronic pain, pp. 141–152. Boston: John Wright.

Spiegel, D. (1988). Dissociation and hypnosis in post-traumatic stress disorders. *Journal
of Traumatic Stress*, **1**, 17–33.

Spiers, P. A., Schomer, D. L., Blume, M. D., & Mesulam, M-Marsel. (1985). In Mesulam, M., *Principles of Behavioral Neurology*, pp. 289–326. Philadelphia: F.A. Davis.

Spindler, H. A., & Reischer, M. A. (1982). Electrodiagnostic studies in the evaluation of
pain. In Hendler, N. H., Long, D. M., & Wise, T. N. (Eds.), *Diagnosis and treatment
of chronic pain*, pp. 53–62. Boston: John Wright.

Spitzer, H., Desimone, R., & Moran, J. (1988). Increased attention enhances both behavioral and neuronal performance. *Science*, **240**, 338–240.

Squire, L. R., & Zola-Morgan, S. (1985). The neuropsychology of memory: New links
between humans and experimental animals. In Olton, D. S., Gamzu, E., & Corkin, S.

D. (Eds.), *Memory Dysfunctions: An Integration of Animal and Human Research from Preclinical and Clinical Perspectives*, pp. 137–149. New York: N.Y. Academy of Science.

Starkstein, S. E., Robinson, R. G., & Price, T. R. (1987). Comparison of cortical and sub-cortical lesions in the production of poststroke mood disorders. *Brain*, **110**, 1045–1059.

Stein, D. G. (1988). In pursuit of new strategies for understanding recovery from brain damage: Problems and perspectives. In Boll, T., & Bryan, B. K. (Eds.), *Clinical Neuropsychology and Brain Function: Research, Measurement, and Practice*, pp. 13–55. Washington, DC: American Psychological Association.

Strub, R. L., & Black, F. W. (1985). *The Mental Status Examination in Neurology*, 2nd ed. Philadelphia: F.A. Davis.

Strub, R. L., & Black, F. W. (1988). *Neurobehavioral Disorders: A Clinical Approach*. Philadephia: F. A. Davis.

Stuss, D. T., & Benson, D. F. (1983). Frontal lobe lesions and behavior. In Kertesz, A. (Ed.), *Localization in Neuropsychology*, pp. 429–454. New York: Academic Press.

Stuss, D. T., & Benson, D. F. (1986). The Frontal Lobes. New York: Raven.

Swisher, L. (1985). Language disorders in children. In Darby, J. (Ed.), *Speech and Language Evaluation in Neurology: Childhood Disorders*, pp. 33–96. New York: Grune & Stratton.

Stuss, D. T., Stethem, L. L., Hugenholtz, M. H., Richard, M. T. (1989). *The Clinical Neuropsychologist*, **3**, 145–156.

Szabon, L., & Groswasser, Z. (1989). Heterotopic bone formation involving wrist and fingers in brain-injured patients: A report of three cases. *Brain Injury*, **3**, 57–61.

Szatmari, P., & Taylor, D. C. (1984). The neurological examination in child psychiatry: A review of its uses. *Canadian Journal of Psychiatry*, **24**, 155–162.

Szeto, H. (1989). Maternal-fetal pharmacokinetics and fetal dose-response relationships. In Hutchings, D. E. (Ed.), *Prenatal Abuse of Licit and Illicit Drugs. Annals of the New York Academy of Sciences*, **562**, 42–55.

Tabaddor, K., Mattis, S., & Zazula, T. (1984). Cognitive sequelae and recovery course after moderate and severe head injury. *Neurosurgery*, **14**, 701–708.

Taylor, G. J. (1984). Alexithymia: Concept, measurement, and implications for treatment. *The American Journal of Psychiatry*, **141**, 725–732.

Teasdale, G., & Mendelow, D. (1984). Pathophysiology of head injuries. In, Brooks, B. (Ed.), *Closed Head Injury: Psychological, Social, and Family Consequences*, pp. 4–36. New York: Oxford University Press.

Terr, L. X. (1985). Children traumatized in small groups. In Eth, S., & Pynoos, R. (Eds.), *Post-Traumtic Stress Disorder in Children*, pp. 45–70.

Thatcher, R. W., Lester, M. L., McAlaster, R., & Horst, R. (1982). Effects of low levels of cadmium aand lead on cognitive functioning in children. *Environmental Health*, **37**(3), 159–165.

Thibault, L. E., & Gennarelli, L. A. (1985). Biomechanics and craniocerebral trauma. In Becker, D. B., & Povlishock, J. T. (Eds.), *Central Nervous System Trauma Status Report*, pp. 379–389. National Institute of Neurological and Communicative Disorders and Stroke, National Institutes of Health.

Thickman, M., & Ranseen, J. D. (1986). Personality changes associated with head trauma: Implications for rehabilitation specialists. *Topics in Acute Care and Trauma Rehabilitation*, **1**(1) 32–37.

Thomas, A., & Chess, S. (1977). *Temperament and development*. New York: Brunner/Mazel.

Thomas, C. B. (1982). Stamina: The thread of human life. *Psychotherapy and Psychosomatics*, **38**, 74–80.

Thompson, R. F. (1988). Brain substrates of learning and memory. In Boll, T., & Bryant, B. K. (Eds.), *Clinical Neuropsychology and Brain Function: Research, Measurement and Practice*, pp. 61–83. Washington, DC: American Psychological Association.

Thomsen, I. G. (1989). Do young patients have worse outcomes after severe blunt head trauma? *Brain Injury*, **3**, 157–162.

Thorndike, R., Hagen, E. P., & Sattler, J. M. (1986). *The Stanford-Binet Intelligence Scale: Fourth Edition. Guide for Administering and Scoring*, 2nd printing. Chicago: Riverside Publishing Co.

Tilson, H. A., & Sparber, S. B. (Eds.). (1987). *Neurotoxicants and Neurobiological Function: Effects of Organoheavy Metals*. New York: Wiley.

Todd, M. M., Fleischer, J. E., & Karagianes, T. (1985). Intracranial pressure monitoring in the post injury patient. *Trauma*, **2**(1), 40–55.

Tornheim, P. (1985). Traumatic edema in head injury. In Becker, D. B., & Povlishock, J. T. (Eds.), *Central Nervous System Trauma Status Report*, pp. 431–432. National Institute of Neurological and Communicative Disorders and Stroke, National Institutes of Health.

Torrens, M. J. (1983). Neurologic and Neurosurgical disorders associated with impotence. In Krane, R. J., Soroky, M. B., & Goldstein, I. (Eds.), *Male Sexual Dysfunction*, pp. 55–61. Boston: Little, Brown.

Touen, B. C. L. (1987). The meaning and value of soft signs in neurology. In Tupper, D. E. (Ed.), *Soft Neurological Signs*, pp. 281–295. New York: Grune & Stratton.

Towbin, A. (1987). Neuropathologic correlates. In Tupper, D. E. (Ed.), *Soft Neurological Signs*, pp. 157–178. New York: Grune & Stratton.

Trauner, D. A., & James, H. E. (1985). Evaluation of coma. In James, H. E., Anas, N. G. & Perkin, R. M. (Eds.), *Brain Insults in Infants and Children*, pp. 173–178. New York: Grune & Stratton.

Trenerry, M. R., Crossen, B., DeBoe, J., & Leber, W. (1989). *Stroop Neuropsychological Screening Test Manual*. Odessa, FL: Psychological Assessment Resources.

Trexler, L. I., & Zappala, G. (1988). Re-examining the determinants of recovery and rehabilitation of memory defects following traumatic brain injury. *Brain Injury*, **2**, 187–203.

Trief, P. M., Elliott, D. J., Stein, N., & Frederickson, B. E. (1987). Functional vs. organic pain: A meaningful distinction? *Journal of Clinical Psychology*, **43**, 219–226.

Trimble, M. R. (1988a). *Biological Psychiatry*. New York: Wiley.

Trimble, M. R. (1988b). Body image and the temporal lobes. *British Journal of Psychiatry*, **153** (Suppl. 2), 12–14.

Tucker, D. M. (1981). Lateral brain function, emotion, and conceptualization. *Psychological Bulletin*, **89**, 19–46.

Tupper, D. E. (1986). Neuropsychological screening and soft signs. In Obrzut, J. E., & Hynd, G. W. (Eds.), *Child Neuropsychology*, Vol. 2, pp. 139–186. Orlando: Academic Press.

Tupper, D. E. (1987). The issues with 'soft' signs. In Tupper, D. E. (Ed.), *Soft Neurological Signs*, pp. 1–16. New York: Grune & Stratton.

Unterberg, A., & Baethmann, A. (1985). Secondary changes in brain biochemistry with brain edema. In James, H. E., Anas, N. G., & Perkin, R. M. (Eds.), *Brain insults in infants and children: Pathophysiology and Management*, pp. 61–73. New York: Grune & Stratton.

Uzzell, B. P., Langfitt, T. W., & Dolinkas, C. A. (1987). Influence of injury severity on quality of survival after head injury. *Surgical Neurology*, **27**, 419–429.

Valciukas, J. A. (1985). The role of the psychologist in occupational neurotoxicology: Apropos of Huszco et al.'s "Psychology and organized labor." *American Psychologist*, **40**, 1053–1054.

Valciukas, J. A., & Lilis, R. (1980). Psychometric techniques in environmental research. *Environmental Research*, **21**, 275–297.

Valciukas, J. A., Lilas, R., Eisinger, J., Blumberg, W. E., Fischbein, A., & Selikoff, I. J. (1978). Behavioral indicators of lead neurotoxicity: Results of a clinical field survey. *International Archives of Occupational and Environmental Health*. **41**, 217–236.

Valciukas, J. A., Lilas, R., Singer, R., Fischbein, A., Anderson, H. A., & Glickman, L. (1980). Lead exposure and behavioral changes: Comparisons of four occupational groups with different levels of lead absorption. *American Journal of Industrial Medicine*, **1**, 421–426.

van der Kolk, B. A. (1984). *Post-Traumatic Stress Disorder: Psychological and Biological Sequelae*. Washington, DC: American Psychiatric Association.

van der Kolk, B. A. (1988) The trauma spectrum: The interaction of biological and social events in the genesis of the trauma response. *Journal of Traumatic Stress*, **1**, 273–290.

van der Kolk, B. A., & Ducey, C. (1984). Clinical implications of the Rorschach in post-traumatic stress disorder. In van der Kolk, B. A. (Ed.), *Post-Traumatic Stress Disorder: Psychological and Biological Sequelae*, pp. 29–42. Washington, DC: American Psychiatric Press.

Van Lancker, D. (1985). Hemispheric contributions to language and communication. In Darby, J. K. (Ed.), *Speech and Language Evaluation in Neurology: Adult Disorders*, pp. 247–295. New York: Grune & Stratton.

Van Praag, H. M., Plutchik, R., & Conte, H. (1986). The serotonin hypothesis of (auto)aggression. In Mann, J. J., & Stanley, M. (Eds.), *Psychobiology of Suicidal Behavior. Annals of the New York Academy of Sciences*, **487**, 150–650.

Van Zomeren, A. H., Brouwer, W. H., & Deelman, G. G. (1984). Attentional deficits: The riddles of selectivity, speed and alertness. In Brooks, N. (Ed.), *Closed Head Injury: Psychological, Social, and Family Consequences*, pp. 74–107. New York: Oxford University Press.

Vargha-Khadam, F., O'Gorman, A. M., & Watters, G. V., (1985). Aphasia and handedness in relation to hemispheric side, age at injury and severity of cerebral lesion during childhood. *Brain*, **108**, 677–696.

Walker, A. E. (1978). The pathology of brain death. In Korein, J. (Ed.), *Brain Death: Interrelated Medical and Social Issues*, pp. 272–280. *Annals of the New York Academy of Science*, **315**

Waller, P. F., Stewart, J. R., Hansen, A. R., Stutts, J. C., Popkin, C. L., & Rodgman, E. A. (1986). The potentiating effects of alcohol on driver injury. *Journal of the American Medical Association*, **256**, 1461–1466.

Walton, J. (1985). *Brain's Diseases of the Nervous System*, 9th ed. New York: Oxford University Press.

Washton, A. M., & Gold, M. S. (1987). *Cocaine: A Clinician's Handbook*. New York: Guilford.

Watkins, E. O. (1976). *The Watkins Bender-Gestalt Scoring System*. Novato, CA: Academic Therapy Publications.

Watson, S. J., Khachaturian, H., Lewis, M. E., & Akil, A. (1986). Chemical neuroanatomy as a basis for biological psychiatry. In *American Handbook of Psychiatry*, 2nd ed., Vol 8: *Biological Psychiatry*, pp. 3–33. New York: Basic Books.

Weber, R. J., & Pert, A. (1989). The periaqueductal gray matter mediates opiate-induced immunosuppression. *Science*, **245**, 188–192.

Wechsler, D. (1981). *Wechsler Adult Intelligence Scale — Revised*. The Psychological Corporation.

Wechsler, D. (1987). *Wechsler Memory Scale-Revised. The Psychological Corporation*.

Weddell, R. A., Trevarthen, C., & Miller, J. D. (1988). Reactions of patients with focal cerebral lesions to success or failure. *Neuropsychologia*, **26**, 373–385.

Weiner, R. L., & Eisenberg, H. M. (1985). Radiographic evaluation of head injury: Key concepts. *Trauma*, **2**(2), 26–39.

Weintraub, S., & Mesulam, M. (1985). Mental state assessment of young and elderly adults in behavioral neurology. In Mesulam, M-Marsel (Ed.), *Principles of Behavioral Neurology*, pp. 76–162. Philadelphia: F.A. Davis.

Weiss, G. H., Salazar, A. M. Vance, S. C., Grafman, J. H., & Jabbari, B. (1986). Predicting posttraumatic epilepsy in penetrating head injury. *Archives of Neurology*, **43**, 771–773.

Weiss, J. M., & Glazer, H. I. (1975). Effects of acute exposure to stressor on subsequent avoidance-escape behavior. *Psychosomatic Medicine*, **37**, 499–502.

Weiss, J. M., Glazer, H. I., Pohorecky, L. A., Brick, J., & Miller, N. E. (1975). Effects of chronic exposure to stressors on avoidance-escape behavior and on brain norepinephrine. *Psychosomatic Medicine*, **37**, 522–534.

Westermeyer, J., & Wahmenholm, K. (1989). Assessing the victimized psychiatric patient. *Hospital and Community Psychiatry*, **40**, 245–249.

Wetherby, A. M. (1985). Speech and language disorders in children—An overview. In Darby, J. K. (Ed.), *Speech and language evaluation in neurology: Childhood disorders*, pp. 3–32. New York: Grune & Stratton.

White, R. F. (1987). Differential diagnosis of probable Alzheimer's disease and solvent encephalopathy in older workers. *The Clinical Neuropsychologist*, **1**, 153–160.

Widerhbolt, J. L., & Bryant, B. R. (1986). *Gray Oral Reading Tests — Revised*. Austin TX: Pro-Ed.

Wilcox, J. A., & Nasrallah, H. A. (1987). Childhood head trauma and psychosis. *Psychiatry Research*. **12**, 303–306.

Willis, W. G. (1988). Neuropsychological diagnosis with children: Actuarial and clinical models. In Tramontana, M. G., & Hooper, S. R. (Eds.), *Assessment Issues in Child Neuropsychology*, pp. 93–111. New York: Plenum.

Willis, W. G., & Widerstrom, A. H. (1986). Neuropsychological development. In Obrzut, J. E., & Huynbd, G. W. (Eds.), *Neuropsychology. I*, pp. 13–53. Orlando, FL: Academic Press.

Wilson, B. C. (1986). An approach to the neuropsychological assessment of the pre-school child with developmental deficits. In Filskov, S. B., & Boll, T. J. (Eds.), *Handbook of Clinical Neuropsychology*, Vol. II, *Dysarthria*. New York: Wiley.

Wilson-Pauwels, L., Akesson, E. J., & Stewart, P. A. (1988). *Cranial Nerves*. Philadelphia: B.C. Decker.

Wolraich, M. L. (1984). Seizure disorders. In Blackman, J. A. (Ed.), *Medical Aspects of Developmental Disabilities in Children Birth to Three*, pp. 215–221. Rockville, MD: Aspen.

Wood, R. (1984). Behaviour disorders following severe brain injury: Their and psychological management. In Brooks, N. (Ed.), *Closed Head Injury: Psychological, Social and Family Consequences*, pp. 195–219. New York: Oxford University Press.

Woodcock, R. W. (1987). *Woodcock Reading Mastery Tests—Rev.* Circle Pines, MN: American Guidance Service.

Woods, B. T. (1987). Impaired speech following early lesions of either hemisphere. *Neuropsychologia*, **25**, 519–525.

Woolf, P. D., Lee, L. A., Hamill, R. W., & McDonald, J. V. (1988). Thyroid test abnormalities in traumatic brain injury: Correlation with neurologic impairment and sympathetic nervous system activation. *The American Journal of Medicine*, **14**, 201–208.

Yamamoto, I., & Sato, O. (1986). Intrauterine development of the skull. In Raimondi, A. J., Choux, M., & Di Rocco, C. (Eds.), *Head Injuries in the Newborn and Infant*, pp. 1–18. New York: Springer-Verlag.

Yarnell, P. R., & Rossie, G. V. (1988). Minor whiplash head injury with major debilitation. *Brain Injury.* **2**, 255–258.

Yeudall L. T. (1980). A neuropsychosocial perspective of persistent juvenile delinquency and criminal behavior: Discussion. *Forensic Psychology and Psychiatry. Annals of the New York Academy of Sciences*, **347**, 349–355.

Ylvisaker, M. (1989). Cognitive and psychosocial outcome following head injury in children. In Hoff, J. T., Anderson, T. D., & Cole, T. M. (Eds.), *Mild to Moderate Head Injury*, pp. 203–216. Boston: Blackwell Scientific Publications.

Young, T., & Lawson, G. W. (1988). Voluntary inhalation of volatile substances. In Lawson, G. W., & Cooperrider, C. A. (Eds.), *Clinical Psychopharmacology*, pp. 251–259. Rockville, MD: Aspen.

Young, T., Lawson, G. W., & Gacano, C. B. (1988). Phencyclidine: A clinical review. In Lawson, G. W., & Cooperrider, C. A. (Eds.), *Clinical Psychopharmacology*, pp. 187–200. Rockville, MD: Aspen.

Young, W. (1987). The post-injury responses in trauma and ischemia: Secondary injury or protective mechanisms? *Central Nervous System Trauma*, **4**(1), 27–42.

Zahn, T. P. (1986). Psychophysiological approaches to psychopathology. In Coles, M. G. H., Donchin, E., & Porges, S. W. (Eds.), *Psychophysiology: Systems, Processes and Applications*, pp. 508–610. New York: Guilford.

Zimmerman, R. A. (1985). CRH secretion is stimulated via pain and other sensory pathways, and emotional stimuli via limbic lobe pathways (Palkovitz, 1987). Computed tomography and head trauma. In James, H. E., Anas, N. G., & Perkin, R. M. (Eds.), *Brain Insults in Infants and Children: Pathophysiology and Management*, pp. 113–124. New York: Grune & Stratton.

Zohn, D. A. (1982). Mechanical (structural) headache. In Hendler, N. H., Long, D. M., & Wise, T. N. (Eds.), *Diagnosis and Treatment of Chronic Pain*, pp. 117–139. Boston: John Wright.

Appendix 1
Postaccident Intake Protocols

This appendix includes

Observations: Used for individuals of all ages.
Intake Interview: Adults.
Personal Injury Checklist.
Parent's Interview.

Some procedures are appended to assist the reader to obtain information efficiently. These are forms I use in my practice: a structured interview form for adults, and a questionnaire that helps ensure that information is not missed due to expressive deficits. During the interview, symptoms that are noted by the victim can be inquired into more fully. There is also a questionnaire for the parents or guardians of children, which also provides a baseline for assessing any impairment or personality problems stemming from an accident. Considerations for a comprehensive neuropsychological examination are included, to plan it, or assess its completeness.

Neuropsychological Observations

Name: Date: Promptness:
Ethnic:
Height   Weight
Accompanied by:
Appearance: Health, cosmetic, dress:
Visible scars, bruises:
Social Quality: Cooperative or resentful; Related/withdrawn
Alertness/Concentration:
   Goal direct/distracted/preoccupied
   Follows/Does not follow/Needs extra instructions:
   Learning of new tasks:

Problem-Solving Style:
   Independent/Need for help/E. must control exam
   Pacing: Fast/Appropriate; Slow
   Standards of performance: Precise/Average; Careless; Bizarre; Primitive
   Flexibility: Gets stuck/Shifts to better/Different response
   Preplanning: Easy ___ Midrange ___ Hard ___ items
   Trial-and-error: Easy ___ Midrange ___ Hard ___
   Reaction to Examiner's Cues:
   Judgment (Awareness of obvious errors): Yes/No
Reaction to Event: Maximizes/Appropriate/Minimizes:
Insight into Impairment:
Emotional Behavior:
   Motivation to do well:
   Depressed/crying:
   Anxious/startle:
   Expressiveness: Spontaneous/Variable/Unexpressive/Holds back
   Expression of anger:
   Mood: Pleasant/Dull/Resentful
   Appropriateness:
Morale: Self-Confident; Apologetic
   Reaction to Difficulty: Persistent; Gives up prematurely.
                    Acknowledges difficulty/Pretends adequacy.
Communication:
   Fluency: Discursive, fluent, adequate, monosyllabic, works but no comment
   Offers/Does not offer: Personal reactions
   Easy/Difficult to understand:
   Comprehends/Does not comprehend examiner:
   Enunciation: Clear/Unclear
Physiological:
   Needs/Does not need excess breaks:
   Pain:
   Autonomic
   Somatic/Sensory
Movement/Coordination Deficit: (Yes/no)
   Uses: One/two hands
   Drops things, breaks pencil, unusual pencil position

Intake Interview: Adult

Background

Name: Date: Preferred Hand:
Date of Birth: Date of Accident:

Address:
Telephone:
Treating Physician?
Attorney, address, telephone:
Where were you born?
At what age did you come to the U.S.?
What is your native language?
At what age did you learn English?
Highest level of education:
High School:

Grades: (High School):		Year Graduated:
(College):		Year Graduated:

Major:
Where Educated?

Married:	Children:

Lives With:

Military Service:	Years:	Highest Rank:

Military Occupation Specialty and duties:
Before the accident, did you have any emotional problems or personal
    counseling?
Were you ever in a hospital for emotional or psychiatric reasons?
Any history of pregnancy or birth problems, early illness, CNS disease? Head
Injury? High fevers? Seizures? Meningitis?
Did you ever have an accident?
Were you ever seriously ill, and/or in the hospital?
Did you have any emotional or physical problems before this accident, that the
accident made worse?
Before the injury did you take any medication?
Did you ever take recreational drugs before __ after __ the accident?
Have you ever had a problem with alcohol?
Have you had more than one accident or other serious injury?

Employment

At what age did you start to work? Did you work continuously?
What was the most skilled job you held before the injury? Job title? How long?
What were your duties?
What was your job at the time of the injury?
Title:
How long?
What were your duties?
What kind of skills are needed to perform this job?
What kind of personality is needed to perform this job?
Did you have to read ( ) write ( ) do calculations ( ) read visual materials,
    e.g., diagrams, charts or maps ( ) make plans ( ) decisions ( ) eye hand
    coordination ( )

Accident

Tell me about the accident:
Did you know the accident would happen, or were you taken by surprise?
Were you dazed or unconscious? For how long? How long was it before you felt
like yourself?
Loss of memory for events before the accident:
Loss of memory for events after the accident:
Did you have any pain?

Disability

Were you in the hospital? How long?
What part of your body was injured?
How long were you disabled after the accident? How long were you unemployed
after the accident?
Did you, or do you now, take any medications, because of the injury?
What treatment have you had since the accident?
Has your health changed after the accident?
If you have not returned to work, is there a reason why?
How long after the accident did you return to work? Did you have any problems
performing your job?
How many jobs have you had since the accident? Are they more skilled, or less
skilled? Do you earn more or less money?
What is your present job? How long on present job?
What kind of skills and/or personality are needed to perform this job?
Do you have any problems performing this job?

Personality Changes and Affective Dysfunction

Do you think about the accident?   How often?
Do you dream about the accident?   How often?
Nightmares?   How often?
When in the last time you had a nightmare or bad dream?
Do you put the accident out of your mind?
Do thoughts about the accident come back often or unexpectedly?
Do you avoid any activities because of bad memories or anxiety?
Do you feel guilty about something connected with your condition?
Compared to before the accident, are your feelings or moods, generally the same,
stronger, or weaker?
Do you hide your feelings?
Do you have difficulty controlling your feelings and actions?
Do you have a problem with your temper?
Do you have sexual problems?
Do you feel like a different person, or not your real self since the accident?
How has your life changed because of the accident?

How do you spend your day?
How has your social life changed because of the accident?
Will your future be different because of the accident?
Did you have any plans that were spoiled because of the accident?
What is the worst effect of the accident?
Does the accident have a special meaning to you?
What plans are you making to improve your condition? Has it improved?
Can you overcome your problems?
Anything else you want to tell me?

Personal Injury Checklist—1

Name: Today's Date:
Since your injury which of the following has bothered you, for the first time, or much more, than before the injury?
            Place a checkmark next to the problem that you have.
___ I have trouble staying awake   (Alertness)
___ I have strange experiences
___ Seizures
___ Blackouts
___ Sometimes I don't feel like a real person
___ Sometimes the world around me doesn't seem real
___ My mind wanders after a short period of time   (Concentration)
___ I get lost
___ I can't tell time as well
___ I don't think as clearly
___ I can't keep two ideas in my mind at once
___ I can't shift from one idea to another
___ I get confused easily
___ I am clumsy when I use my hands   (Sensorimotor)
___ I can't use my body as well (walk, sports, take care of my home)
___ My hands shake
___ I fall a lot
___ My muscles feel stiff and I can't move them easily
     (I have problems with my senses)
___ Dizzy spells   ___ Seeing
___ Smell   ___ Hearing
___ Taste   ___ Sense of touch
___ Too sensitive to light___ Too sensitive to noise
___ I bump into things   ___ Too sensitive to noise
___ I lose my balance
___ I don't know what something is by how it feels
     (There have been changes in my body) (Visceral/Physiological)

___ I have less energy/get tired easily   ___ Arms and legs feel heavy
___ I get sick more often   _____
___ I have sexual problems   (Less desire: ___) (Poor control: ___)
                             (Frigidity: ___) (No erection: ___)
___ Eating: More ___ Less ___   ___ Loss of appetite
___ Weight: More ___ Less ___   (How many pounds different
                                              since accident? _____

___ Sleep: More ___ Less ___
___ Bowels: The Runs ___   Constipation ___
___ Sweating more   ___ Higher blood pressure
___ Rapid heart beat   ___ Urinate too frequently
___ Menstrual problems   ___ Hair loss
___ Headaches   ___ Cold hands
___ Other medical problems: ___ Pains (Where?) _____
___ I don't learn new things as well as before (Mental ability)
___ When I do something, ___ It turns out badly   or ___ I make mistakes
___ I don't think I am as smart as before
___ It is hard for me to solve problems I could do at one time
___ I have to search for words and names   (Memory)
___ I forget the first part of a sentence before somebody gets to the end.
___ I don't remember how to do things I learned recently
___ I don't remember—events ___ —facts ___ that happened recently
___ People tell me I forget what we have just spoken about
___ I have forgotten how to do things I used to do very well
___ Learning something new is hard because I forget it so easily
___ I do not know when I make simple mistakes   (Reduced efficiency)
___ I don't make plans as well
___ Others have to tell me what to do
___ It is hard to correct mistakes
___ I often don't finish doing something I start to do
___ If I start to do something one way, I continue even if it is wrong
 _ I am slower in my thinking ( ) actions ( )
___ I start something new before I finish something else
___ There are things to do and I don't get started
___ I can't put ideas into words the way I would like to   (Communications)
___ Other people don't understand me
___ I don't speak words clearly
___ I don't understand other people
___ Sometimes I don't talk because it might be wrong
___ Arithmetic and calculations   ___ Reading   (Adaptive)
___ Typing   ___ Writing   ___ Studying
___ Driving
___ Using my eyes to read maps, do puzzles, read blueprints and diagrams
___ Taking care of myself: Underline the problem   (Functional)
       (Bathing, dressing, hygiene, eating)

___ Taking care of my home (cooking, cleaning, repair)
___ Taking care of my family
___ Handling money (budget, shopping, banking)
___ Shopping (food, clothing, household)
___ Use of my time (planning, scheduling, awareness)
___ Getting around (trains, busses, driving, how to get to places)
___ Using public places (library, church, clubs, movies, theatres)
___ Enjoying myself (hobbies, sports, games, reading)
___ I can't go back to work
___ I can't do my work as well as I used to
___ I am very sad, or cry too easily   (Affect)
___ Sometimes I'm so depressed I can't get out of bed in the morning
___ I think of how I might die
___ Nervousness ( ) or panic ( ): What bothers you? _____
___ My feelings are not as deep as before
___ I feel guilty about surviving the accident
___ My moods swing from high to low for no reason
___ My feelings are out of control
___ I have problems with anger—too irritable ( ) lose my temper ( )
___ I don't understand why others react to me the way they do
___ I don't understand other people's feelings
___ People tell me I keep doing things they dislike over and over
___ I don't start ( ) or don't finish ( ) tasks because I am discourged
___ I keep thinking about how I wish things should be better
___ I think about or have attempted suicide
___ I feel hopeless that my life will ever be better or enjoyable
___ It is hard to be with people—Who? (family, friends, strangers)   (Social)
___ I feel more lonely
___ I don't feel interested in being with my family or friends
___ Other people don't like me as much as before
___ I am embarrassed about my condition (_____)
___ I think that a lot of people are against me
___ I have fewer close friends
___ I make visits or receive visitors much less often
___ I feel strange and think that people look at me for that reason
___ I think about the accident   (Event)
             All The Time ___ Often ___ Sometimes ___ Never ___
___ It doesn't take much to make me think of my injury and get nervous
___ I have flashbacks about the accident
___ I have had dreams about the accident at the time of the accident:
         Now: All   Most of the
                      Time   ___ Often ___ Sometimes ___ Never ___
___ If you dream, are these dreams nightmares? Yes: ___ No ___
___ I avoid situations that remind me about my condition or of the accident
___ It is important to find out why this happened to me

__ I do not feel like the same person   (Identity)
__ I think that I am less attractive. How?
__ I feel that I have been damaged
__ Other people tell me that I have changed. How? _____
__ It is easier for me to be hurt than before
__ Since the accident I don't have as clear an idea as to who I am
__ I need somebody to take care of me
                                                                                              (Can't enjoy life)
__ I no longer enjoy work ( ) studies ( ) family ( ) friends ( ) leisure
     time ( ) hobbies ( )
__ My life has lost meaning (How?) _____
__ My future has been damaged (How?) _____
__ I hardly ever enjoy myself or feel pleasure
__ Since the accident it is hard for me to be interested in anything
__ I am bored more often than before the accident

Go Back and Make Sure that You Have Not Left Anything Out.
Place a line underneath any problem that you want to talk about.

Parent's Interview

Child's Name: Date:
Address:
Telephone:
Respondent:
Attorney:
Date of Injury?
Height: Weight: Preferred Handed:
Where and when was the child born?
When did the child come to the U.S.?
Has the child lived for any period of time outside the U.S.?
Has the child lived for any time outside the home?
In addition to yourself and your child, who else lives at home?
If there are other children, do they have any problems?
If the parents are separated, when did this occur?
Father's Occupation:
Mother's Occupation:

Pregnancy

Did Mother use alcohol?
Did Mother use drugs?
Did Mother smoke?
Any health problems?

Any birth problems?
Birth Weight?

Development

Walked?
Bladder trained?
Bowel trained?
Began to have friends?
Personality before the age of school?
Any visual problems?
Any hearing problems?
Any speech problems?
Behavioral problems before school?

Cognitive Development

Native language?
Age learned English?
Age used single words?
Age used sentences?
Age learned to write?
Age learned simple calculations?
How many words does your child know know?
Give me an example of one sentence that your child spoke in the last 24 hours?

Education

Age entered school?
Age in kindergarten?
Age in first grade?
Ever left back?
Ever in special education?
Present grade?
Where did the child study?
What is your child's worst subject?
What is your child's best subject?

Health

(Before Accident) *Age of illness?*

After-effects?
Any serious illness?

Ever hospitalized?
Ever take medicines?
Ever hit head?
Meningitis, high fever, seizures?
Has there been a change of preferred hand?
Visual problems?
Hearing Problems?
Other health problems?
Any other accidents, frightening events, or family problems that could have interfered with your child's ability to study or get along with others?

Accident

Describe the accident:
Was the child dazed or unconscious? How long?
Was the child nervous? How long?
Was the child taken to the hospital? How long?
Are there any scars?
Has the child had seizures?
Does the child complain of pain?
Does the child complain of headaches? How often? Where are they? How described?
Was the child given any medicines for seizures, headaches, other pains, nervousness, or depression?
For how long?
Are any of these medicine being taken now?
Are there health problems that happened for the first time after the accident?
Bad dreams or nightmares?
When did you become concerned about the child?
What did you see that made you feel something was wrong?

How Has the Child's Personality Changed?

Is your child more or less emotional than before the accident?
Does your child express his or her feelings when he is happy, angry or sad, or does he or she hold them back?
Does your child seem unnaturally unemotional?
Is your child very nervous?
Does your child avoid certain kinds of activities because of fear?
Does your child avoid activities/places that remind him or her of the accident?
Does your child have bad dreams, nightmares?
Is your child easily frightened?
Has your child lost control over temper or other feelings?

Do you think your child's emotional reactions are normal?
   Too strong? Too weak?
   Lose temper? Cry too easily?
   Frightened easily? Reaction is strange?
How does your child get along with other people?
   Family?
   Friends and other children?
   Strangers?
   School? Does the teacher complain about behavior?

School and Homework

Are school records available?
Have the school records been requested?
Does your child learn normally?
Does your child study normally?
Does your child concentrate or continue work in a normal way?
Does your child give up too easily?
Does your child forget things in school or at home too easily?
Have the school grades changed?

Overview

What is the worst effect of the accident?
Anything else you want to tell me?

Appendix 2
Some Sensorimotor
Assessment Procedures

The examiner notes the preferred hand, and draws conclusions modified by age, sex, occupation, health, and constitution (height and body build).

Smedley Hand Dynamometer (Stoelting, Chicago) for Grip Strength

Norms for both sexes are available from 6 to 18. The author uses a 2 year deviation in equivalent age between the hands as an indicator of impairment of one hand. The cause of impairment may be ipsilateral or contralateral depending on the site of neurological damage.

Pocket Smell Test (Sensonics, Haddonfield, NJ)

Three odors are released by scratching with a pencil; the patient chooses from four printed alternatives. The examiner asks the patient first whether anything is smelled, then elicits the patient's identification. The examiner must distinguish between inability to detect odors, and loss of memory associating an odor with its stimulus.

Visual Fields to the Periphery by Confrontation

With one eye closed, a finger is moved from the center of vision into each quadrant, i.e., left, right, up, down. The examiner observes whether there are any gross deficits in the visual fields, taking into account that the nose, forehead, and lower cheekbone somewhat restrict the field. This is a very rough assessment, far inferior to arc perimetry described below. If there is evidence of field deficits, this is verified by referring the patient to an ophthalmologist with a request for automated visual fields.

Arc Perimeter (Stoelting, Chicago)

This procedure takes about 25–30 minutes. This device has a chin rest, a mirror directly ahead, and a semicircle marked every 10°. It is rotated 360° for each eye, with the other eye covered. A white (or colored) disk at the end of a baton is moved from the center or periphery of vision to the other extreme of the visual field, with one eye closed (a surgical eye patch is used for sanitary reasons). The visual fields are recorded on a standard diagram for each eye. Particular patterns of deficits can be related to damage in the visual tracts and optic radiation (lateral geniculate to occipital cortex) (see Bajandas & Kline, 1987, for a thorough explication with diagrams). The patient can be referred for automated visual fields.

Test of Bilateral Directed Tapping

This is an unpublished measure of tapping speed and control, devised by me. It comprises four quadrants on an ordinary sheet of 8½ × 11 inch paper. Each quadrant is divided into ½ inch squares, arranged in 10 rows and 7 columns. The patient is directed to place the first tap into a box (upper left of each quadrant) with a circle; the patient uses a red china marking pencil, and the paper is supported by an appropriate sized glass plate, which offers resilience so that the pencil bounces upwards. Trials 1 and 3 are with the preferred hand and 2 and 4 with the non-preferred hand: 15 seconds/trial are offered. The taps for preferred and non-preferred hands are compared, with equality to +25% advantage for the preferred hand considered normal range. Ability to follow instructions, accuracy of tapping, wrist motion and handling of pencil, strength and accuracy of tapping with each hand, and relative speed compared to age-group, etc. are observed. This is useful for individuals age 6 and up. (The author will provide available norms.)

Bead Stringing

A box of differently shaped beads with a hole drilled through them and a shoelace with a knot near one end are provided. The instructions are to string 10 beads of any kind as rapidly as possible. Observations are made as to efficiency of handling the string and beads (e.g., whether the materials are left on the table or raised completely, whether instructions to stop at 10 are remembered or forgotten); the reason for lack of compliance is recorded. The usual range is 35 to 55 seconds.

Examination of Extraocular Movements

A finger is tracked vertically and horizontally in front of the face, and whether the eyes follow smoothly and synchronously is observed. A finger is held steady in front of the face, and the patient is observed to keep the eyes directed on the finger while the head moves left and right, and then up and down. Symmetry and smoothness of directed gaze are observed.

Vestibularocular Reflex

A finger is rotated in each direction in front of the eyes (both are open). The smoothness of the tracking response is observed. The patient is asked whether this stimulation causes dizziness. A high proportion of patients who state that they are dizzy show deficits of balance.

Tests of Balance

Caution is exerted that the examiner, spouse, or parent is nearby. The patient is asked to do toe–heel walking (place heel in front of the other toe); the same exercise is done with eyes closed; children are asked to skip; to stand on each leg separately while the examiner counts to 10; the patient stands with eyes closed while the examiner counts to 20.

Accommodation to Light

With the room darkened, a small flashlight is directed into each pupil. The degree and equality of constriction for each pupil are observed.

Convergence on an Approaching Target

A finger is moved from about arms length to 6 inches in front of the eye, and the point at which a single image is seen as two images is observed. With adequate convergence, no breakup occurs, or it occurs at 6 inches or less.

Gait

The patient is asked to walk some distance and to return, at a rapid pace. The position in which the body is held, whether the feet are apart or together, and freedom of movement of arms and legs are observed.

Stereognosis or Identifying Objects by Touch

This is performed with the eyes closed, and four different coins are placed in each hand to identify (a quarter, nickel, dime, and penny). Beginning about age 7 or 8 the patient can be expected to accurately identify such familiar objects. The coins are placed in random order for alternate hands. If there are no errors, the procedure is stopped after 4 different coins are identified with each hand. If there is more than one error after four trials with each hand, the procedure is repeated. The number of right- and left-hand errors is compared. The results can offer evidence for peripheral or central deficits, depending on the entire pattern of sensorimotor functioning.

Kinesthesis

Awareness of the location of the limbs in space is tested for each arm. A finger is placed in front of the patient's face, eyes open. The patient is told that the finger will not move. The patient is directed to close his eyes, to hold his hands on his lap, then to touch his own nose, his knee, the examiner's finger in space, his nose again. Observed is the accuracy in touching the examiner's finger and his own nose. The procedure is then repeated for the other hand. Significant differences in kinesthetic control can be observed between arms.

Vibration

A 128 cps tuning fork is applied to each knee in turn, and then to one of the bones of the wrist. The fork vibrates for some time so that it can be touched left–right–right–left relatively rapidly giving the patient the opportunity to compare each side. The patient is asked whether the stimulus is felt, and whether there is any differences between the limb.

Hearing

Pitch forks of frequencies 128, 256, 512, 1024, and 2048 cps are available from medical supply stores. They are struck on a hard object, and with the patient facing away from the examiner, held at the vertex (above the center of the head). The patient is asked whether he hears anything. Then the fork is rotated over to each side of the head, and the patient is asked whether the sound is the same or different. If there is a deficit on one side, the vibrating fork is applied to the temporal bone behind the ear. The reader is reminded that this will stimulate the auditory branch of the eighth cranial nerve directly, differentiating between "air conduction," or problems stemming from the tympanic membrane or bones of the middle ear, and "bone conduction," with deficits stemming from dysfunction of the auditory nerve directly.

Appendix 3
Neuropsychological Use of the Rorschach Inkblot Test: Stress-Related Response

I compared over 160 TBI patients (ambulatory) with 49 individuals referred for stress reactions (rape, harassment, false arrest, etc.). Two features seemed to distinguish the groups, i.e., the reduced productivity and creativity after TBI. There is considerable overlap between the Rorschachs of severely stressed individuals and brain-damaged individuals, i.e., the stressed individual shows signs of reduced cognitive efficiency. This is discussed in Chapters 9 (Intellectual Functioning) and 15 (Stress).

The brain-damaged individual does not have the spontaneous self-expression so often observed in the unimpaired individual. The impaired individual will often stop after the first response. The number of responses (R) most reliably differentiated the TBI and Stress (ST) groups. A reliable differentiating factor is the "good response," i.e., one that is accurate and totally lacking in any vagueness (Rg). Another measure of cognitive difficulty and reduced productivity is rejection (rej, see above). Reduced creativity and verbal facility is revealed by reduced Originals of good form (O+), and total content categories (TCC).

Of interest is the fact that extended form accuracy (F+% involving all determinants) did not differentiate between stressed and brain-damaged individuals (77% for both groups). Unreliable differences are obtained for number of accurate or inaccurate responses integrating the entire inkblot, number of Populars (P), and proportion of total easy responses (Human + Animal %).

Perseverations (inappropriate repetition of a response) appeared primarily in the TBI group, but were very rare (Table A.1).

Rorschach Stress-Related Content

Content offers diagnostic information, as well as attitudes toward the self, toward being impaired, and therapeutic considerations including attitude toward the future, presence of depression, anxiety, anger, and hopelessness.

TABLE A.1. Quantitative comparison of brain-injured and stress subjects.

	TBI		ST			
	X	SD	X	SD	Diff	P
R	14.5	5.0	18.0	5.6	−3.5	.000
Rg	8.7	3.8	11.3	4.7	−2.6	.001
O+	1.6	2.4	3.2	3.5	−1.6	.006
ExF+%	76.7	13.9	77.2	16.6	−0.5	NS
Rej	0.9	1.5	0.3	0.7	+0.6	.002
TCC	5.9	2.5	7.4	3.1	+1.5	.006

The Experience of Anxiety

Personalized Experience of Aggression by Rorschach Figure

"Death confronting me; death with a knife in my head, there is nothing I can do, there are electric charges coming off his body; standing over me, jumping out of the page; coming toward me with outstretched hands; looking at me, gives me an eerie feeling; eyes staring, its going to attack you, frightful. A giant getting smaller as you are standing down looking up at it, as though he caught somebody running around his house; King Kong walking toward you; a monster hanging over me, trying to hit me with a ray; standing high over me, jumping out of the page; coming toward me with outstretched hands; tiger rug, it appalls me; angry faces looking directly at me; looks like my friends, because they turned their backs on me; death confronting me; when you see something like this you know it is the end; makes me feel real bad; yukky, it's dangerous; color disturbs me; I don't like bats, always coming after you; mounted bear rug, I'd be afraid of it; coming toward me with outstretched hands; I'm a little thing, its trying to hit me; looking at me, gives me an eerie feeling; you see it in a scary movie; raising its ears, frightening."

Identical Event Is Reported and Identified with a Reenactment of Trauma

[Woman who was caught in the explosion of inflammatory shavings she tried to stuff in an incinerator:] "It reminds me of a person, body hands, clothes around it. I think of me. I think of fire around it. I have a dress on. Arms in the air, I see the fire, she got caught on fire. (Mood?) Numb scared. X-Ray of somebody's back. [The victim of a fall] Two people hanging by the edge of a cliff." [Girl injured in an amusement park ride with another girl, who had nightmares of the cage cutting her body in half:] "Siamese twins. Want to get away from each other. Your body, how it would look from the inside;" [Auto accident victim] "looks like my car accident. Things splattered around and crushed like bodies, or a war or battle; looks like my car accident."

Ongoing Realistic Danger

Human Aggressors

"Arguing; getting ready to fight; faces with gaping jaws; looming over somebody; just caught somebody doing something; lifting someone in his arms; gloating; conjuring up something; pulling something apart; coming at each other, going to fight; swinging a baby; stomping; trying to beat up someone; faces with gaping jaws; looming over somebody; beat up."

Animal Aggressors

"Bears climbing on the lady; trying to bite; scavanging; snapping at its prey; showing their teeth; mouth wide open in anger; attacking; coming, crawling at you; eyes staring, its going to attack you, frightful; a spider with jaws, going to attack; they have something in their mouth, and it is bleeding, dangling down, alive; trying to kill; pigs' masks, looking at one another, grinning; facing each other, having a confrontation; scavenging; snapping at its prey; mouth open in anger; going to attack; bats coming after you."

Distanced but Ongoing Danger

Animal-Like Aggressors

"Dragon pushing out fire or smoke; monster from outerspace, about to be blown up; Godzilla running away in fear; ferocious demon-serpent [with religious association of a Saint] stepping on me. Pigs' masks grinning, facing each other, having a confrontation."

Anticipated Danger

"Deer smelling the air to see if there is anybody around; Something is dripping, hanging on a thread, ready to fall; fly, he came down and he sniffed food."

Denial of Danger

"Nice guy, a decent character, nice guy doesn't make you hurt; someone with big feet" [with threat denied]; monster from outer space, about to be blown up; Godzilla running away in fear; wolf, not necessarily ready to pounce on anything; someone with big feet [a threatening image, while the subject denied any mood in the figure]; somebody putting hands with mittens over the eyes from the back, just a game."

Neutral Activity

"Looking, lifting, standing, flying."

Pleasant, Constructive, Cooperative

"Two bears kissing; angels dancing."

Identity

Process of Victimization or Destruction

Living Victim

A 12-year-old boy, victim of an auto accident: "Two birds smashing into each other; splattered cat, got run over . . . Rat is running; falling out of the sky, alive at the moment, when he hits the ground he's going to be dead; a bat got beat up, trying to do something with his wings and he don't have the strength; cat howling; caught by a hunter and killed; tiger trying to kill a mouse."

Inanimate Object Being Destroyed or Out of Control

(Burning; force of gravity): "Fire in a car; force of gravity; ripping it apart; flame; oil shooting out of the ground, color makes it look like oil or tar."

Identity as a Victim

Mutilated (Cosmetically, Anatomically Deteriorated; Damaged)

External appearance: "Ugly face, disturbing, even my face" (a man who required rhinoplasty after an auto accident); "two feet, I can't even wear high heeled shoes; a skull or somebody's face, I was thinking of the hole in my head" [5-year-old struck by a car); "worn out heels"; (A man, age 20, who had been in a coma for many days): "Man after a long day's work, sad eyes, drawn-out face . . . panting like a dog, tongue hanging out . . . depressed, tired, weary, worn out; skull, guy who died in the atomic explosion."

Internal Anatomy

"Tissue; blood; X-Ray; accident victim; that is damaged, broken, dead; wheat hanging off a stalk; kidney, blood coming out of the cut."

Dead Organisms

"Deteriorating leaf; an organ spattered with blood; insects like dead, upside down; dinosaur is dead. Mice are crawling on him to see if they could get meat; bat died, somebody killed it and threw it out the window; bones, broke apart when somebody threw it out the window."

Helpless, Vulnerable, Appealing for Help

"Two hands praying; holding on for dear life; a body in the middle, hands reaching out; crying for help with their hands up; holding up her hands, she has problems; orchid, delicate and fragile, cut off."

Still Struggling

"Holding on for dear life; struggling; wants to get the hell out of there; crabs trying to survive."

Defeated—The Battle is Lost

"Picking up the body, a pair of hands, pieces laying around, they had a fight over something; pulling something apart; lying in a hospital; man's head used as a decoration for an animal skin; insects like dead, upside down."

Loss of Control

"Swinging; balancing; whirling around; spinning; pirouetting; blindfolded, being helped on the side by two tigers; off balance, like they're tugging or something; two heads from Fantasia, trying to meet to kiss; two flying elephants, spinning around."

Reduced Self-Esteem

(Seen by a 12-year-old girl): "Old people."

Weltanschauung

Search for the Meaning of Life

"A woman reaching, her hands, searching for answers."

One's World or Adaptation Has Been Destroyed

The world is no longer experienced as a place that is nurturant, or where one can cope. "Volcano, explosion" are signs of disintegration experienced within one's personality.

Man-Made Dangerous Events

Examples are accidents, weapons, explosions. "Nuclear bomb, white is melting rocks; rockets and planes: simulation of a stealth bomber; rocket; missile, flames coming out, smoke pouring up, the ignition, in motion; fireworks exploding or bursting; explosion with all the dust going up; oil shooting out of the ground; something is dripping, hanging on a thread, ready to fall."

Overwhelming Natural Forces, World Is Being Destroyed

"Volcanos erupting, spitting out fire or flame; fire—a lot of smoke, forest fire, thick smoke beneath the trees; storms—storm clouds, sometimes clouds get real black, tornado, with a lot of dust, going to be a storm, dark clouds, here it is really going to rain."

The World Is Dangerous

Nonmoving

Bee; wasp; spider; weapon, etc.

Animate

"Close-up of a fly, checking it out, viewing for the kill."

Reactive

Dysphoric Mood

(Directly expressed by patient, or inferrable by the examiner): "Sad; weird; contempt ('laughing at'); scared; shocked; voodoo; a lot of stuff flying; not a friendly one, the color black makes it look that way; gray clouds, a gloomy day; deer smelling the air to see if there is anybody around [anticipation of danger].

Suicidal Fantasy

"I had a vision of heavenly hands; God giving people a hand up to heaven."

Guilt

"Praying to God."

Hopelessness

"Frozen in ice. Stuck in the spaceship forever; spider trapped in slime."

Defenses

Denial of Damage

"Celebrated Oriental sitting on a thrown; Eiffel tower covered with decorations to celebrate Bastille day; giant man, resting, he's not hurt; Person in a funny costume, happy; somebody putting hands with mittens over the eyes from the back; just a game, she's blocking everything out."

Consciously Conceals Damage/Impairment from Others

"Mask. (?) I won't let others see my problems; Eyeglasses (?) Anyone who wears 'shades' is hiding."

Restititutive Maneuvers

Compensation for Weakness/Unconscious Denial of Damage

"Guardian angel watching over them" (A woman who denied anxiety subsequent to an accident that temporarily threatened her vision).

Rebirth Fantasy

"Firmament, newness coming forth."

Wish-Fulfilling Fantasy

"Problems, I guess; hopeful; spiritual creatures from the mood, good and bad; lake near my parents' home; castle on a hill where they shoot bows and arrows [auto accident victim whose head broke the windshield and tends to stay home]; hopeful spiritual creatures from the mood; an old woman who is taking care of the child; two people dancing, carrying bowling bags and curtsying to each other, happy; lights in a diskotheque; two girls on a rocking horse, happy; Spanish dancer, hair in the air, feels sexy, kicking leg up in the air."

Grandiosity

"Castle; Flyhead trying to kill Spiderman; spaceship, bad guys build it with guns, flying off."

Release Phenomena

"Red looks like ink. That's a strong image to me. I'm more sensitive and more touchy."

Satisfactory Pre-Morbid Adjustment

Pleasant content. "Guitar with sounds coming out."

Awareness of Cognitive Impairment

"I hope you don't think I'm crazy; I can't figure it out; it's like a nightmare; it doesn't make sense; I can't tie the top to the bottom; it's like the going on in my head, I can't do anything about it; Salvatore Dali; Fantasia; I wish you could tell me later what these pictures are; I didn't see anything at all so I said a raccoon; it has a dog's face but it is a bat; it doesn't look like anything to me; somebody drew something and you're supposed to use your imagination; I don't know what I'm supposed to be seeing in these things."

Social Status

Interactive

"Two women waving goodbye, a sad picture; two men trying to rescue each other; two men climbing down a mountain holding hands, afraid of falling."

Isolated

"Alien from another planet; [A woman with complaints of changed identity and empty figure drawings] Birds . . . I don't know what they are. They are not people."

Object of Contempt (e.g., for Facial Scars)

"Face, snickering; trophy under glass; man has his tongue sticking out."

Forced to Be on Good Behavior

"Two French poodles . . . posing like in a dog show, they look well-groomed" (a man who was arrested after being provoked into giving a bribe, no physical injury)."

Concealment

"African Mask."

Appendix 4
Treatment of the Sequelae of Head Trauma

ARTHUR GREENSPAN, M.D.

Most head injury patients suffer from numerous somatic and emotional complaints. They frequently have multiple injuries, such as neck, back injuries, and injuries to the limbs. One must never forget that it is important to treat the whole patient, not just a symptom or a cluster of symptoms. Very often medicines must be combined to be effective. A single drug is often insufficient in patients with multiple complaints.

Another important factor is that the drugs usually have to be titrated; the dose must be adjusted upward or downward to have the desired result. A common mistake is to give the right drug in the wrong dose, with little or no benefit, and then to move along to the next drug and have the same problem. When two drugs are appropriately combined, however, they may have an excellent therapeutic affect. This can apply to two, three, or more drugs at one time. Thus, as with other medical problems, the treatment of head injury patients is part science, and part art and experience.

First, I would like to deal with the problem of sleep disturbance, because this occurs commonly in head injury patients, and illustrates the principles of titration. Characteristically, patients with head injuries suffer from numerous sleep difficulties. Many complain that it takes them at least an hour to fall asleep. They also complain of multiple awakenings throughout the night, and of early morning awakening with an inability to fall back to sleep. Each of these symptoms represents an opportunity for the astute physician to intervene appropriately with the right combination of medicine. Very often, a patient who is unable to initially fall asleep in less than 2 hours, requires an antianxiety drug—this disturbance frequently is due to tension or anxiety.

A type of antianxiety medication that is most effective is a major tranquilizer, such as a Phenothiazine. Usually, only a low dose is required. Drugs such as Trilafon (perphenazine) 4 mg, Stelazine (trifluoperazine) 2 to 5 mg, and Compazine (prochlorperazine) 10 mg are often helpful. In addition, in some cases, a minor tranquilizer such as Librium (chlordiazepoxide), Valium (diazepam), or Xanax (alprazolam), in modest amounts, is also helpful. In both the major and minor tranquilizers, numerous other medications are available, the ones mentioned are merely a few of the more popular ones.

The initial dose of major tranquilizers (phenothiazines), should be at a relatively low level. The dose should be gradually built up. For example, a patient who complains that it takes 4 hours to fall asleep at night, is given Stelzaine (trifluoperazine 2 mg) to start. After a week, the patient reports that it takes 2½ to 3 hours to fall asleep; the Stelazine (trifluoperazine) is now increased to 4 mg. If in a week, it only takes 1 hour to fall asleep, the Stelazine (trifluoperazine) is then increased to 5 or 6 mg. The patient is now able to fall asleep within 15 or 20 minutes, which is a normal lapse of time. Interestingly enough, the patient's anxiety has abated almost completely at the same time and tension is reduced. Thus, the titration accomplished two things—sleep and the lessening of anxiety.

When it comes to multiple and early morning awakenings, a similar situation arises. However, the use of an antidepressant, e.g., a tricyclic drug such as Elavil (amitriptylene), Tofranil (imipramine), Pamelor (nortriptylene), and Norpramine (desipramine) is often useful.

When the patient states that he wakes up at three or four in the morning and cannot get back to sleep again, one can start with 10 mg of Pamelor (nortriptylene) at bedtime. If he still wakes up a little bit later, the dose is increased to 20 mg. If he sleeps until 6 A.M., the dose is increased to 30 mg. He then states he sleeps the whole night, and his depression has started to clear up at the same time. Thus, by titrating the medication, he can eliminate the sleep disturbance on both ends: difficulty in falling asleep and early morning awakening. At the same time, anxiety and depression are reduced. This is a key to successfully treating the head injury patient, and it also applies in general to many psychiatric disturbances.

In many other nontraumatic psychiatric or emotional disturbances, the use of sleeping pills is generally not necessary and often not indicated. When a patient takes a sedative, such as a barbiturate or similar drug, he may get several hours of sleep; wake up feeling drugged, having a hangover, and still anxious and depressed. He may complain that he feels terrible, even though he has had 3 or 4 hours of sleep. Therefore, the use of sedating drugs that do not calm anxiety or depression is generally not beneficial.

Another problem occurs when patients complain that whenever they roll over, they are awakened by pain in some body part. In a case like this, the sleep disturbance can be treated effectively only if the antidepressant and antianxiety medication is combined with a pain medication, such as a nonsteroidal anti-inflammatory drug and/or analgesic drug, and a muscle relaxant.

In a few cases, the entire sleep disturbance is due to pain. The simple use of pain- and muscle-relaxant medication may be sufficient; the use of other drugs may not be necessary. In the case of the person who cannot sleep because of headache or other pain, it should be remembered that many pain clinics utilize antidepressant and antianxiety medications for the treatment of pain. These drugs, particularly at low dosages, have an analgesic effect separate from their antidepressant and antianxiety effects, so that pain is often reduced dramatically with the use of these medications. The dose is usually about one-quarter or one-third of the amount used in emotional illness, such as depression.

Headaches

The control of headache in head injury patients represents a challenge to the clinician (see Chapter 4). There are both medical and nonmedical approaches to headache treatment. In recent years, use of biofeedback training sessions has become a helpful adjunct to the use of medication, and is widely used at present in the treatment of head injury patients, who do not wish to take medication or who wish to take as little medication as possible. Naturally, biofeedback has its limitations and does not work for everyone. However, it helps many patients substantially.

Concerning medication, numerous analgesic drugs—the most simple being derivatives of aspirin and Tylenol (acetaminophen)—are very often sufficient in cases of mild to moderate head injury. However, many patients have severe, recurring, pounding headaches, and require stronger medications. The use of Darvon (propoxyphene), Tylenol (acetaminophen) with codeine as well as other combination drugs such as Vicodin, Fiorinal, and Fioricet, and numerous other pain and headache preparations is widely known. The use of strong narcotic drugs is generally not necessary and generally not indicated, as it can have such adverse effects as addiction and depression.

The above mentioned psychotropic medications, such as antidepressants and major and minor tranquilizers, are extremely useful in the treatment of headache. In addition, beta-blockers, calcium channel blockers, nonsteroidal antiinflammatory drugs, and many others can be used effectively in the control of headache.

Although steroid medications have been used in the treatment of headache due to head trauma, they are usually reserved for the early stages of injury immediately following the head trauma, when they may be useful in reducing cerebral edema.

In certain posttraumatic headaches, local anesthetic blocking agents, which are injected at the site of pain, or trigger point injections may be useful. Very often the trigger points are located in the neck, the back of the skull, or the trapezius musculature. Another popular treatment of headache includes the use of Ergot preparations such as Cafergot, Ergot Medihaler, Ergomar, and so on.

Less often used, but very effective, are the antiseizure medications. Many of these medications such as Tegretol (carbamazepine) and Dilantin (phenytoin) have been used successfully in severe pain control.

The use of muscle relaxants is particularly helpful in headache control if spasm of the neck muscles or the scalp muscles occurs. Some of these drugs include Flexeril (cyclobenzaprine), Parafon (chlorzoxazone), and Soma (carisoprodol).

In cases where headache is due largely to muscle spasm and tension in the neck musculature, physiotherapy such as T.E.N.S. treatment (Transcutaneous Electrical Nerve Stimulation) is quite beneficial. Moist heat and other forms of physiotherapy to muscles in spasm are often also useful.

Another important factor is that certain headaches may be associated with an increase in blood pressure following the trauma. This is fairly common in dark-skinned people. It is well known that black people are more prone to hypertension. Very often the hypertension is first diagnosed after a head trauma. Naturally, the treatment of high blood pressure consists of a large variety of antihypertensive medications, which should be prescribed by the patient's own family doctor or internist.

Many clinicians overlook a variety of home remedies that patients use, such as linaments, analgesic creams, hot packs, cold packs, and ointments. Since many of these home remedies are often beneficial, the treating physician should not disapprove of them or overlook their use.

Occasionally, the clinician comes across a patient who has previous history of headache. This condition is exacerbated by the head injury. In this case, other psychotropic medications, such as MAO inhibitors and lithium carbonate, have been found useful.

It should be noted that certain headache preparations contain mild doses of butalbital or phenobarbital. These drugs are occasionally helpful in the treatment of headaches.

The treatment of headache is wide ranging and, unfortunately, no single drug or combination of drugs works on all patients. The treatment must be individualized. The clinician must be creative and willing to try drugs that are not necessarily familiar. Virtually all of the above mentioned drugs are safe and nonaddicting when used judiciously and carefully. Obviously, excessive dosage should be avoided. In case of unresponsiveness, the patient should be referred to a headache clinic or a specialist in the field of head trauma or headache.

Altered States of Consciousness or Awareness and Seizure Disorders

Altered states of consciousness and seizures are common after head trauma (see Chapter 6). It is useful to divide these problems into immediate and later occurring disturbances. Immediate problems occurring minutes or hours after a head injury are well covered in books and journals of emergency medicine and neurosurgery. These problems are generally dealt with in the hospital. A clinician using this book will most likely encounter patients who have been discharged from a hospital or emergency room, and whose level of awareness is sufficient to function outside of an institution.

Loss of consciousness is common immediately following, or shortly after, a head injury. Prolonged unconscious states, stupor, and coma lasting days or weeks have a poor prognosis, although cases of remarkable recovery have often been noted.

Prolonged seizures immediately following a head injury carry an ominous prognosis. Patients whose level of awareness varies from time to time, or who experience fainting spells, blackouts, syncope, seizures, and so on, deserve the benefit of an appropriate clinical workup, including MRI, CAT scan, cervical X-rays, angiography, evoked potential studies. Referral may be necessary to an ear specialist to discern differences in injuries to the inner ear and brain stem (Chapter 7). An EEG and/or computerized EEG are often helpful in discerning brain dysfunctions.

A clinician having to deal with these problems faces a formidable task. Fainting spells and blackouts are often dealt with as minor forms of seizure activity. Frequently, they respond to antiseizure drugs, such as Dilantin (phenytoin), Tegretol (carbamazepine), Depakene (valproic acid), and Phenobarbital.

Major seizure disorders may occur at any time following a head trauma. Both minor and major head injuries are prone to seizure disorders. Naturally, more serious head injuries tend to develop seizure problems more frequently. Because seizures may occur at any time after a head injury, months, and occasionally, years may go by before the first seizures is noted. Occasionally, in cases involving litigation, the case may be long settled prior to the onset of seizures. Reactivation of a previously dormant childhood seizure disorder occasionally occurs.

Patient compliance with taking appropriate doses of medication is often a problem, and tests of blood levels of the antiseizure medication are often required on a regular basis.

Seizures following a head injury are generally controllable, but occasionally may be prolonged, frequent, and severe. In cases of intractible seizure activity, neurosurgical procedures may be required to extricate scar tissue from the cerebral cortex. Although it is generally safe to use antidepressant and antianxiety medication and major tranquilizers on head injury patients, high doses of these drugs may lower the seizure threshold. Because high doses of these drugs are not necessary in this patient population, this rarely presents a problem.

Minor seizure activity, such as brief absences or brief bouts of syncope, are often readily controlled by such minor tranquilizers as Valium (diazepam), Tranxene (chlorazepate), Klonapin (clonazepam), and Phenobarbital.

Other states of altered awareness that are quite common include patients complaining of confusion, the inability to think straight, getting lost, or being forgetful; an inability to concentrate, and numerous cognitive disturbances. They are described extensively elsewhere in this book. Generally, they persist for months and sometimes years; often they clear up spontaneously. They may be difficult to treat. Cognitive rehabilitative therapy is often useful in these cases.

Diminished blood flow to the mid- and hind-brain occasionally occurs in middle aged or elderly patients, particularly when the vertebrobasilar circulation is affected. This occurs readily in cases where arthritis of the cervical spine is prominent with osteophyte formation impinging on the vertebral arteries.

It is well known that intracranial bleeding is a serious complication of head trauma and, as mentioned above, this must be ruled out with the appropriate MRI or CT scan.

Anxiety Disturbances

Anxiety disturbances are common following trauma of any sort, but are particularly common after a head injury (see Chapter 15). The anxiety level is frequently correlated with disturbances in the sleep pattern, particularly in the early part of the night. The patient frequently complains of difficulty falling asleep, very often of several hours duration. The more severe the anxiety or tension, the longer it takes to fall asleep. This is a very important factor in determining the level of patient dysfunction and very useful in determining the efficacy of the treatment of the anxiety, whether it be psychotherapy, biofeedback, medication, or any other form of treatment.

As the anxiety and tension diminishes, the sleep pattern tends to return gradually toward normal, meaning that the patient falls asleep within 15 to 20 minutes.

Numerous medications are available for the treatment of anxiety and tension. The major tranquilizers, such as Phenothiazine and other similar drugs, in low doses are frequently beneficial in reducing anxiety. The minor tranquilizers, such as Valium (diiazepam), Librium (chlordiazepoxide), Xanax (alprazolam), Tranxene (chlorazepate), and Mebrobamate, are also frequently useful in reducing tension and anxiety. On occasion, a major tranquilizer can be used together with a minor tranquilizer, particularly if the patient suffers from anxiety, tension, and headache.

Biofeedback therapy has proved, in recent years, to be extremely helpful in the treatment of tension and anxiety following head trauma. Psychotherapy in its many variations has also proved to be effective in controlling anxiety and, naturally, the combination of any of these modalities is both safe and effective.

The question as to why head injury victims suffer from anxiety is an interesting one. In recent years, many investigators have come to the realization that a great deal of anxiety and depression is psychophysiological in nature. This means that the centers of the brain that control emotion have been jarred and that mood swings and anxiety are due to actual brain dysfunction, not merely a psychological reaction to the realization that one has been injured seriously and that one's life style has been compromised. No doubt, the realization that one has sustained a serious injury is a contributing factor, but it should no longer be viewed as the sole or major factor in anxiety or depression resulting from head trauma.

Depression, like anxiety, is often associated with disturbances in sleep. However, these disturbances occur more frequently in the middle of the night or early in the morning. Again, the use of appropriate treatment, be it psychotherapy or medication, is often associated with diminished sleep disturbance. As the sleep disturbance returns to normal, the patient frequently reports that the depression has been markedly reduced. Other problems commonly associated with depression are memory disturbances and anorexia.

Many patients are also agitated (Chapter 13). They cannot sleep, eat, or concentrate, and are nervous and forgetful. This cluster of symptoms, along with vertigo, is commonly labeled "postconcussion syndrome." Unfortunately, postconcussion syndrome is not necessarily a benign condition, as many clinicians formerly believed. There is frequently subtle brain damage and loss of judgment, diminished ability to plan ahead, diminished tolerance to alcohol, aggressive outbursts, irritability, anger, family dysfunction, separation and divorce, numerous other psychological problems, job problems, family problems, school problems, and work problems. The problem of postconcussion syndrome is a global dysfunction that unfortunately does not go away in 2 or 3 months, as used to be believed. The symptoms may persist for many months, or even years. In many cases of moderate to severe injury, the symptoms may be permanent.

Several classes of drugs are available for the treatment of depression. However, it should be realized that if a depressed person is agitated, an antidepressant alone will not suffice. An antianxiety drug must be provided at the same time. The classes of antidepressants include tricyclic and tetracyclic antidepressants, MAO inhibitor drugs, and lithium carbonate. These drugs represent the major groups of antidepressants. The most frequently useful antidepressant drugs are the tricyclic ones, particularly the nonsedating members of that family, such as Pamelor (nortriptylene) and Norpramine (desipramine).

In cases where the sleep disturbance is pronounced, more sedating members of this family are often useful, such as Elavil (amitriptylene) and Tofranil (imipramine). These drugs again are often beneficial where headaches are pronounced. They have a remarkable pain reducing effect which is recognized in pain clinics worldwide.

Vertigo and Dizziness

Vertigo and dizziness are not identical. Vertigo is generally due to injury of the middle or internal ear (labyrinth) (Chapter 7). Occasionally, a concussion of the labyrinth may be diagnosed by a ear specialist. Vertigo may be due to damage to the nucleus of the vestibular portion of the eight-cranial nerves in the brainstem. Approximately 40 to 45 percent of cases of vertigo are due to ear damage or associated brainstem damage.

In other cases, the vertebrobasilar artery insufficiency may result in bouts of dizziness. This is common in cases of whiplash associated with arthritis of the cervical spine. Some cases of dizziness are associated with a transient drop in blood pressure. This can occur when a head injury patient changes position from lying to standing or from sitting to standing too rapidly. This is known as orthostatic hypotension, and is not true vertigo.

Other patients with head injuries feel faint at times for no apparent reason. As mentioned previously, syncopal attacks and blackouts are quite common among head injury patients.

Numerous medications are helpful in the treatment of vertigo and dizziness. Psychotropic medication is often helpful. Other drugs that frequently help are Antivert (neclizine), Marezine (cyclizine), Buclidin (buclizine), and Dramamine (dimenhydrinate); transdermscopalamine patches that are placed behind the ear are often helpful.

True vertigo due to ear injury or brainstem injury is characterized by a sensation of the room spinning. Dizziness, on the other hand, which may be due to other causes, generally does not manifest this symptom. This is useful in the differential diagnosis of true vertigo versus dizziness.

Many cases of vertigo are associated with nausea, and drugs that reduce nausea are often beneficial. A few of these drugs are Tigan (trimethobenzamide), Compazine (prochlorperazine), and Bellergal-S (bellafoline, ergotamine, and phenobarbital).

The treatment of dizzy spells and vertigo requires patience, as this symptom may persist for a prolonged period of time, often months or years, following the accident. This is generally followed by a gradual improvement as the patient's overall health improves with time (Chapter 18).

Further Reading

For further information on Titration of neuroleptic drugs for anxiety, depression and insomnia see:

Baloh, R., & Honrubia, V. (1990). *Clinical Neurophysiology of the Vestibular System,* 2nd ed. Philadelphia: F.A. Davis Co.

Becker, D., & Gudeman, S. (1989). *Textbook of Head Injury.* Philadelphia: W.B. Saunders Co.

Currier, R., DeJong, R., & Crowell, R. (1990). *Yearbook of Neurology & Neurosurgery.* Chicago: Yearbook Medical Publishers.

Detre, T., & Jarecki, H. (1971). *Modern Psychiatric Treatment.* New York: Lippincott.

Kaplan, H., & Sadock, B. (1989). *Comprehensive Textbook of Psychiatry,* 5th ed. Baltimore: Williams & Wilkins.

Talbott, J., Hales, R., & Yudofsky, S. (1988). *Textbook of Psychiatry.* Washington, D.C.: The American Psychiatric Press.

Wall, P., & Melzack, R. (1989). *Textbook of Pain,* 2nd ed. New York: Churchill Livingstone.

Index